Drug Therapy
and
the Elderly

D1275518

The Jones and Bartlett Series in Nursing

Adult Emergency Nursing Procedures, Proehl

Basic Steps in Planning Nursing Research: From Questions to Proposals, Fourth Edition, Brink/Wood

Biotherapy: A Comprehensive Overview, Rieger

Bloodborne Pathogens, National Safety Council

Bone Marrow Transplantation, Whedon

Cancer Chemotherapy, Barton Burke et al.

Cancer Nursing: Principles and Practice, Third Edition, Groenwald et al.

A Challenge for Living, Corless et al.

Chemotherapy Care Plans, Barton Burke et al.

Chronic Illness: Impact and Interventions, Third Edition, Lubkin

Comprehensive Cancer Nursing Review, Groenwald et al.

Comprehensive Cancer Nursing Review, Groenwald et al.

Comprehensive Perioperative Nursing Review, Fairchild et al.

Desk Reference for Critical Care Nursing, Wright/Shelton

Drugs and Protocols Common to Prehospital and Emergency Care, Cummings

Drug Therapy and the Elderly, Swonger/Burbank

Dying, Death, and Bereavement: Theoretical Perspectives and Other Ways of Knowing, Corless et al.

Essentials of Oxygenation, Ahrens/Rutherford

Fundamentals of Nursing Research, Brockopp/Hastings-Tolsma

Grant Application Writer's Handbook, Reif-Lehrer

Handbook of Oncology Nursing, Second Edition, Gross/Johnson

Health Policy and Nursing: Crisis and Reform in the U.S. Health Care Delivery System, Harrington/Estes

Human Aging and Chronic Disease, Kart et al.

Human Development, Fourth Edition, Freiberg

Intravenous Therapy, Nentwich

Introductory Management and Leadership for Clinical Nurses, Swansburg

Management and Leadership for Nurse Managers, Swansburg

Mastering the New Medical Terminology, Second Edition, Stanfield/Hui

Mathematics for Health Professionals, Third Edition, Whisler

Medical Instrumentation for Nurses and Allied Health-Care Professionals, Aston/Brown

Medical Terminology with Vikki Wetle, RN, MA, Video Series, Wetle

Memory Bank for Chemotherapy, Second Edition, Preston/Wilfinger

Memory Bank for Critical Care, Third Edition, Ervin

Memory Bank for Hemodynamic Monitoring, Second Edition, Ervin/Long

Memory Bank for HIV Medications, Wilkes

Memory Bank for Intravenous Therapy, Second Edition, Weinstein

Memory Bank for Medications, Second Edition, Kostin/Sieloff

The Nation's Health, Fourth Edition, Lee/Estes

New Dimensions in Women's Health, Alexander/LaRosa

Nursing and the Disabled, Fraley

Nursing Staff Development, Swansburg

Nutrition and Diet Therapy, Second Edition, Stanfield

Oncology Nursing Drug Reference, Wilkes et al.

Oncology Nursing Homecare Handbook, Barton Burke

Oncology Nursing in the Ambulatory Setting, Buchsel/Yarbro

Oncology Nursing Society's Instruments for Clinical Nursing Research, Frank-Stromborg

Oxygen Administration, National Safety Council

Perioperative Nursing, Fairchild

Perioperative Patient Care, Third Edition, Kneedler/Dodge

Perspectives on Death and Dying, Fulton/Metress

Primary Care of Women and Children with HIV Infection: A Multidisciplinary Approach, Kelly et al.

Ready Reference for Critical Care, Strawn/Stewart

Understanding/Responding, Second Edition, Long

Women's Health Development, McElmurry et al.

Working with Older Adults, Third Edition, Burnside/Schmidt

Drug Therapy and the Elderly

Alvin K. Swonger, PHD

College of Pharmacy
University of Rhode Island

Patricia M. Burbank, RN, DNSC

College of Nursing
University of Rhode Island

Jones and Bartlett Publishers
Sudbury, Massachusetts

Boston   Toronto   London   Singapore

World Headquarters

Jones and Bartlett Publishers
40 Tall Pine Drive
Sudbury, MA 01776
978-443-5000
info@jbpub.com
www.jbpub.com

Jones and Bartlett Publishers International
Barb House, Barb Mews
London W6 7PA
UK

Library of Congress Cataloging-in-Publication Data
Swonger, Alvin K.
    Drug therapy and the elderly/Alvin K. Swonger, Patricia M.
Burbank.
        p. cm.
    Includes bibliographical references and index.
    ISBN 0-86720-716-7
    1. Geriatric pharmacology.   I. Burbank, Patricia M.   II. Title.
RC953.7.S93   1995
615.5′8′0846—dc20
DNLM/DLC
for Library of Congress   94-29758
                                                                CIP

The selection and dosage of drugs presented in this book are in accord with standards accepted at the time of publication. The authors and publisher have made every effort to provide accurate information. However, research, clinical practice, and government regulations often change the accepted standard in this field. Before administering any drug, the reader is advised to check the manufacturer's product information sheet for the most up-to-date recommendations on dosage, precautions, and contraindications. This is especially important in the case of drugs that are new or seldom used.

Acquisitions Editor	Jan Wall
Production Editor	Mary Cervantes Sanger
Editorial Production Service	John A. Servideo
Manufacturing Buyer	Dana L. Cerrito
Typesetting	Sunrise Composition
Cover Design	Hannus Design Associates
Cover Printing	Malloy Lithographing, Inc.
Printing and Binding	Malloy Lithographing, Inc.

Printed in the United States of America
99 98   10 9 8 7 6 5 4 3 2

*To all our friends and relatives
who find themselves
in
their golden years*

Contents

Preface

Many times in recent years, each of us has said to students at the University of Rhode Island that the single biggest problem in current medical practice in the United States may well be the failure to adjust doses of medications to fit the special requirements of the elderly. Despite a flood of literature detailing the necessity for dosage reductions for many medications used by the elderly, the all-too-common practice continues to be one of routine prescription for elderly clients of doses that were designed for young and middle age adults and that were determined through studies that excluded older patients. This book aims to help in the process of correcting that erroneous practice as well as improving other aspects of health care delivery for the elderly—with principal emphasis on drug therapy. We hope that all health care professionals who are knowledgeable about the special issues pertaining to use of drugs by the elderly will act as their advocates, working with physicians to optimize their drug therapy.

Standard drug reference sources, such as the *Physicians' Desk Reference* and *Facts and Comparisons,* often provide documentation regarding drug cautions or contraindications that pertain to elderly clients or the disorders from which they most frequently suffer. Such drug information resources also provide special dosing information pertaining to elderly individuals, but only for a small percentage of the medications frequently used by the elderly. This book provides the most thorough compilation currently available of all the specific information health care providers need to know to successfully facilitate drug therapy for elderly clients specifically.

Drug Therapy and the Elderly is divided into three parts, the first two introductory in nature and the third consisting of a complete drug handbook for each of the major classes of drugs commonly used by elderly clients. The first unit provides an introduction to gerontology in two chapters, one highlighting biochemical and physiological aspects of aging and the other the sociological issues.

The second part provides the principles that need to guide drug therapy for the elderly. The ideas developed in this part provide the conceptual framework for rational therapeutics for the elderly. The five chapters in this unit deal with the demographic patterns of drug use by the elderly, changes in how drugs act as people age, adverse effects that are particularly prevalent for the elderly, how health care professionals can contribute to enhancing drug therapy for elderly persons, and the legal and ethical considerations that need to guide health care support for the elderly.

The third part applies the principles developed in the second part to each of the major drug categories most widely used by the elderly. The selection of topics was determined in part by an analysis of which drugs are most widely used in practice by older Americans. Each chapter in this unit begins with a concise review of the pathophysiology that is relevant to the drug groups to be considered in that chapter. The drug discussions in each chapter follow a consistent format designed to help the reader use *Drug Therapy and the Elderly* as a reference tool to guide delivery of health care services. Each drug topic includes *Clinical Indications in the Elderly, Altered Pharmacokinetics or Pharmacodynamics in the Elderly, Adverse Effects and Contraindications in the Elderly, Interactions in the Elderly,* and *Administration in the Elderly.* Under the last of these headings, specific recommendations are included regarding drug doses for the elderly, to the extent that these have been adequately determined at the time of publication.

With the addition of approximately 30 new drugs every year in the United States as well as added knowledge about older drugs, the complexity of drug information is expanding at an incredible rate. Although the expansion of our knowledge about drugs provides some valuable new opportunities for helping clients maintain or improve their health, the tremendous volume of that information is also threatening to overwhelm even the most conscientious health care providers, not to mention consumers. The need, therefore, is for drug information resources that focus on specific aspects of drug therapy, such as the effective use of drugs for the elderly. *Drug Therapy and the Elderly* is intended to serve that purpose.

Acknowledgments

Drug Therapy and the Elderly began its life when Jan Wall of Jones and Bartlett Publishers approached us with the idea for a book devoted expressly to the issues of drug therapy that pertain to older persons. While many at Jones and Bartlett were instrumental in bringing this book to fruition, we want especially to acknowledge John Servideo, who skillfully edited the manuscript.

Professor Burbank also wishes to thank Ruth Milbank for review and editorial comments on portions of the manuscript and Professor Swonger extends his appreciation to his department colleagues and Provost Beverly Swan, who supported his request for a sabbatical leave to work on the project. Elsie Swonger provided the illustrations that are original to this work.

Both authors want especially to thank their respective families for the love and support they so generously provide. Our love and gratitude go to:

Amanda Burbank
Elsie Swonger
Krish, Jeff, and Jaelyn Johnson
Joline, Matt, and Alina Swonger

Finally, we extend our deep gratitude to those who are the subjects of this book, our elders, for all that they have taught us about their needs, their love of life, and about living with dignity and grace.

CHAPTER 1

Biochemical and Physiological Characteristics of Aging

WHY DO WE AGE?

Why do people age? Surely you will not be surprised that such a momentous question does not lend itself, at this stage of knowledge, to a concise answer. It is a question that will continue, for some time, to generate more questions than answers, more theory than established mechanisms.

One safe observation to begin with is that aging is universal to all species, though the rate of aging among species varies tremendously. Even restricting consideration to mammalian species, one observes an approximately 80-fold range in maximum life span potential (MLSP). Humans, with an MLSP of about 120 years have the longest life span among mammals, while mice, at an average of 3.5 years, have one of the shorter ones. MLSP appears to be a genetically coded species characteristic that can only be marginally altered by any known manipulation of environment or lifestyle. Although average life expectancy for humans has increased dramatically in the last two millenia—from about 20 years to about 73 years in the present-day United States—this change reflects a decrease in premature mortality from disease and, especially, childhood infections, and has not been accompanied by a significant increase in the maximum ages achieved by society's eldest members. Individual persons and even certain family groups may differ in the chronological age at which the familiar signs of aging become evident, but less so after age 70 than before. Even in a society obsessed with looking young, it becomes difficult to mask the effects of aging beyond a point.

So, aging is something we share with all living creatures. One might even be tempted to suggest parallels between aging of living organisms and inanimate machines, such as the automobile, but differences are apparent and, indeed, instructive. If an automobile is taken straight off the assembly line and stored safely away, perhaps in a vacuum container, and never used, one can reasonably expect the vehicle will be "like new" even many years later. Machines age mainly as a direct function of level of use, though diligent care may have a modest ameliorating effect. By contrast, the aging of biologic organisms appears to include two distinct components: (1) a genetically preprogrammed sequence of physiological changes that proceed throughout life largely independent of level of activity (at least within the normal range) and (2) a deterioration of specific vital organ functions as a result of wear-and-tear or disease. While the second of these contributions may fundamentally resemble what happens to machines, the first is unique to living organisms. Some gerontologists carefully distinguish between these two factors that contribute change with age by reserving the term *aging* for the preprogrammed, maturative component and employing the term *senescence* for the wear-and-tear factor. Whatever the terminology, the important thing is to recognize that the overall pattern of changes with age is the combined influence of tissue use and disease superimposed on genetically regulated life phase changes.

MLSP among mammalian species correlates with several measurable parameters, notably (1) brain weight, (2) time required for sexual maturation of the individual member of the species, and (3) the number of cell replications programmed for tissue systems that exhibit finite mitotic potential. MLSP also correlates inversely with fecundity—the number of potential offspring that a female member of the species can average per year. Thus, mice, with an MSLP of about 3.5 to 4 years, have low brain weight and reach sexual maturity rapidly. Their fibroblasts have a doubling capacity of 14–28 replications before proliferative capacity declines sharply. A female mouse might produce 100 offspring in a year. Humans, with an MLSP of about 120 years, have a much larger brain weight and require more than a decade to reach sexual maturity. A human female is limited to approximately one offspring per year. Human fibroblasts can replicate an average of 40–60 times before proliferative capacity drops off. Why does MLSP correlate with these particular parameters? The answer is provided by the theory of evolution.

MLSP, as a species characteristic, must be amenable to adaptation since it clearly varies somewhat for individuals within each species. The great variation in the magnitude of MLSP values for various species makes clear that MLSP is a species characteristic that does evolve. Under what circumstances would an increase in MLSP favor species survival and when might it, in fact, work against survival? Extended survival of the individual is most likely to correlate with viability of the species for any species that either has a long latency to sexual maturity or that invests more than is typical in protection, nurturance, or the education of its young by mature members of the population. It is important, in this context, to remember that evolution operates in a manner so as to maximize likelihood of survival of the species, via transfer of the germ-seed from generation to generation. The average length of survival of the individual, on the other hand, will be influenced by evolution only to the extent that it contributes to passing of the genetic material to subsequent generations. For many species, the individual's contribution to survival of the species practically ends when reproductive capacity ends. If the species is one that further invests in continuity of the germ-line by having developed tactics for raising of the young, survival of mature individuals will continue to correlate with viability of the species throughout the parental life phase. This will be most obviously the case for those species that have evolved intelligence as a mechanism of survival (hence the correlation of MLSP with brain weight) and which transfer a great deal of information from parent to offspring during formative years.

Why wouldn't an extension of MLSP always contribute to added viability of a species? When both the years of reproductive capability and the years of parenting have passed by, continued survival of the elderly individuals of a species no longer significantly affects the survival of the species. In fact, for species that exist in habitats with significant limitations on food or space, further extensions of MLSP for the species might even work against species survival by increasing competition for resources from nonreproductive older individuals. Thus, evolutionary pressure operates to promote a life span in each species that is both adequately long but not excessively long for the needs of the species. Aging and its ultimate consequence—death—are, in fact, requisite to species survival.

MLSP is not only an adaptable characteristic of species, but, according to the fossil record, it is a characteristic that can adapt rapidly. Anthropological studies suggest, for example, that the changes in cranial capacity of early hominids evolved in a relatively brief time span. Genetic control of MLSP appears to rest with a relatively small percentage—perhaps no more than 7%—of the total complement of genes, an estimate based on the observation that changes in bodily appearance and physiologic activities that accompany aging are events controlled by no more than about that fraction of the genetic material. Mutations from time to time at any of these sites would cause a degree of variability in MLSP within each species, allowing the operation of natural selection to ensure a near optimum MSLP for each species.

Genetic control of aging appears to be achieved nonuniformly. Some tissues of the body could continue to function well for much longer periods of time. The genetic strategy for limiting life-span appears instead to focus on particular tissues sometimes called the "hot-spots" for aging. The loci for age-related changes are mainly the tissues with cells that have finite doubling capacity—neuronal, bone, myocardial, and reproductive cells. These tissues are focal points for the anatomical changes of aging.

With respect to the wear-and-tear component of the changes that accompany longevity, there are many theories as to how time takes its toll on physiological tissue. Genes may mutate intrinsically at a finite rate or damage may accumulate to DNA or DNA polymerases. That damage may be brought about by the action of free-radicals, slow viruses, or genetic amplifications or deletions. Genetic material that is thus altered may exhibit increased antigenicity, triggering autoimmune attack against the tissue. As damage to the genetic materials accumulates, protein synthesis becomes less reliable, resulting in diminished protein turnover or synthesis of faulty proteins. More complete discussions of the theories of aging can be sought elsewhere (Martin, 1985; Hayflick, 1985; Lamy, 1988).

THE ANATOMY OF AGING

Many of the anatomical aspects of aging are superficial and, therefore, a familiar part of life in human society. Older people are, on average, smaller in stature. This is partly due to the fact that women survive longer on average than men and therefore constitute a disproportionate fraction of the geriatric population. It is also partly due to the fact that mean height of humans—at least those in the United States—has been increasing over the decades, as evidenced by the observation that college freshman are now 1–2 inches taller on average than were previous generations. Historical and archeological records likewise indicate that colonial Americans were shorter on average. This trend toward greater height is probably attributable to improvements in nutrition. Yet not withstanding these population factors, it is also evident that individual women and men are smaller in their 90s than they were in their 70s. Height declines after age 50 at an estimated rate of 1.2 cm per 20 years. Most loss of height is attributable to shortening of the spinal column, brought about by a thinning of each disk of the spinal column and increased curvature of the spine. The long bones of the limbs, by contrast, do not undergo appreciable shortening. Arm span, for example, remains unchanged. The elderly therefore have the appearance of extremities that are long relative to their trunks. This trend is further exacerbated by postural changes in the elderly—a tendency toward slight flexion of the knees and hips.

Another change relating to the skeletal structure is a continuing enlargement of the skull. Head circumference is 2% greater for those age 65 than those age 20. Although the masto-occipital suture begins closure at about age 30, the parietomastoid suture of the cranium does not fully close until near age 80. Bone growth continues to some extent into the 80s at other sites as well, including ribs and pelvis, both of which broaden. At the same time, however, developing osteoarthritis reduces bone mass, so that the tendency is for bones at these growth sites to become wider but weaker. Osteoporosis, which is a gradual loss of bone matrix, is a very nearly universal aspect of aging, though it is relatively greater for females than males, for whites than blacks, and for small persons than larger ones.

Average weight is lower among elderly persons than among young adults, but excessive weight works less against longevity than many people tend to assume. Between 65 and 74 years of age, the percentage of both men and women who are overweight is as high or higher than for young adults. However, the percentage of overweight males and females declines in each decade thereafter. At the same time, the percentage of males and females who are underweight gradually increases between ages 65 and 97. Most elderly individuals therefore reached their maximum weight at an earlier stage of life—at age 42 on average. Average weight declines among the elderly, more so for men than women. Unfortunately, this decline in average weight is probably more due to loss of muscle mass than reduction in fatty tissue.

Another change of aging is alteration in patterns of body hair distribution, though there are major differences by race and gender. White males not only have considerably more body hair than males of oriental or native

American ancestry, but also reach peak hirsutism earlier in life and begin graying more quickly. Male-pattern baldness, a genetic inheritance from the mother, affects many white men as they age. White men may develop hairiness of the ears. White women are prone to facial hirsutism of the chin or upper lip as they age, but this almost never occurs in oriental women. Growth of hair that occurs at puberty as secondary sexual characteristics begins to reverse with aging. Axillary and pubic hair loss occurs in both men and women, but more in women than men and more for oriental women than caucasian women.

One of the most widely recognized anatomical changes of aging is wrinkling of the face. The natural lines of facial expressions deepen even during young adulthood and become increasingly evident with passage of years. Frown lines may develop beside the nose, crow's feet may form as radiations from the lateral canthus, the nasolabial groove may deepen as a result of smiling, or the chin groove may deepen. Wrinkling of the face is the result of loss of fat and elastic fibers in the facial skin. Loss of elasticity may also cause elongation of the face. Facial complexion may become ashen due to reduced perfusion of facial capillaries.

Internally, most major organs decline in size in elderly persons, even in the absence of disease. This occurs, for example, for the brain, kidneys, eyes, vocal cords, fat deposits, and striated muscles. Although a decrease in use may be partly involved in the involution of striated muscle tissue, it can hardly be viewed as a significant factor for such continuously used organs as the eyes and kidneys. The heart, lungs, and prostate gland are exceptions to the general trend toward involution, becoming larger or maintaining their size during aging.

Some of these anatomical correlates of aging resemble changes brought about by certain disorders and thus can either mask or exacerbate disease-related problems. Wrinkling of the skin, for example, can also be caused by excessive exposure to solar radiation. In fact, the solar exposure factor is so pronounced that wrinkling is a poor indicator of chronological age. The pale appearance of the face of the elderly person may suggest anemia, it may be exacerbated by anemia, or it might mask identification of anemia. Changes in body hair patterns might suggest an endocrine disorder if the effects of aging are not taken properly into account.

PHYSIOLOGICAL CHANGES OF AGING

Physiological changes occur in all major organ systems with aging (Figure 1.1). Collectively, these changes impact on health and vitality and some also affect responsiveness of medications, as discussed in Chapter 4.

The Central Nervous System

Changes in the central nervous system due to aging have been well-documented. At the level of gross brain morphology, there is a decrease in both brain volume and brain weight. The loss of brain weight is only partly

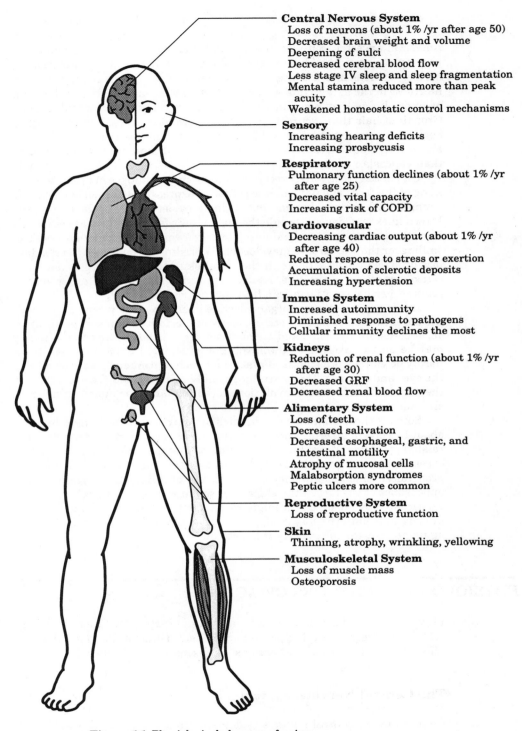

Central Nervous System
Loss of neurons (about 1% /yr after age 50)
Decreased brain weight and volume
Deepening of sulci
Decreased cerebral blood flow
Less stage IV sleep and sleep fragmentation
Mental stamina reduced more than peak
 acuity
Weakened homeostatic control mechanisms

Sensory
Increasing hearing deficits
Increasing prosbycusis

Respiratory
Pulmonary function declines (about 1% /yr
 after age 25)
Decreased vital capacity
Increasing risk of COPD

Cardiovascular
Decreasing cardiac output (about 1% /yr
 after age 40)
Reduced response to stress or exertion
Accumulation of sclerotic deposits
Increasing hypertension

Immune System
Increased autoimmunity
Diminished response to pathogens
Cellular immunity declines the most

Kidneys
Reduction of renal function (about 1% /yr
 after age 30)
Decreased GRF
Decreased renal blood flow

Alimentary System
Loss of teeth
Decreased salivation
Decreased esophageal, gastric, and
 intestinal motility
Atrophy of mucosal cells
Malabsorption syndromes
Peptic ulcers more common

Reproductive System
Loss of reproductive function

Skin
Thinning, atrophy, wrinkling, yellowing

Musculoskeletal System
Loss of muscle mass
Osteoporosis

Figure 1.1 Physiological changes of aging.

accounted for by loss of water content (dehydration), also entailing a loss of cellular constituents such as protein, lipids, and nucleic acids. Apparently the absolute number of neurons in the brain slowly declines, more so in some brain regions than others. Glucose utilization by the brain slowly declines as well, and cranial vascular beds exhibit increased resistance to blood flow. Pigments called lipofuscins accumulate causing the gray color of brain tissue to deepen.

At the neuron level, damage gradually accumulates to cellular nucleic acids, resulting in increased errors in transcriptional and translational activity. The result is increased production of faulty proteins that are unable or less able to conduct cellular functions. Energy resources also decline as nerve cells become increasingly resistant to insulin, diminishing glucose uptake. Synthesis of neurotransmitters, needed for intercellular communication across the synapses, declines due either to diminished energy resources, faulty synthetic enzymes, or both. The normally highly organized structure of the neuron may deteriorate: the intricate network of microtubules that extend along the axon may become tangled or the nerve terminal may come under autoimmune attack.

The result of the accumulation of such changes can include changes in perception, memory, cognition, and consciousness in elderly persons. A degree of hearing loss is virtually inevitable with aging, but varies in extent from person to person. Changes in visual function often occur, but can often be managed with eyeglasses. Even the physiochemical inputs to the brain, such as those that stimulate sensations of thirst and hunger, tend to be muted with age. Inattention to these signals that serve fluid and energy homeostasis may contribute to dehydration or weight loss.

Memory function is often less affected than is commonly supposed even among the elderly themselves. Decreases in acquisition of new information often have more to do with impaired sensory systems or attention than with any change in memory function. The elderly generally exhibit more reduction in mental stamina than in peak acuity and may require more time to complete a learning task than would a younger person.

The Endocrine System

The endocrine system is, in some respects, less affected by aging than other major organ systems in that declines in catabolism of hormones tend to substantially offset declines in production. This is the case for testosterone, cortisol, aldosterone, and thyroxine, for example. The result is that circulating levels of these hormones remain about the same in older individuals compared to younger adults, in the absence of specific endocrine disorders. Pancreatic production of insulin, however, often declines with age resulting in decreased glucose tolerance if not frank diabetes.

The Cardiovascular and Renal Systems

Cardiac output, in the absence of congestive heart failure, is maintained better among the elderly than might be imagined, but there is an essentially linear reduction in efficiency in its pumping action with each year after age 30. As the cardiac muscle ages, there is a gradual increase in afterload—the amount of blood that remains in the ventricle after each heart beat. The aged heart also responds differently during periods of elevated requirements for blood flow. In older persons, the heart increases end-diastolic pressure and stroke volume to meet increased demand, whereas in younger persons, increases in heart rate provide for increases in demand. The conductile system of the heart also gradually deteriorates rendering it more susceptible to drugs that depress conductance of cardiac impulses.

Renal function declines at a rate of about 1% per year after age 30, significantly affecting both general health and drug elimination. Nephrons gradually shrivel; some nephrons undergo necrosis and are supplanted by scar tissue. By age 85, the number of nephrons is likely to be half what it was at age 25.

The Respiratory System

The respiratory system is also subject to age-related changes in function. The airways often narrow. The lungs begin to lose some of their elasticity, and the chest wall itself becomes more rigid. Alveolar surface area declines. All of these changes reduce pulmonary function and may culminate in diminished oxygenation of blood.

The Host Defense Systems

Many gerontologists and physiologists view the aging of the immune system as having special relevance in the mechanisms of aging. The human host is in constant contact with viral, bacterial, and fungal pathogens and, many believe, aberrant host cells with carcinogenic potential, as well. The host defense systems—the immune system and the reticuloendothelial system—act vigorously to hold potential onslaughts in check and to maintain the health and survival of the host as long as possible. The whole system rests on the sophisticated ability of the host defense systems to recognize the difference between host tissue and foreign or aberrant cells and to launch a vigorous attack against the intruders. Failure to provide an adequately vigorous defense results in infectious disorders or cancerous growths, while failure to recognize self culminates in autoimmunity. It is a delicate balancing act in the best of circumstances, but made greatly more difficult by the changes in the defense systems with aging.

While it is beyond the scope of the current discussion to detail the operation of the host defense mechanisms, the reader is briefly reminded that the immune system includes two major components: cellular immunity, provided by T lymphocytes, and humoral immunity, provided by B lymphocytes. The latter depend somewhat on the former for guidance, and both direct the work of the phagocytic scavenger cells, macrophages and neutrophils, of the reticuloendothelial system. Although the number of circulating white blood cells remains about constant throughout life, nevertheless evidence indicates that there is a progressive decline in function of both the B lymphocytes and T lymphocytes after reproductive maturity. T lymphocytes, though originating as bone marrow stem cells, migrate during human infancy to the thymus gland, where they mature to provide the endowment of T lymphocytes. Though stem cells retain proliferative capacity throughout a human lifetime, the mature T lymphocytes have finite doubling capacity. The thymus gland, moreover, undergoes involution at pubescence. Thus, this system of T lymphocyte production seems expressly designed to provide optimum host defense capability during the reproductive period and for a finite period thereafter.

The Gastrointestinal System

The gastrointestinal system undergoes a general involution during aging. The mucosal lining thins as it becomes less cellular. Liver, pancreatic, and gastric enzymes and gastric acid are all secreted in smaller quantities in the elderly, but so too is the protective mucus. Consequently, digestion may be impaired or, conversely, chronic gastritis or peptic ulcers may develop. Gastric emptying time increases as well, by as much as 2–3 fold, slowing the rate of movement of ingested substances into the intestines. Intestinal motility decreases as well, resulting in the constipation that is so common among the elderly. Blood flow to the alimentary tract decreases by as much as 50% as the competition from other tissues for cardiac output increases. The elderly are more likely to suffer nutritional deficiencies than their younger counterparts, in part because changes in alimentary function promote malabsorption and partly because changing life circumstances, such as living alone or institutionalization, may disrupt good nutritional habits developed during early stages of life.

CONCLUSION

Anatomical and physiological changes occur in nearly every part of the body with aging. These changes affect outward appearance as well as the function of each major organ system. These changes provide the context for the health status of elderly persons as well as the actions of drugs that they require.

REFERENCES AND RECOMMENDED READINGS

Hayflick L: The aging phenomenon, in O'Malley K. and Waddington JL (eds): *Therapeutics in the elderly,* New York, Elsevier, 1985, pp. 3–12.
Jarvik LF, Matsuyama SS: Genetic aspects of aging, in Rossman: *Clin. Geriatr.,* Philadelphia, Lippincott, 1986, pp. 68–93.

Lamy PP: Introduction to the aging process, in Delafuente, Stewart: *Therapeutics in the Elderly,* Baltimore, Williams & Wilkins, 1988, pp. 3–22.

Latham KR, Johnson LR: Aging at the cellular level, in Rossman: *Clin. Geriatr.,* Philadelphia, Lippincott, 1986, pp. 31–56.

Martin GM: Current views on the biology of aging, in Butler RN, Bearn AG (eds): *The Aging Process: Therapeutic Implications,* New York, Raven Press, 1985, pp. 21–31.

Meier DE: The cell biology of aging, in Cassel, Walsh (eds): *Geriatric Medicine,* Springer-Verlag, 1984, pp. 3–12.

Rossman I: The anatomy of aging, in Rossman: *Clin. Geriatr.,* Philadelphia, Lippincott, 1986, pp. 3–22.

Rowe JW: Physiologic changes with age and their clinical relevance, in Butler RN, Bearn AG (eds): *The Aging Process: Therapeutic Implications,* New York, Raven Press, 1985, pp. 41–49.

Weksler ME: Biologic basis and clinical significance of immune senescence, in Rossman: *Clin. Geriatr.,* Philadelphia, Lippincott, 1986, pp. 57–67.

CHAPTER 2

Psychosocial Aspects of Aging

Human beings can best be understood as whole persons who have physiological, psychological, social, and spiritual aspects. These elements can be examined separately, but only with the understanding that they are interdependent and interact within the context of the whole person.

Since understanding of human beings can best be promoted within a holistic framework, it is essential to integrate the psychosocial and physical aspects of aging. The individual's psychological state and general outlook on life influence his or her health status as well as daily activities such as health behaviors. Because of this close relationship with physical health, psychosocial and spiritual well-being have relevance for medication-taking behaviors, the need for medications, and the effects of these medications.

This chapter explores understanding older people through descriptions of common life experiences, transitions, and losses. The potential for personal growth through these events is discussed, as well as theoretical perspectives for understanding the impact of medications during these times.

STEREOTYPES OF AGING IN AMERICA

The percent of older people in the United States is growing at a rapid rate. Persons over age 65 currently comprise 12.6% of the population, with that number expected to grow to 22% by the year 2030 (Bureau of Census, 1989). The fastest growing segment of the population is the 85 and older age group. Although some changes in culture can be noted as the result of the new demographics, our society continues to be youth-oriented. Looking and acting young while being a contributing member of society, usually through some form of paid employment, is highly valued.

Unfortunately, negative attitudes toward the elderly are common. The "systematic stereotyping and discrimination against people because they are old" is "ageism" (Butler, 1987, p. 22). Negative stereotypes usually produce negative attitudes, and negative attitudes foster negative stereo-types in a circular relationship (Palmore, 1990). Education to correct the negative stereotypes and myths about what the elderly are really like is imperative in order to begin to change negative attitudes.

Health care professionals are not immune to ageism and negative atti-tudes toward elderly or toward caring for them. Research studies have consis-tently found negative attitudes among health care professionals to be similar to those in the general population (Campbell, 1971; Gunter, 1971; Kayser & Minnergerode, 1975; Reif, 1982). Although it has not been clearly shown that such attitudes directly affect behaviors, it has been suggested that some nurses holding negative attitudes toward older people may engage in behav-iors that are physically or psychologically detrimental to older patients (Pen-ner, Ludenia, & Mead, 1984; Brands, 1975). Fortunately, educational courses or programs have been found to have an effect on reducing negative attitudes among nurses in several studies (Gunter, 1971; Tobiason et al., 1979).

Table 2.1 The Palmore Facts on Aging Quiz: Part 1 (FAQ1) (From Palmore EB: *Ageism: Negative and Positive*. New York, Springer, 1990, pp. 183–184. © 1990 Springer Publishing Company, Inc. Used by permission.)

1. The majority of old people (age 65+) are senile (have defective memory, are disoriented, or demented).
2. The five senses (sight, hearing, taste, touch, and smell) all tend to weaken in old age.
3. The majority of old people have no interest in, nor capacity for, sexual relations.
4. Lung vital capacity tends to decline in old age.
5. The majority of old people feel miserable most of the time.
6. Physical strength tends to decline in old age.
7. More than one-tenth of the aged are living in long-stay institutions (such as nursing homes, mental hospitals, homes for the aged, etc.).
8. Aged drivers have fewer accidents per driver than those under age 65.
9. Older workers usually cannot work as effectively as younger workers.
10. Over three-fourths of the aged are healthy enough to carry out their normal activities.
11. The majority of old people are unable to adapt to change.
12. Old people usually take longer to learn something new.
13. It is difficult for the average old person to learn something new.
14. Older people tend to react slower than younger people.
15. In general, old people tend to be pretty much alike.
16. The majority of old people say they are seldom bored.
17. The majority of old people are socially isolated.
18. Older workers have fewer accidents than younger workers.
19. Over 15% of the population are now age 65 or over.
20. The majority of medical practitioners tend to give low priority to the aged.
21. The majority of old people have incomes below the poverty line (as defined by the federal government).
22. The majority of old people are working or would like to have some kind of work to do (including housework and volunteer work).
23. Old people tend to become more religious as they age.
24. The majority of old people say they are seldom irritated or angry.
25. The health and economic status of old people will be about the same or worse in the year 2000 (compared to younger people).

Because part of people's self image is a reflection of how people perceive themselves as being viewed by others, health care professionals' attitudes toward elderly are very important. If nurses convey a feeling that they do not really want to be caring for a particular older patient, that patient may feel a loss of self-worth. Repeated experiences contributing to low self-esteem may translate into decreased motivation to maintain one's health status, including taking one's medication as prescribed.

Palmore's *Facts on Aging Quiz* (Table 2.1) is helpful in identifying commonly held myths about older people. Comparing one's answers with the "correct answers" can help recognize stereotypes related to older people.

DESCRIPTION OF THE ELDERLY POPULATION

Although there is much individual variation among older people, knowledge of the elderly as a group can help to dispel myths about aging and to change negative attitudes about the elderly. Demographic statistics indicate that the majority of people over age 65 in this country are retired, female, have adult children living within close proximity, have an average of four chronic illnesses but no functional limitations, live in rural areas, drive cars, have enough income to meet their needs, and take an average of two to four prescription drugs. Most older women are widowed and live alone, while the majority of older men are married and live with their spouses. About half have a high school education (Tables 2.2, 2.3, 2.4).

Table 2.2 Population by sex, by living area, by marital status, and by age (U.S. Census, 1990)

		65–74 Years	(%)	75–84 Years	(%)	85 and older	(%)
Gender	male	7,941,613	(10.4)	3,765,862	(8.5)	857,698	(1.8)
	female	10,164,945	(14.7)	6,289,246	(10.9)	2,222,467	(3.8)
Living in:							
Metropolitan	male	5,853,753	(9.8)	2,698,326	(8.1)	608,809	(1.7)
area	female	7,597,700	(14.8)	4,620,746	(10.4)	1,624,843	(3.5)
Rural area	male	2,087,860	(12.4)	1,067,536	(10.1)	248,889	(2.3)
	female	2,567,245	(16.9)	1,668,500	(12.4)	597,624	(4.5)
Marital status							
Male	never						
	married	392,314	(4.9)	181,886	(4.8)	44,693	(5.2)
	married	6,287,518	(79.2)	2,674,385	(71.0)	436,769	(50.9)
	separated	113,819	(1.4)	39,825	(1.1)	7,092	(0.9)
	widowed	701,651	(8.8)	732,438	(19.4)	347,413	(40.5)
	divorced	446,311	(5.6)	137,328	(3.6)	21,731	(2.5)
Female	never						
	married	489,966	(4.8)	379,334	(6.0)	156,644	(7.0)
	married	5,253,888	(51.7)	1,768,765	(28.1)	195,365	(8.8)
	separated	129,986	(1.3)	42,309	(0.7)	7,548	(0.3)
	widowed	3,587,808	(35.3)	3,832,368	(60.9)	1,805,814	(81.3)
	divorced	703,297	(6.9)	266,470	(4.2)	57,096	(2.6)

Table 2.3 Persons in household and in group quarters by age and sex (U.S. census, 1990)

		65–74 Years	(%)	75–84 Years	(%)	85 and older	(%)
Living in *(total pop.)*	household	17,770,393	(98.1)	9,384,175	(93.3)	2,306,398	(74.9)
	institution-alized	284,107	(1.6)	636,138	(6.3)	755,817	(24.5)
	other persons	52,058	(0.3)	34,795	(0.3)	17,950	(0.6)
Male in	household	7,794,360	(98.1)	3,579,040	(95.0)	714,074	(83.3)
	institution-alized	121,615	(1.5)	176,775	(4.7)	140,151	(16.3)
	other persons	25,638	(0.3)	10,047	(0.3)	3,473	(0.4)
Female in	household	9,976,033	(98.1)	5,805,135	(92.3)	1,592,324	(71.6)
	institution-alized	162,492	(1.6)	459,363	(7.3)	615,666	(27.7)
	other persons	26,420	(0.3)	24,748	(0.4)	14,477	(0.7)

Table 2.4 Persons in household by relationship to householder by age and sex (U.S. Census, 1990)

		65–74 Years	(%)	75–84 Years	(%)	85 and older	(%)
Relationship to *householder*	householder (total)	7,043,104	(90.4)	3,180,847	(88.9)	590,639	(82.7)
Male	family house-holder (total)	5,935,417	(76.2)	2,452,506	(68.5)	371,651	(52.0)
	with married spouse	5,691,856	(73.0)	2,322,944	(64.9)	333,278	(46.7)
	nonfamily householder (total)	1,107,687	(14.2)	728,341	(20.4)	218,988	(30.7)
	living alone	1,008,447	(12.9)	685,775	(19.2)	208,392	(29.2)
	relatives of householder (total)	623,743	(8.0)	345,137	(9.6)	108,849	(15.2)
	spouse	364,868	(4.7)	171,594	(4.8)	30,551	(4.3)
	child	17,586	(0.2)	818	(–)	17	(–)
	other relatives	241,289	(3.1)	172,725	(4.8)	78,281	(11.0)
	nonrelatives of householder in family households	46,936	(0.6)	19,945	(0.6)	6,829	(1.0)
	in nonfamily households	80,577	(1.0)	33,111	(0.9)	7,757	(1.1)
Relationship to *householder* *Female*	householder (total)	4,473,478	(44.8)	3,606,026	(62.1)	1,078,607	(67.7)
	family house-holder (total)	1,244,730	(12.5)	632,209	(10.9)	164,925	(10.4)

Table 2.4 Continued

		65–74 Years	(%)	75–84 Years	(%)	85 and older	(%)
Female (cont.)	with married						
	spouse	317,902	(3.2)	118,052	(2.0)	12,021	(0.8)
	nonfamily householder						
	(total)	3,228,748	(32.4)	2,973,817	(51.2)	913,682	(57.4)
	living alone	3,122,786	(31.3)	2,909,526	(50.1)	889,919	(55.9)
	relatives of householder						
	(total)	5,374,530	(53.9)	2,124,791	(36.6)	482,454	(30.3)
	spouse	4,729,789	(47.4)	1,497,891	(25.8)	132,671	(8.3)
	child	29,575	(0.3)	2,549	(–)	61	(–)
	other relatives	615,166	(6.2)	624,351	(10.8)	349,722	(22.0)
	nonrelatives of householder in family						
	households	40,666	(0.4)	27,721	(0.5)	15,874	(1.0)
	in nonfamily households	87,359	(0.9)	46,597	(0.8)	15,389	(1.0)

Regarding psychological and cognitive status of older adults, the majority have no difficulty with long- or short-term memory and have no cognitive deficits. Only 4% of those age 65–75 and 25% of those over 80 years of age are estimated to have some cognitive dysfunction defined as dementia (Wills, 1993). Acquisition of new knowledge and skills is unaffected for healthy older people, although they tend not to learn as well as younger people when stressed or when time pressure is present. Less than 10% of elderly living in the community have significant mental illness (Palmore, 1990). Most older people are not bored or lonely, and most feel either useful or would like some useful work to do. Research on happiness or life satisfaction indicates that there are not significant differences in life satisfaction between older adults and those in younger age groups. Instead, happiness later in life seems to depend on happiness earlier in life. Personality in later life can generally be characterized as a continuation of earlier general approaches to life. Happiness and successful adjustment early in life seems to be predictive of happiness and adjustment in one's later years.

Older people as a group are very heterogeneous. This means that there is wide variation among those who are over age 65. They are more dissimilar to each other than any other age group. Therefore, generalizations about older people as a group should be undertaken with caution. Each individual should be carefully assessed, rather than making assumptions about what a person is like from group characteristics or stereotypes. Statistics summarize frequent or common characteristics of the population of older adults, but care must be taken to remember that there is a wide range of potential characteristics within a statistical picture.

LIFE EXPERIENCE AND TRANSITIONS

Transitions occur throughout the life cycle. Early life transitions, such as going to nursery school or kindergarten for the first time, and those of adolescence, such as graduating from high school, are viewed positively and as important developmental milestones. Often life transitions such as marriage are accompanied by much celebration. Transitions such as moving, changing jobs, and having babies are all viewed positively if they meet society's expectations of improvement in one's social status. Bridges (1980) identified three stages for all kinds of transition, whether desired or dreaded, chosen or imposed: (1) ending of the old; (2) a period of confusion and distress, and (3) new beginnings. Regardless of the desirability of the transition, a person must say good-bye to the former lifestyle before the transition can occur. No matter how happy the transition may be, such as having a long-awaited baby or a carefree life, some other phase of life for which there may be great nostalgia is ending. This needs to be recognized as a loss. In the second stage, a period of readjustment occurs, which is usually characterized by confusion and distress. If the adjustment is successful, new beginnings with potential for growth and renewal can occur in the third stage.

An examination of the differences between age groups shows how the experience of aging is one of living with transitions (Tables 2.2–2.4). Often these transitions include moving from employment to retirement, from one home to another (usually smaller), from being active to less active, from health to chronic illness, from being married to being widowed, and from extensive social networks to smaller circles of family and friends. Such transitions are defined as losses within our society and are often viewed negatively. Successful aging requires coping with these losses and accepting one's new life situation positively. One must acknowledge the ending of part of life, often a cherished part, go through a period of distress and adjustment, and begin again to create a meaningful life.

Life transitions are experienced differently by different people. The death of a spouse, for instance, is not always a devastating experience. For some whose marriages have been extremely difficult and oppressive, death of a spouse may bring a change in lifestyle that allows creativity and self-actualization for the first time. For some, retirement may mean freedom to do what they have longed to do all their lives. For others, it may be a loss of the central purpose and meaning in their lives. The same life transition may have a variety of meanings for different people.

Also, a single life transition may have multiple meanings for a given person. An example of this might be a husband, whose wife has become ill, and who is forced into a caregiver role for the first time in his life. For him, this may mean grieving the loss of his former role in which he was cared for by his wife. However, he may also discover a sense of meaning and pleasure in his caregiver role, being able to give to the person who had given so much to him over the years. Since the same transition can have so many possible meanings, it is extremely important to assess the actual meanings of the transition for each individual case.

The responses older people have to life transitions and the outcomes or paths their lives take are determined by their personalities and their personal and social resources. There are many theories and frameworks available to help understand and explain the personalities and behaviors of older persons. Since the purpose of this book is to present information about aspects of aging that relate to medication use and effects, this discussion will include theories and perspectives most applicable for understanding drug-related issues. Two relevant theories which give us insight into psychosocial aspects of elderly are Erikson's developmental stage theory and Maslow's hierarchy of needs theory. Both of these approaches were developed to promote understanding of behavior across the life span, not specifically older people, but both have much to offer in this area.

Erikson (1963) proposed a developmental theory which gives insight into life perspectives as a whole. He identified eight chronological stages of life and tasks associated with each stage. The last stage of life, old age, is concerned with ego integrity versus despair. The task for older people is to review their lives and determine if they are satisfied with the way their lives were lived. Feelings about and responses to past life transitions are called forth and evaluated in terms of how well the older person feels he or she adjusted to the transitions. Integrity derives from the person being generally satisfied with this evaluation of his or her life. If, however, people look back over their lives and are disappointed, feeling that there is no longer any time or possibility for change and with no chance for new beginnings, despair may result. This may bring feelings of anger and contempt for oneself as well as for others. Erikson's theory places importance on the experiences of an entire lifetime as determining whether old age will bring opportunities for contentment and growth or despair and restriction of human potential. This theory emphasizes the importance of the older person's whole life perspective rather than focusing on the immediate situation in her or his life.

Maslow (1968) viewed human beings as motivated to meet five levels of needs. He identified a hierarchical pattern in the shape of a pyramid (Figure 2.1) defining lower level needs on the pyramid as stronger motivators than higher level needs near the top of the pyramid. He believed that the most basic needs for all human beings are the biological needs such as respiration, circulation, nutrition, elimination, sleep, activity, rest, and comfort. Safety and security needs including sensory function, environmental safety, and legal and economic protection are next. If these most basic two levels of need are met, the need for belonging and love, for communication and relationships of all kinds, and sexuality, become of prime importance. Next self-esteem, derived from effective coping, intelligence, and maintaining autonomy and control, becomes the active motivational force. At the peak is self-actualization, which involves living a meaningful and enriching life, creativity, growth, legacies, and transcendence. Although Maslow has viewed these needs as hierarchical, with top level needs not able to be met without the lowest level needs being satisfied, it seems that some older adults are able to achieve self-actualization and fulfillment in the face of compromised physiological integrity, pain, and even without experiencing safety and security. Maslow, in his studies of self-actualized people, did not

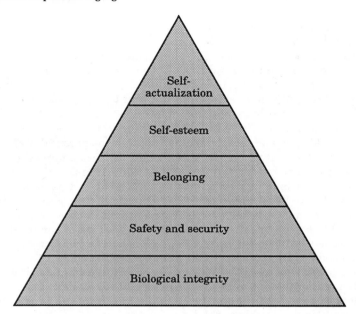

Figure 2.1 Maslow's hierarchy of needs.

find any young adults who had achieved self-actualization. Perhaps the experience of aging is essential to bring enough life transitions and potential growth experiences to enable older people to become fulfilled and self-actualized human beings.

Some of the common life transitions experienced by elderly bring about unmet needs. For instance, the grief response associated with the death of a spouse may affect every level of need. In the first level, body function may be disturbed as the person experiences physical symptoms associated with acute grief. Needs of safety and security, belonging and love go unmet as the primary person who met these needs is gone. A major person who probably contributed to self-esteem is lost and life patterns and the ability to self-actualize are threatened. Other life transitions may affect other levels; however, according to Maslow, if lower level needs are not met, it is not possible to meet the higher level needs. A change in one's health status may make it impossible to meet the most basic needs of physiological integrity. Retirement may threaten the need for safety and security if it brings with it a threat to financial security. If finances are not a problem, a loss of self-esteem may result if a person's self-image is strongly attached to his or her job.

One useful way of viewing personal responses to life transitions can be found in the stress-coping model. In the stress-coping model, life transitions outlined above are viewed as stressors that precipitate stress responses that can have a harmful effect on physiological and psychosocial health. The individual must then respond to the stressor, usually calling forth previously used, successful coping mechanisms to apply to this new situation. For many older people, several major life transitions may occur within a relatively short period of time. For instance, an older man may retire, move to Florida with his wife, and discover he has diabetes and heart disease all in the same year.

Day-to-day hassles also cause stress in peoples' lives. Older people often have more difficulties with daily hassles than do younger people, as changes in their health status and living situations may make activities of daily living more difficult to accomplish. Daily hassles combined with stress from major life transitions make coping with stress even more difficult for the older person.

Three types of factors determine how successfully stress from life transitions and daily hassles will be handled. The first, **characteristics of the individual,** include the meaning the person attaches to the event, past history of successful use of coping mechanisms, existing level of stress, health status, and general outlook on life. The second, **external characteristics,** include supports that have a buffering effect on the stress level such as the support of friends and family and activity level. The third, **characteristics of the stressor(s),** include such factors as magnitude, length of time since the occurrence, number of stressful events experienced, and whether the event was expected or not.

Stress responses include both physical and psychological signs and symptoms. The stressed individual may experience feelings such as anxiety, restlessness, withdrawal, lack of interest, depression, or anger. Cognitive abilities may also be affected as forgetfulness, errors in judgment, preoccupation, lack of concentration, and orientation toward the past may predominate. Physical signs and symptoms such as increased heart rate and elevated blood pressure, difficulty breathing, perspiration, tremors, and tight muscles occur quickly in response to stress. Other physical symptoms are more generalized such as loss of appetite, sleep disturbances, and fatigue. Because the function of the immune system changes with age as well as in response to stressors, it is to be expected that the incidence of diseases related to immune system function would increase among older people. More research is needed to explore this relationship.

Human beings have the capacity to encounter stressful life situations or transitions and to utilize them as growth experiences. In this personal growth perspective, life transitions are viewed as natural occurrences within the life path. As natural parts of life, all transitions can be viewed as having potential, at least, to be growth producing, enabling the individual to progress in his or her growth toward wholeness. Difficult experiences can either be viewed as devastating set backs or as challenges to conquer, from which to learn and grow. Some personal characteristics are, in effect, resources which are helpful in promoting these experiences as growth producing for the older person. These include good health and good physical condition, a sense of some degree of control over life events, self-awareness and self-esteem, flexibility, tolerance, the support of family and friends including having a confidante, and a spiritual belief in a supreme power. Nurses and other health professionals can use a battery of questions (Table 2.5) to assess the older person's self-image and other psychosocial factors.

Table 2.5 Questions for assessing self-perception and life transition

Introduction
- I'd like to get to know you better. Tell me a little about yourself.

Activity pattern
- What kinds of things do you do on a typical day? (Elicit data regarding life space, friends, social contacts, spheres of interest.)
- Have you noticed any changes in your daily activities or social contacts?
- Has your activity level changed as you have grown older?

Life transitions
- Have you had any major changes in your life this past year? (If yes, what were they?)
- How did you feel about each of these?
- How are you coping with these?
- How have you coped in the past with similar changes?

Self-image
- Can you share with me your feelings about growing older?
- What is the best part of getting older for you?
- What is the most difficult part of getting older for you?
- How do you feel about your health now?
- Have any changes occurred in your health that you think about a lot?

Self-perception
- How do you feel about yourself? Do you feel comfortable with the way you look and feel?
- How would you describe yourself to another person? (physical appearance and personality)
- What would you describe as your strengths and weaknesses?
- Are there things you would like to change about yourself? Describe them.
- Are you pleased with your life so far? Describe.
- Do you have future goals you would like to achieve?
- Do you have something or things so important in your life that they give your life meaning? If yes, what are they? If no, please describe your life at this time.

Adapted from Mezey, Raukhorst, & Stokes, 1980; Burbank, 1993.

Life transitions are generally thought of as primarily influencing an older persons' psychological outlook on life, but these transitions also have an impact on overall health status and daily living. Every aspect of life can be changed, including the older persons' need for medications, the way the drug interacts with or affects their bodies, and their ability or motivation to take the drug appropriately.

The interaction between drugs and psychosocial issues for older people must be viewed from two perspectives: the effect of psychosocial factors on drug-taking behaviors and drug responses and the effect of drugs on psycho-social functioning. Since effects of medications on cognition and emotions will be discussed elsewhere, the focus here is on the effect of psychosocial factors on drug-taking behaviors and responses to drugs.

If an elderly person is experiencing despair and a loss of ego integrity because of a negative assessment of his or her life (following Erikson's theory), life may not seem worth living any more. That older person may become depressed and lose interest in life. Medications intended to prolong his or her life and health may seem contrary to his or her goals. Medications that are expensive or do not give any positive relief of symptoms may be even more difficult to justify. Taking medications to promote life is perceived as self-defeating. Suicide rates are higher for older adults than any other age group, with males over age 80 having the highest rates. It is impossible to determine how many older people contribute to their own deaths or declines in health by failing to take their medications as prescribed. This possibility certainly needs to be considered when caring for an older person who seems depressed or dissatisfied with life.

The interaction between psychosocial factors and the effects of medications is difficult to assess, but one for which there is much evidence. Understanding these responses is complicated by the introduction of age-related changes that alter physiological responses. Further adding to the confusion, the physiological effects of a drug enter the picture. Lastly, most elderly people take multiple medications and have several chronic diseases making it very difficult to identify the individual effects of age changes, disease, stress response, and medications. These are factors that contribute to the difficulties associated with elderly and drugs.

Many medications influence cognitive or affective functioning, positively or negatively. Such effects can be intended effects, side effects, or toxic effects and will be discussed in later chapters. It is important to remember that the relationship between drugs and psychosocial aspects is a reciprocal and complex one. Potential negative influences of drugs may impact any of these areas according to Maslow's hierarchy of needs (Figure 2.2).

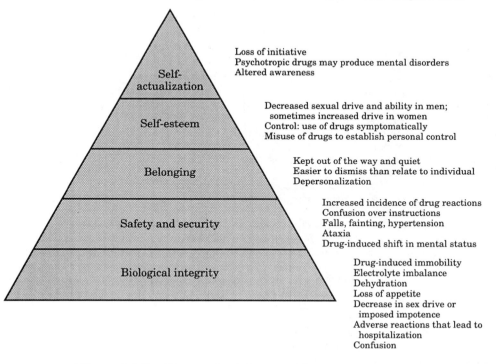

Figure 2.2 Possible negative influence of drugs on the hierarchy of needs. (From Ebersole, P. and Hess P., *Toward healthy aging: Human needs and nursing response, 4th ed.*, St. Louis, Mosby, 1994, p. 308. Reprinted with permission.)

CONCLUSION

In summary, psychosocial issues for older persons are complex because older people are a very diverse group. Common stereotypes of older Americans need to be dispelled by accurate information. The stage of ego integrity versus despair in Erikson's developmental theory is one useful way for developing a broader life view of older people. Likewise, Maslow's hierarchy of needs can help provide a more specific understanding of the needs and motivations of older adults. Life transitions, which occur with greater frequency and bring more stress in old age, pose a threat to ego integrity and to meeting needs at all levels. Recognition of common stress responses and coping behaviors and resources lends insight into the psychosocial issues of the elderly. Finally, the psychosocial issues of aging have significant implications for drug-taking behavior and medication responses among the elderly. A holistic approach when assessing and interacting with older people is therefore necessary for effective drug therapy and clinical care.

REFERENCES AND RECOMMENDED READINGS

Brands A: Factors influencing geriatric nursing practice in the drug therapy regimen of aged patients in selected nursing homes. *Dissertation Abstracts,* 1975; 36:3.

Bridges W: *Transitions: Making sense of life's changes.* Reading, MA; Addison-Wesley, 1980.

Burbank PM: Assessing the meaning of life among older clients: An exploratory study. *Journal of Gerontological Nursing,* 1993; 18(9):19–28.

Butler R: Ageism, in Maddox G. (ed.): *The encyclopedia of aging.* New York; Springer, 1987.

Campbell ME: Study of the attitudes of nursing personnel toward the geriatric patient. *Nursing Research,* 1971; 20(2):147–151.

Ebersole P, Hess P: *Toward healthy aging: Human need and nursing response.* St. Louis; Mosby, 1985.

Erikson E: *Childhood and society,* ed 3. New York; Norton, 1963.

Gunter LM: Students' attitudes toward geriatric nursing. *Nursing Outlook,* 1971; 19:466–469.

Kayser JS, Minnergerode F: Increasing students' interest in working with aged patients. *Nursing Research,* 1975; 24:23–26.

Maslow AH: *Toward a psychology of being.* New York; Van Nostrand Reinhold, 1968.

Mezey MD, Raukhorst LH, Stokes SA: Health assessment of the older individual. New York, Springer, 1980.

Palmore E: *The facts on aging quiz.* New York, Springer, 1988.

Palmore EB: *Ageism: Negative and positive.* New York, Springer, 1990.

Penner LA, Ludenia K, Mead G: Staff attitudes with image or reality? *Journal of Gerontological Nursing,* 1984; 10:110–117.

Reif L: The critical need for nurses in long-term care: Implications for geriatric education. *Gerontology and Geriatric Education,* 1982; 3:145–153.

Tobiason SJ, Knudson F, Stengel JC, Giss M: Positive attitudes toward aging: The aged teach the young. *Journal of Geriatric Nursing,* 1979; 5:18–23.

CHAPTER 3

An Overview
of Drug Use
and Misuse
among the Elderly

Older people are the fastest growing age group in the United States, and they use more medications than any other age group. This extensive use of medications is due not only to the increased prevalence of chronic illnesses among this population, but also to inappropriate prescriptions and misuse of prescribed and over-the-counter drugs. Medications present special problems for older persons because of their altered physiology and responses to drugs. This will be discussed in more detail in Chapters 4 and 5.

Older people are at increased risk for drug-related illness (Colt & Shapiro, 1989), accounting for an estimated 5–23% of hospital admissions, 1–5% of office visits, and 1/1000 deaths (Nolan & O'Malley, 1988). A recent report found that 40% of hospital admissions for drug-related illness in older persons were related to noncompliance with the medication regimen (Col, Fanale, & Kronholm, 1990). Because older people take a greater number of drugs; are more likely to misuse drugs; and have a greater probability of side effects, toxic effects, and drug interactions; there is great need for close attention to the area of drugs and the elderly.

Drugs can provide great relief and control of symptoms related to many chronic diseases and can play an extremely important role in promoting health, prolonging life, and improving the quality of life. However, the potential for drugs to have adverse effects on health, disease, and quality of life is also greater for older people. The purpose of this chapter is to increase understanding about drug use and misuse by the elderly. The chapter presents information about demographic changes, which indicate the rapid growth of the older age population; discusses the extent and types of medications used by the elderly; and outlines areas of misuse of drugs both by physicians caring for older persons and by older individuals themselves. The issue of noncompliance is discussed in more detail in Chapter 6.

DEMOGRAPHICS

The classification and definition of "elderly" as people over age 65 was determined arbitrarily in 1935 when the Social Security Act was passed. It has no physiological or social basis; nothing magical happens at age 65 to make a person old. However, most data are available using this age as a marker for older adults. Therefore, the terms *older adults* or *elderly* will be used to refer to those aged 65 and older throughout this book.

The population in the United States is 249 million, with 18 million people between the ages of 65–74 and 13 million aged seventy-five and older. Those over 85 years of age number 3 million (Bureau of the Census, 1990). The elderly are the fastest growing age group in the United States, and are expected to continue to grow faster than any other age group. While the population under age 65 grows by only about 12% per year, those over 65 years of age increase by more than 20%. The 75 and over age group increases in even greater increments, by nearly 40% each year (Tables 3.1, 3.2, Figure 3.1).

Population projections for future years indicate an increase in percent of elderly in the population from 12% in 1990 to 13% in the year 2000, 20% by 2025, and 22% by 2050. Unless there is a new baby boom, these demographic changes are expected to stabilize, resulting in a population in the United States where all generations and age groups are approximately the same size (Table 3.3).

Table 3.1 Estimated Population Increase from 1975 to 2050

Age (yrs)	Percent increase
All ages	50.2
0–19	17.3
20–64	57.8
65–74	122.8
75+	138.1

Source: US Census Population Reports, Series P-25 No. 470.

Table 3.2 Elderly Population in the United States

Year	Total no. (in millions)	% of total 75 yrs and over
1900	3.1	29
1940	9.0	
1965	18.5	
1970		38
1975	22.4	
2000*	31.8	45
2030*	55.0	

*Projected.
Source: US Census Population Reports, Series P-25, No. 470.

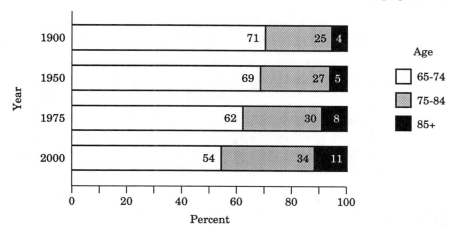

Figure 3.1 Changing demographic characteristics of the elderly. Lamy, PP (1980). *Prescribing for the elderly.* Littleton, MA: PSG Publishing.

Table 3.3 Population Projection: United States

	Population in millions			
	1975	**2000**	**2025**	**2050**
All ages	213	264	302	320
0–19	75	80	84	88
20–64	116	154	173	183
65–74	22	30	45	49
75+	8.4	13	16	20

Source: US Census Population Reports, Series P-25 No. 470.

In 1900, life expectancy at birth was 49 years, increasing to 68 years by 1950. Now a white female born in 1975 has a life expectancy of 77.2 years. It is postulated that life expectancy may increase up to 100 years within the next 20 years.

There is wide variation in life expectancy by gender and race. Across all races, females have a longer life expectancy than males. At present, the life expectancies of both African Americans and Native Americans are significantly less than for white Americans. This is due mainly to diseases that have not been adequately controlled in minority groups. Other factors include socioeconomic issues and problems of access to health care.

Life expectancy is increased by controlling diseases and promoting health through preventive measures and healthful living. Despite rapid advances in medicine and technology, only 2.4 years have been added to the average life expectancy since 1950. Studies indicate that lifestyle changes will most likely be required if further increases in life expectancy are to be realized. Changes that might increase life expectancy include getting 7–8 hours of sleep each night, eating well-balanced meals, exercising regularly, refraining from smoking, consuming no more than moderate amounts of alcohol, and having a positive mental attitude. Current self-help literature and the media now focus on these health-promoting lifestyle changes to minimize disease and improve health.

Since lifestyle changes have already been implemented by some, it is anticipated that the older generations of the future will enjoy better health status with fewer limitations from chronic diseases than the current cohort of elderly. If this does occur, despite the increase in numbers of elderly, the need for medications will be postponed to a later age. Until those who have adopted healthier lifestyles join the older generation, it is expected that prescription and over-the-counter medication use will increase as the older population increases.

HEALTH STATUS

Most people are able to carry on their normal activities and functioning up to the age of 75. After age 75, the effects of chronic disease have a greater impact, and problems of ill health and dependency become more prevalent. Only about 9% of the elderly, however, report their health as poor, and most consider themselves to be in good or excellent health (Lamy, 1980).

The major causes of death among those over age 65 are, in order of decreasing frequency, heart disease, malignant neoplasms, cerebrovascular disease, chronic obstructive pulmonary disease (COPD), influenza and pneumonia, diabetes mellitus, accidents and their complications, cirrhosis of the liver, and suicide. Table 3.4 shows the rates according to age group. It should be noted that all of these diseases are chronic and often require long-term medication and treatment except for influenza and pneumonia which are time-limited.

Approximately 80% of older persons have at least one chronic disease, with an average of four per person. The most common chronic illnesses for older adults can be found in Table 3.5, which shows the differences between elderly under and over age seventy-five. Of these chronic conditions, arthritis, hypertension, heart conditions, orthopedic problems, and diabetes

Table 3.4 Leading Causes of Death for Persons 65 Years of Age and Older (in thousands)

Cause	65–74 yrs	75–84 yrs	85+ yrs
Heart disease	180.8	239.0	199.3
Malignant neoplasms	146.8	116.6	44.7
Cerebrovascular diseases	28.4	52.0	48.9
Chronic obstructive pulmonary diseases	25.9	26.7	10.1
Pneumonia/influenza	10.2	22.0	28.7
Diabetes mellitus	10.3	11.0	5.9
Accidents and adverse effects	8.5	9.6	7.0
Chronic liver disease, cirrhosis	6.5	2.9	0.6
Suicide	3.4	2.3	0.6

From US Department of Commerce. Statistical abstract of the US. 110th ed. Washington, DC: Bureau of the Census, 1990:49.

Table 3.5 Rates of Chronic Illness in Adults by Age (per 1000 Population)

	18–44 yrs	45–64 yrs	65–74 yrs	75+ yrs
Arthritis	52.8	273.3	463.6	511.9
Hypertension	61.8	252.0	392.4	337.0
Hearing impairments	54.1	135.6	264.7	348.0
Heart conditions	40.7	126.1	284.7	322.2
Chronic sinusitis	149.5	192.1	154.0	131.4
Visual impairments	29.3	47.3	56.3	111.2
Orthopedic problems	135.4	155.0	154.9	182.0
Diabetes	11.9	56.4	98.3	98.2
Varicose veins	26.8	54.1	82.5	64.8
Hemorrhoids	46.9	79.7	74.1	73.1

From US Department of Commerce. Statistical Abstract of the US. 110th ed. Washington, DC: Bureau of the Census, 1990:118.

require the most long-term and intensive medication management. Two of these chronic diseases, heart conditions and arthritis, cause the greatest amount of activity limitation among older persons, each affecting about 23% of the older population (Lamy, 1980).

Functional status, or the ability to carry out usual activities of daily living, is a more accurate indicator of health status than is the number of chronic diseases. By looking at functional status indicators, the ability of the older person to be independent and perform necessary activities can be more appropriately assessed. Functional ability, which encompasses physical, psychological, and social domains, is usually evaluated by examining activities of daily living (ADLs). These include basic self-care, hygiene, and instrumental activities of daily living (IADLs), such as tasks necessary to run a household.

In a large national sample of nearly 28,000 people over age 65 living in the community, difficulty with one or more ADLs or IADLs was found to increase as age of subjects increased. This study found 12.9% of the respondents had difficulty with at least one ADL. The greatest difficulty among this sample was with bathing (8.9%), followed by walking (7.7%), bed and chair transfer (5.9%), and dressing (5.1%). They reported the least difficulty with toileting (3.5%) and eating (1.1%) (Leon & Lair, 1990).

Among noninstitutionalized elderly, 17.5% reported difficulty with at least one IADL (Leon & Lair, 1990). Getting around the community caused difficulty for 13.5% of this population. Shopping was difficult for 11%, and doing light housework was difficult for 10.1%. Other difficult tasks were preparing meals (7.5%), handling money (6.3%), and using the telephone (4.4%).

Women over 85 had more difficulty with ADLs (38.4%) and IADLs (56.4%) than men (26.3% and 50.5%). African-American elderly were more likely than whites to report having difficulty with both ADLs and IADLs, but IADLs were more difficult than ADLs for all age groups. Older people who lived with a spouse reported less difficulty with ADLs or IADLs on the average than those who lived alone or with other relatives (Leon & Lair, 1990).

DRUG USE

Use of both prescribed and over-the-counter drugs is known to be high among older adults; however, it is difficult to obtain accurate statistics on drug use. According to Lamy, 85% of elderly living in the community receive prescribed drugs (Lamy, 1980). The number of prescribed medications increases dramatically with age and is greater for females than males in every age category (Figure 3.2).

Information on the prescribing patterns of approximately 225,000 physicians was obtained in the National Ambulatory Medical Care Survey conducted in 1980. This survey provided data on more than 380 million patient visits, including drugs prescribed by diagnosis and other patient characteristics. According to this study, physicians prescribed medications

Figure 3.2 Number of acquisitions of prescribed medicine per person per year, by sex and age. Lamy, PP (1980). *Prescribing for the elderly.* Littleton, MA: PSG Publishing.

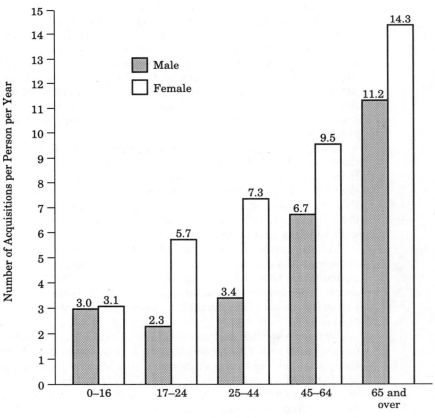

during more than 80% of visits by persons age 65 and older. Rates ranged from an average of 1.93 medications per visit by general and family practice physicians to 2.24 medications among internists. Cardiovascular drugs were prescribed most often (21% of all prescriptions), then central nervous system medications (18%), and fluid and electrolyte balance medications (14%). Digoxin was the pharmaceutical used most often for persons over 65 (5.1% of all drugs prescribed), followed by furosemide (3%). Physicians prescribed one or more medications in 88% of visits for essential hypertension (National Center for Health Statistics, 1982).

A somewhat different picture of medication use emerges in long-term care facilities. It was estimated that almost 95% of patients in long-term care facilities receive drugs (Lamy, 1980) with an average number of 3.3 medications per patient (Kalchthaler et al., 1977). The most frequently prescribed medications were analgesics (51% of patients), antihypertensives (46%), cardiovascular drugs (41%), and antimicrobials (39%) (Kalchthaler et al., 1977). The appropriateness of this extent of drug usage in long-term care facilities needs further assessment (Cooper, 1978).

Polypharmacy is the prescription of multiple medications. Multiple drug regimens can be justified when clients suffer from more than one disorder, when different drugs relieve different symptoms of a disease, or when one drug improves the benefit of another. In practice, however, multiple drug regimens are often too complicated or lack adequate rationale for each individual drug. Elderly with multiple chronic conditions often have more than one physician, which can lead to poorly coordinated care. Medications given to relieve nonspecific symptomatology or the side effects of other medications are thought to be the major factors contributing to adverse drug reactions resulting from polypharmacy (German & Burton, 1990). When prescribing patterns were examined by the number of medications per visit and diagnosis, data showed that patients with ischemic heart disease received 2.5 drugs per visit; those with hypertension 1.85 drugs, and persons with osteoarthritis 1.72 drugs, for patients with obesity 1.86, for those with diabetes 1.83, and for persons visiting a physician's office for a general medical exam 0.41. The highest proportion of those receiving 3 or more drugs were individuals with ischemic heart disease (52.4%), followed by people with diabetes (36.1%), neurotic/depressive disorders (32.2%), and hypertension (28.1%) (National Center for Health Statistics, 1983).

Final decisions have not yet been made in the current deliberations on health care reform, so it is impossible to speculate regarding the effect that reforms will have on medication use among the elderly. One change that seems imminent, however, is the move toward primary care providers, that is, physicians and nonphysician health care professionals such as nurse practitioners who will deliver primary care to patients. This may have a positive effect on the health of clients by reducing the likelihood that polypharmacy of the same medication will be prescribed by different physicians. Although there is a paucity of information on the prescribing patterns of nonphysician providers, one study which examined prescribing behaviors of 156 nurse practitioners concluded that their prescribing patterns were more conservative than those of physicians and were appropriate for the medical diagnoses (Holland, Batey, & Dawson, 1985).

Over-the-counter (OTC) or nonprescription drugs are also widely used by elderly. These drugs are convenient, often less expensive than prescription drugs, and do not require the time and expense of a doctor's visit. Although research in this area has been lacking, the studies that have been conducted show that the elderly frequently use many nonprescription drugs and usually do not consult their physician about using these drugs. In a Canadian study, 54% of males and 80.8% of females over age 59 used over-the-counter drugs (Chaiton et al., 1976). In Washington, D.C., Over-the-counter drugs were used by more than two-thirds of elderly ambulatory patients. The most commonly used OTC drugs appear to be vitamins, analgesics, cough and cold remedies, laxatives, and antacids.

Drug costs are also of concern for older individuals. It has been estimated that 20% of out-of-pocket expenses for the elderly population are for medicine (National Council on Aging, 1970). This is a significant proportion of their expenditures, especially since many of them are on fixed incomes with limited resources. Average costs of prescribed medications according to activity limitation increase dramatically as limitations increase (Lamy, 1980).

DRUG MISUSE

Effective use of prescription drugs depends on accurate diagnosis of client problems, drug selection, appropriateness of dose, accurate follow-up evaluation, and correct assessment of the effectiveness of the medication regimen. Effective use of over-the-counter drugs requires the same steps except the person "diagnosing" the problem and "prescribing" the drugs is the individual or family caregivers. Drug misuse consists of problems in any of these areas, as well as problems of noncompliance, of sharing or saving drugs, and improper storage of drugs. For prescription drugs, the problems can be related to either the physician or the client, and sometimes both are at fault. Over-the-counter drugs present special concerns for older people and will be discussed in a subsequent section.

Physician-Centered Problems

Many physicians, as well as other health professionals, have **negative attitudes** about caring for older people. Such negative attitudes may result in less attention or follow-up of older clients. Thus, there is an increased potential for drug problems resulting from misdiagnosis, inappropriate dosing, lack of education about adverse effects, or inadequate instructions regarding how to take the drug.

Pathology may manifest with greater variation in older people than in younger people; therefore, **accurate diagnosis** may be more difficult for some physicians. Studies have found that physicians frequently underestimate subtle cognitive impairment or disability in elderly clients (Calkins et al., 1985; Canadian Task Force, 1991). This often results in prescription of medication regimens which these clients are unable to follow. In addition, the multiple chronic diseases and altered physiology usually require downward adjustment of doses to lower amounts. This makes **appropriate dosing** more difficult. There is little consistent evidence that the physicians' age, years of experience, or level of education affect prescribing behaviors (Christensen & Bush, 1981). One study that assessed physicians' knowledge about prescribing for the elderly found that their mean knowledge was significantly lower than the minimum score determined by a panel of experts (Ferry, Lamy, & Becker, 1985). Physicians who depend primarily on drug advertising and who do not attend continuing education courses are especially likely to have an inadequate understanding of prescribing for the elderly.

Appropriate use of medications is fostered by **client education** when the drug is first prescribed, including information about the purposes, correct doses, times, side effects, and any special instructions. Drug education is seldom provided or sought by clients in physicians' offices because of time constraints. Pharmacists are available to provide education when the prescription is filled, but, in practice, information is unlikely to be given unless clients seek this information. Later, inadequate **follow-up** by the physician may result from negative attitudes toward older clients and chronic illness. The assumption may be made that older clients with several chronic illnesses will continue to deteriorate in health status. Too often, physicians assume that the current group of prescribed medications will have to be continued for the rest of the client's life. This attitude does not foster frequent review, change, reduction in the number of drugs, or reduction of doses that may be required as the older person's physiology changes.

Another problem that is related to physicians but beyond their control is that clients sometimes go to several different physicians at the same time, usually for different problems. Clients do not always tell one doctor that they are seeing another doctor, possibly because of fear they will be perceived as disloyal. One result is that different doctors may prescribe the same drug using different names (such as generic and a brand name drug), so the client does not recognize them as the same drug. Unless the client has both prescriptions filled at the same pharmacy and one where a record is kept of all the client's drugs, the person may end up taking a double dose of the drug without knowing it. Serious complications can result.

Physician-centered problems can be improved through education that impacts attitudes and updates them on diagnosing and prescribing the latest drug therapy for the elderly. Good nursing care in the office setting should include clear client education, both verbally and in writing, about all aspects of medication use. The nurse should also act as an advocate for the client with the physician to assist the client in getting the best care possible. Older clients are sometimes reluctant to ask doctors questions and need to be encouraged to do so. Making a list of questions prior to the office visit sometimes helps older persons organize their thoughts. Since the elderly have complex problems, they need to be educated to be responsible and knowledgeable consumers of drug therapy.

Client-Centered Problems

Client-centered problems can be categorized as intentional and unintentional problems. Review of available evidence suggests that many elderly patients lack knowledge about their medication regimens, lack understanding of drug purpose, and have little knowledge of the potential side effects of their medications (German & Burton, 1989). **Unintentional problems** include those resulting from inadequate knowledge about drug dose or special instructions, forgetting to take a dose, taking the drug at the wrong time, or confusion about the medication instructions because of cognitive deficits. **Intentional problems** involve not taking the drug as directed because of side effects, adjusting the dosage to fit symptoms or perceived needs, sharing drugs with others who have similar diseases or symptoms, taking less of the drug to save money, or taking too much or too little of a drug in an attempt to end one's life. Saving medications for later use, frequently past the expiration date, and storing drugs in places where they are exposed to moisture, heat and/or light also causes difficulties. Many times medication errors result from a combination of unintentional and intentional problems.

Underuse of prescription drugs is the most common deviation from adherence to drug regimens; overuse or abuse are rarely reported as problematic among the elderly. Difficulty opening bottles, especially childproof containers, because of functional limitations can contribute to problems of underusage (German & Burton, 1989).

Use of nonprescription drugs can contribute to problems among older adults for many reasons. Elders may not take the drug as recommended because of inability to read the small print, in the directions or in the package insert, listing contraindications and side effects. They may have selected the drug without recognizing the symptom as an indicator of a more serious problem requiring medical attention. For instance, they may take an antacid to relieve pain they think is from heartburn, when it is, in effect, cardiac-related pain. The OTC medication may interact adversely with prescription medications they are already taking. There may be a tendency to over medicate because OTC drugs are thought to be less potent and less harmful than prescription medications. Use of OTC drugs may mask signs and symptoms and confuse a physician's diagnosis, if patients do not tell the doctor they are taking the drug. Although OTC drugs can be very beneficial, they also can cause many problems for older people.

CONCLUSION

This chapter has reviewed drug use and problems of misuse among older people in the United States. Demographic data indicating the proportion of elderly in the population together with projections for future growth and data showing the high degree of drug use among older adults demonstrate that the use of medications will increase dramatically in future years. Problems associated with medication use among the elderly are also expected to increase accordingly. A discussion of current drug use among older people identified types of drugs most frequently prescribed, problems with multiple drug prescriptions, over-the-counter drugs, and drug costs.

Misuse of medications arises from both physician-centered problems and client-centered problems. Among problems attributed to physicians are negative attitudes toward elderly, difficulty making accurate diagnoses and giving appropriate prescriptions, and insufficient client education and follow-up. The tendency of clients to use several physicians without communicating that information also causes difficulties such as drug over-prescription.

Client-centered problems include unintentional errors such as forgetting to take a dose or misunderstanding the instructions concerning the drug. Intentional problems such as not taking the drug because of side effects, self-regulation of the dosage, sharing drugs with others, and not taking the drug to save money most often result in underuse of medications. Functional limitations can also make opening drug containers difficult.

Often, both physician and client-centered problems occur for an older person, which, when combined with compromised physical status from age changes and disease states, make medication use an especially difficult problem. Knowledge about the intricate interrelationships among these problems can help the health care professional better serve older clients and become more aware of the necessity for careful assessment and monitoring. With improvements in client advocacy and education, the health of older people can be promoted by reducing adverse effects from drug misuse.

REFERENCES AND RECOMMENDED READINGS

Calkins DR, Rubenstein LV, Cleary PD, et al.: Failure of physicians to recognize functional disability in ambulatory patients. *Annals of Internal Medicine,* 1985; 114:451–454.

Canadian Task Force on the Periodic Health Examination. Periodic health examination, 1991 update no. 1: Screening for cognitive impairment in the elderly. *Canadian Medical Association Journal,* 1991. 144:425–431.

Chaitan A, Spitzer WO, Roberts RS, et al.: Patterns of medical drug use—a community focus. *Canadian Medical Association Journal,* 1976; 114:33.

Christensen DB, & Bush PJ: Drug prescribing: Patterns, problems and proposals. *Social Science Medicine,* 1981; 15:343–355.

Col N, Fanale JE, & Kronholm P: The role of medication noncompliance and adverse drug reactions in hospitalization of the elderly. *Archives of Internal Medicine,* 1990; 150:841–845.

Colt HG, & Shapiro AP: Drug-induced illness as a cause for admission to a community hospital. *Journal of the American Geriatrics Society,* 1989; 37:323–326.

Cooper JW, Jr: Drug therapy in the elderly. *American Pharmaceutical Association,* 1978; N518(7).

Ferry ME, Lamy PP, & Becker LM: Physicians' knowledge of prescribing for the elderly: A study of primary care physicians. *Journal of the American Geriatric Society,* 1985; 33:616–621.

German PS, & Burton LC: Medication and the elderly: Issues of prescription and use. *Journal of Aging and Health,* 1990; 1(1):4–34.

Holland JM, Batey MB, & Dawson K: Nurse practitioner prescribing patterns: Drug therapy and client health problems. *Journal of Ambulatory Care Management,* 1985; 8:44–53.

Kalchthaler T, Coccaro E, & Lichtiger S: Incidence of polypharmacy in a long-term care facility. *Journal of American Geriatrics Society,* 1977; 25:308–313.

Lamy PP: *Prescribing for the elderly.* Littleton, MA: PSG Publishing, 1980.

Leon J, & Lair T: *Functional status of non-institutionalized elderly: Estimates of ADL and IADL difficulties,* DDHS Pub. No. (PHS) 90–3462, Agency for Health Care Policy and Research. Rockville, MD: Public Health Service, 1990.

Lundin DV: Medication taking behavior of the elderly: A pilot study. *Drug Intelligence and Clinical Pharmacy,* 1978; 12:518.

National Center for Health Statistics & Cypress BK: Medication therapy in office visits for selected diagnosis: The National Ambulatory Medical Care Survey, U.S., 1980. *Vital & Health Statistics,* Series 13–, No. 71. DHHS Pub. No. (PHS) 83–1732. Public Health Service. Washington, DC: U.S. Government Printing Office, 1983.

National Center for Health Statistics & Cypress BK: Drug utilization in office visits to primary care physicians: The National Ambulatory Medical Care Survey, 1980. *Vital & Health Statistics,* 86, DDHS Pub. No. (PHS) 82–1250. Hyattsville, MD: Public Health Service, 1982.

National Council on Aging. *The golden years: A tarnished myth.* Washington, DC: National Council on Aging, 1978.

Nolan L, & O'Malley K: Prescribing for the elderly part I: Sensitivity of the elderly to adverse drug reactions. *Journal of the American Geriatrics Society,* 1988; 36:142–147.

US Bureau of the Census. *General population statistics.* Economics and Statistics Administration. Washington, DC: US Department of Commerce Census Bureau, 1990.

CHAPTER 4

Altered Pharmacokinetics and Pharmacodynamics in Geriatric Patients

In spite of the fact that people age 65 and older already comprise more than 10% of the population in the United States, in spite of the inevitability that the percentage of Americans over 65 will increase dramatically in the decades ahead, and in spite of the fact that those over 65 take a high proportion of the drugs used by the entire population, elderly patients seldom enjoy the safeguard of taking drugs that have been specifically tested in people of their own age group. Although the Federal Drug Administration is taking steps to rectify the relative dearth of information regarding drug effects unique to older Americans, the fact remains that most drugs in current clinical practice, even those most used in the elderly, have never been specifically evaluated for age-dependent differences in clinical pharmacology. Nevertheless, the evidence that does exist clearly demonstrates that the elderly do respond differently than younger people to many, perhaps even most, medications. Often the differences are quantitative in nature, that is, the effects are similar but occur at lower (or less often, higher) doses. Occasionally the differences are even qualitative, with unique responses occurring in the elderly that do not occur in younger patients. Elderly individuals not only respond differently than younger patients to drugs, but their responses are also more variable and less predictable. Aging, it seems, does not impact to the same extent or at the same rate on all of us. Rational and effective use of medications in the elderly is complicated by several of the changes that occur with aging (Figure 4.1):

1. age-dependent changes in how the body handles drugs, or pharmacokinetics;
2. the frequent presence of chronic diseases that alter pharmacokinetics or which are themselves altered by drug therapy; and
3. age-dependent changes in tissue response to drugs, or pharmacodynamics.

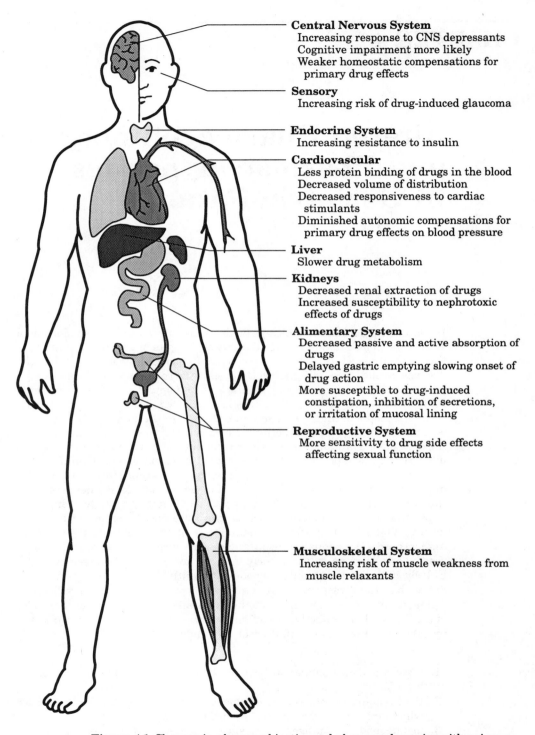

Central Nervous System
Increasing response to CNS depressants
Cognitive impairment more likely
Weaker homeostatic compensations for
primary drug effects

Sensory
Increasing risk of drug-induced glaucoma

Endocrine System
Increasing resistance to insulin

Cardiovascular
Less protein binding of drugs in the blood
Decreased volume of distribution
Decreased responsiveness to cardiac
stimulants
Diminished autonomic compensations for
primary drug effects on blood pressure

Liver
Slower drug metabolism

Kidneys
Decreased renal extraction of drugs
Increased susceptibility to nephrotoxic
effects of drugs

Alimentary System
Decreased passive and active absorption of
drugs
Delayed gastric emptying slowing onset of
drug action
More susceptible to drug-induced
constipation, inhibition of secretions,
or irritation of mucosal lining

Reproductive System
More sensitivity to drug side effects
affecting sexual function

Musculoskeletal System
Increasing risk of muscle weakness from
muscle relaxants

Figure 4.1 Changes in pharmacokinetics and pharmacodynamics with aging.

ALTERED PHARMACOKINETICS IN OLDER PERSONS

Pharmacokinetics refers to the way in which the body and its physiological mechanisms deal with an administered drug. The pharmacokinetic phase of drug action begins when a drug has dissolved in a body fluid after administration and it ends when the drug has been inactivated by metabolism and/or excretion. The ultimate interest in pharmacotherapeutics is how the drug affects bodily health and disease processes (i.e., pharmacodynamics), but pharmacokinetics takes the opposite vantage point—how the body impacts on the drug. Pharmacokinetics is important, ultimately, because pharmacokinetics greatly influences the extent to which the drug will be available at its site of action to produce its characteristic clinical effects. For convenience, pharmacokinetics is divided into three phases: absorption, distribution, and inactivation (the last of which includes metabolism and elimination). So, pharmacokinetics is the study of how the body absorbs a drug into the bloodstream, distributes it to its site of action and elsewhere, and finally inactivates it. Each of the three phases of pharmacokinetics is subject to changes with aging; such changes are referred to as age-dependent kinetics (Table 4.1). An understanding of how the body's ability to handle drugs changes with age is absolutely prerequisite if drug therapy for the elderly is to be rational and compassionate.

Absorption

Absorption is the process by which a drug moves from its original site of application into the bloodstream and lymphatic system—the **central compartment** of circulating fluids. Most drugs act at a site that is different from the one to which they are applied. For example, a psychotropic drug taken orally ultimately acts on the brain but comes into initial contact with the physiological systems in the alimentary tract. Before such a drug can reach its site of action, it must first move into the central compartment for distribution throughout the body. The only exceptions to this rule are the relatively small number of drugs that can be applied directly to their desired site of action, for example, a dermatological agent applied to the skin. Even then, the site of action is likely to be below the surface of the skin in the deep layers of the epidermis, so some absorption may still be required. Drugs that are applied directly to their site of action are called **topical** medications; all other drugs require systemic absorption for effectiveness. Drugs that are given by injection (intramuscular, subcutaneous, etc.) require absorption, with the sole exception of drugs given intravenously, because these drugs are applied directly to the central compartment.

When a drug requires systemic absorption, two natural questions to ask are how completely and how quickly is the drug absorbed. The answer to the first question will be a major determinant of the extent of effect of the drug on the body. The answer to the second question will be a major factor influencing how quickly the client's response will begin. Either of these questions can be answered empirically by monitoring changing plasma

Table 4.1 Age-dependent Drug Kinetics and Dynamics

Effects may be increased by		Effects may be decreased by	
Decreased renal extraction		**Decreased plasma binding permitting**	
Ampicillin	Lithium	**increased extraction**	
Atenolol	Nadolol	Phenytoin	
Digoxin	Penicillin		
Disopyramide	Practolol	**Decreased active absorption**	
Doxycycline	Procainamide	Calcium	
Flecainide	Quinidine	Galactose	
Gentamicin	Streptomycin	Thiamine	
Kanamycin	Tetracycline		
		Decreased passive absorption	
Decreased hepatic extraction		Most drugs but not much	
Acetaminophen	Phenobarbital		
Amobarbital	Phenylbutazone	**Increased volume of distribution**	
Benzodiazepines (if	Propoxyphene	**for fat-soluble drugs**	
oxidized)	Propranolol	Chlordiazepoxide	
Labetalol	Quinidine	Diazepam	
Lidocaine	Theophylline		
Meperidine	Tricyclic	**More breakdown in stomach if gastric**	
Meprobamate	antidepressants	**emptying time delayed**	
Metoprolol	Verapamil	Penicillin	
Morphine	Warfarin		
		Decreased tissue responsivity	
Decreased plasma protein binding		Amphetamine	
Digoxin	Salicylates	Isoproterenol	
Meperidine	Sulfonamides	Norepinephrine	
Phenylbutazone	Warfarin	Quinidine	
Quinidine			
Decreased red blood cell binding			
Acetazolamide	Meperidine		
Decreased volume of distribution for			
water-soluable drugs			
Ethanol			
Propicillin			
Less breakdown of acid-labile drugs in			
stomach due to hypochlorhydria			
Penicillin			
Increased tissue responsivity			
Anticholinergics	Benzodiazepines		
Antihistamines	CNS depressants		
Barbiturates	Digitalis		
(paradoxical	Hypotensive agents		
excitation)	Lidocaine		

concentrations over time after administration of a drug. Drugs given by injection will always be completely absorbed ultimately, but will vary in how rapidly they are absorbed. Drugs given orally may be only partially absorbed, the rest being excreted with the feces. The mucosal membranes along the entire length of the gastrointestinal system provide a surface for absorption; the thin epithelial wall together with the high rate of blood flow in adjacent blood vessels provides circumstances generally favorable to rapid absorption. However, specific conditions in the stomach and intestines can play an important role in modifying both extent and speed of absorption for drugs given orally.

In the stomach, for example, the digestive fluids are highly acidic. The low pH of stomach fluids promotes rapid absorption of weak acids by keeping these drugs in a nonionized form, but inhibits absorption of weak bases by promoting their ionization. Stomach acids can actually break down certain drugs before they ever have a chance to be absorbed. Such drugs (e.g., penicillin) are referred to as acid labile. Older people usually have lower rates of acid secretion in the stomach (hypochlorhydria), even in the absence of specific gastrointestinal disorder, and therefore absorption of acid labile drugs may actually improve in the elderly. Foods present in the stomach may bind to or sequester drugs, thereby reducing their absorption.

In any event, the stomach provides a much smaller surface area for absorption than do the intestines. The longer a drug spends in the stomach, the slower will be its absorption. The stomach functions as a kind of temporary reservoir for ingested foods, beverages, and drugs. These substances do not pass through continuously but are, instead, periodically flushed out into the duodenum, the initial segment of the small intestines. The time between flushes is called **gastric emptying time** and it is an important determinant of how quickly drugs act. A long gastric emptying time (slow gastric emptying rate) means that the drug spends a lot of time in the stomach where absorption is relatively slow. There are a lot of factors that alter gastric emptying time, some of which are more common among the aged: gastric ulcers, hypothyroidism, pyloric obstruction, or use of aspirin, anticholinergic, or sympathomimetic medications. Other factors that occur independent of age but influence gastric emptying time are pain, hot meals, high fat foods, low stomach pH, vigorous exercise, and lying on the left side. The time that a medication remains in the stomach along with other contents can range from 15 minutes to 7 hours. Any factor that delays gastric emptying will delay onset of drug action, though there will be little effect on ultimate total absorption.

Gastric emptying time is prolonged in the elderly for at least two reasons. First, acid secretion is less (hypochlorhydria), resulting in a higher gastric pH and delayed emptying. Second, activity of the sphincters that control emptying is diminished. As a result, elderly persons may respond a bit more slowly to orally administered drugs than do others.

In the intestines, absorption proceeds rapidly for most drugs. The pH in the intestines is higher, so weak bases are less ionized and absorbed faster here, while weak acids fare less well. Some drugs are metabolized to a significant degree in the intestines, either by the intestinal flora or by enzymes in mucosal cells. Either way, a portion of the administered dose is destroyed before ever becoming available for therapeutic action. A few drugs are only slowly absorbed even in the intestines, and, for these drugs, the rate of intestinal motility can be important. For example, propranolol, a very slowly absorbed drug, barely has enough time to get fully absorbed in the best of circumstances; if the individual is experiencing diarrhea, the drug will pass through the intestines more rapidly and a higher portion than usual will be lost in the feces. Conversely, the time available for absorption will be longer than usual for those clients suffering from constipation.

Aging is associated with a general involution of the alimentary tract. The effective surface area of the intestines decreases with age and there is a loss of mucosal cells. Blood flow in the vessels surrounding the intestines may decline reducing the rate of removal for newly absorbed substances into the bloodstream. Drugs and nutrients that require active involvement of mucosal cells for absorption (e.g., calcium, iron, thiamine, vitamin B_{12}) are less rapidly absorbed by elderly persons.

Elderly individuals are much more likely to use laxatives or antacids. Both of these classes of drugs can impact on absorption of other drugs used concurrently. Laxatives increase intestinal motility and will decrease absorption of slowly absorbed drugs. Some elderly clients actually develop nutritional deficits from long-term use of laxatives, depriving their alimentary system of sufficient time to absorb required nutrients. Antacids have an especially significant effect on absorption of other drugs, forming complexes with many drugs (e.g., digoxin, tetracyclines, vitamin A, chlordiazepoxide) that cannot be absorbed. Most drugs should not be taken within an hour before or two hours after the client takes an antacid.

Overall, the elderly are likely to absorb many drugs less quickly and less completely than younger persons do. Onset and total drug availability at the site of action may therefore be less; however, pharmacokinetic changes in inactivation for the elderly, discussed below, often more than offset the influence of diminished absorption of drug availability.

Distribution

Distribution refers to the rapid movement of drug molecules through the bloodstream and lymphatic system, which follows immediately after the absorptive phase. Once a drug enters the central compartment, it is available rapidly for penetration into various tissues. The rate at which drug penetrates a tissue from the central compartment varies from tissue to tissue and as a result of drug properties and physiological conditions. Some tissues are protected by rather restrictive barriers—the brain by the **blood-brain barrier,** and fetal tissue, during pregnancy, by the **placental barrier.** Fat tissue will rapidly take up drugs that are lipophilic; that is, drugs that are highly soluble in fatty media. Hydrophilic drugs, ones that dissolve better in water than in fat, will penetrate fat tissue only slowly if at all.

Tissues that have low blood supply (i.e., poorly perfused tissues) will take up drug at a slower rate. The decrease in cardiac output that accompanies aging gradually changes the regional distribution of blood flow in the body, reducing blood flow to the alimentary tract and nephrourinary system in favor of the more immediately crucial flow to the cerebrum and heart. As a result, delivery of drug molecules to the liver and kidneys is slower, delaying inactivation of many drugs.

The total volume of body tissues that a given drug is able to ultimately penetrate is that drug's **volume of distribution.** The volume of the plasma in an average person is approximately 3 liters, so drugs that have a measured volume of distribution approximating that value can be assumed to remain mainly in the bloodstream. The total volume of extracellular fluid for the average person is about 12 liters, so drugs with values higher than that must penetrate at least some tissue cells and may have an intracellular site of action. Elderly persons have from 10–15% less total body water than adults at age 30, so whatever portion of an administered water-soluble drug reaches the central compartment will be distributed into a smaller volume. Hence, it will have to be more concentrated. Elderly people, on the other hand, have a higher percentage body fat, on average, than younger adults, so fat-soluble drugs are more extensively stored in older people and accumulate to a greater extent. This may be part of the reason that many drugs that act on the brain, drugs typically with high fat solubility, have exaggerated effects in the elderly.

One of the most important facets of distribution is the binding of many drugs to proteins, mainly albumin proteins, contained in the blood. Drugs with this ability circulate through the bloodstream partly bound and partly unbound, the relative size of these two pools being different but characteristic for every drug. Only the unbound pool of the drug is available for most pharmacokinetic activities and to exert the characteristic effects of the drug, but whenever part of the unbound pool is eliminated or metabolized, it is replenished from the pool of a protein-bound drug because binding is reversible and the two pools exist in a kind of equilibrium. Older people usually have a lower level of proteins in the blood and hence fewer drug binding sites. Drugs that are highly protein bound in younger clients will be less so in older people, so that the unbound fraction will be relatively larger in relation to the bound fraction. This means that the drug will have a stronger effect while it is present, but that it will also be more rapidly eliminated by renal excretion, if renal filtration is a major part of its overall inactivation. Binding sites for certain drugs (for example, meperidine and acetazolamide) are found on the surfaces of red blood cells, and older people also have fewer of these on average.

The number of binding sites available on blood proteins is finite, so that some drugs will saturate the available sites at concentrations in the range of those used for clinical purposes. Interactions will occur between two drugs that compete for the same binding sites if either one of them is at all close to the concentration that saturates the available sites. Older people are more susceptible to such interactions because they start with fewer binding sites, which are therefore more readily saturable.

Inactivation

Drugs are inactivated by either metabolism or excretion, or a combination of the two. Most metabolism is accomplished by the liver, while most excretion is accomplished by the kidneys. Some drugs are removed so efficiently from

Table 4.2 Some Drugs Requiring Dosage Adjustment in the Elderly in Proportion to Renal Dysfunction

Antimicrobials	***Anti-inflammatory drugs***
Aminoglycosides	Allopurinol
Cephalosporins	Gold salts
Ethambutol	Sulindac
Methenamine	***Antidiabetic drugs***
Nitrofurantoin	Chlorpropamide
Penicillins	
Sulfonamides	***Psychotropics***
Tetracyclines	Amantadine
	Carbamazepine
Cardiovascular drugs	Diazepam
Atenolol	Flurazepam
Clonidine	Lithium
Digoxin	Meperidine
Disopyramide	
Felodipine	***Antiulcer drug***
Flecainide	Cimetidine
Guanabenz	
Methyldopa	
Nadolol	
Nifedipine	
Procainamide	
Propafenone	
Thiazide diuretics	

the blood by the liver that immediately after absorption, when the newly absorbed drug passes the liver via the portal vein, a substantial portion of the drug may be extracted from the blood in this first pass. Drugs subject to this kind of rapid removal are said to undergo substantial **first-pass extraction.** Elderly people have reduced blood flow in this part of the circulation, so first-pass extraction is less evident. Drugs, such as propranolol, subject to considerable first-pass extraction in young adults, can have an exaggerated effect in older clients. Even drugs not subject to very much first-pass extraction will be delivered less rapidly to the liver in older people because of reduced mesenteric blood flow, with the result that metabolism will be slower (Table 4.1). However, drugs that are highly bound to plasma proteins in young clients may actually be more available to the liver for an elderly client, because a higher fraction of the drug resides in the extractable unbound pool.

Inactivation of drugs by renal excretion is equally subject to change with aging. In fact, changes in kidney function are probably the single most important example of age-dependent kinetics. After age 30 or so, renal function declines by an average annual rate of 1% or about 6–10% per decade. Sixty-six percent of healthy elderly have evidence of impaired renal function, which is, of course, exacerbated in those with renal disease. The decline in renal function is evident both in diminished renal blood flow and in a reduced glomerular filtration rate (GFR). GFR is often used as the simplest and most direct assessment of renal function, so a reduction in

GFR is an important loss of capacity. Other facets of renal functions, such as the ability to concentrate urine in the tubules and the active secretory mechanisms also decline with age. The result is that nearly all drugs that are inactivated primarily by renal excretion will persist longer in the blood of older individuals than in younger ones. Renal clearance of digoxin, for example, is 52% less in elderly persons than in young individuals. Digoxin is a drug used by more than 20% of elderly persons in nursing homes, and the commonplace instances of digoxin toxicity (estimated at about 23%) may be in large measure related to the altered renal extraction. Some of the other drugs primarily inactivated by renal elimination are listed in Table 4.2. Doses of these drugs should be adjusted in elderly individuals in proportion to the change in glomerular filtration rate.

DRUG INTERACTIONS WITH CHRONIC DISEASES COMMON TO OLDER INDIVIDUALS

Another factor that may alter response to drug therapy in older persons is the likely presence of chronic disease: 85% of those over age 65 have at least one chronic ailment and 50% have more than one such problem. The presence of such ailments is relevant to drug therapy in several respects:

1. Drugs used for one disorder may exacerbate another disorder.
2. Drug inactivation may be altered by disorders of the kidney or liver.
3. Drug absorption may be altered by disorders of the gastrointestinal system or other organ systems for drugs applied topically.
4. Drug distribution may be altered by ailments, such as congestive heart failure, dehydration, or edema, that alter volume of distribution.
5. The likelihood of drug-drug interactions will be increased by the necessity for multidrug regimens for multiple disorders.
6. Adverse reactions to medication may be overlooked if mistaken for manifestations of some preexisting chronic disease.

The first of these possibilities reflects the influence that drug therapy might have on disease states, while the other five reflect the ways that presence of disease states might alter drug therapy. Some of the most common ways in which drugs can exacerbate existing diseases are summarized in Table 4.3. Most of these potential hazards are written into the **contraindications** and **cautions** in each drug's supporting documentation. Those involved in providing clinical services to elderly clients need to evaluate each drug being contemplated for addition to a regimen in terms of the client's total health picture rather than as an independent intervention.

The effects of preexisting disease on drug action are just as evident and varied (Table 4.4). Any of the three phases of pharmacokinetics—absorption, distribution, or inactivation—can be impacted by disease. After oral administration of drugs, gastric emptying time is delayed by pyloric obstruction or stenosis, gastric ulcers, achlorhydria, hypothyroidism, or diabetic gastroparesis. This may not reduce total absorption but will slow absorp-

Table 4.3 Common Examples of Exacerbation of Preexisting Conditions by Drugs

Disease	Exacerbating Drugs
Anemia due to folic acid deficiency	Triamterene, trimethoprim, oral contraceptives, methotrexate, antiepileptic drugs
Anxiety	Antiasthmatic drugs, caffeine
Asthma	Beta-2 blockers, cholinomimetics, neuromuscular blockers, cephalosporins, penicillins, sulfonamides, estrogens, aspirin, indomethacin, phenothiazines, verapamil
Blood dyscrasias	Neuroleptics, lithium, antidepressants, antiepileptics
Chronic obstructive pulmonary disease	Narcotics, neuromuscular blockers
Chronic organic brain syndromes	Lithium, sedative-hypnotics, any other depressant drug
Conduction blocks	Tricyclic antidepressants, antidysrhythmic drugs, cardiac glycosides
Congestive heart failure	Beta-blockers, drugs with salt load, antidysrhythmic drugs
Depression and symptoms of excess depression (e.g., ataxia, drowsiness, confusion)	Antiadrenergic antihypertensives, beta-blockers, sedative-hypnotics, antiepileptic drugs, alpha-blockers
Diabetes mellitus	Beta-2 blockers, alpha-agonists, disopyramide
Dysrhythmias	Lithium, anticholinergic drugs*, levodopa, beta-agonists, digoxin and other cardiotonics
Epilepsy/seizure disorders	Antidepressant, neuroleptics, narcotics, nalidixic acid, sedative-hypnotics (withdrawal phase), levodopa, dopamine agonists, cholinomimetics
Esophageal reflux	Anticholinergic drugs
Glaucoma	Anticholinergic drugs, levodopa, benzodiazepines, alpha-agonists, corticosteroids, disopyramide, reserpine
Gout	Thiazide or high-ceiling diuretics
Hearing impairment	High-ceiling diuretics, cisplatin, nitrogen mustards, aminoglycosides
Hypertension	Drugs providing salt load, carbamazepine, corticosteroids, sulfonylureas, estrogens
Hypoplastic anemia	Antineoplastics, gold compounds, aspirin, cardiac glycosides, chlorthiazide, methyldopa, penicillin, phenytoin, sulfonamides, sulfonylureas
Hypotension	Neuroleptics, narcotics especially meperidine, neuromuscular blockers
Hypothyroidism	Lithium, alpha-blockers
Intestinal obstructions	Anticholinergic drugs, narcotics, cholinomimetics
Liver disease	Valproic acid, hydantoins, clonazepam, propylthiouracil
Myasthenia gravis	Lithium, oxazolidones, corticosteroids, type-1A antidysrhythmic drugs, aminoglycosides

Table 4.3 Continued

Disease	Exacerbating Drugs
Osteoporosis	Corticosteroids, aluminum containing antacids
Parkinson's disease	Neuroleptics, cholinomimetics, reserpine
Peptic ulcer or gastritis	Nonsteroidal anti-inflammatory drugs, chloral hydrate, alpha-blockers, cholinomimetics, corticosteroids, sympatholytic antihypertensive drugs, methylxanthines
Peripheral vascular disorders	Levodopa, dopamine agonists, alpha-agonists
Psychosis	Levodopa, corticosteroids
Tardive dyskinesias	Anticholinergic drugs
Thromboembolic disorders	Estrogens, progestins
Urinary retention/prostatic hypertrophy	Anticholinergic drugs, benzodiazepines, narcotics, alpha-agonists, sympatholytic antihypertensive drugs

*Includes most neuroleptics, most antidepressants, many antihistamines, as well as drugs specifically designated as anticholinergics.

Table 4.4 Diseases and Other Physiological Conditions That Impact on Pharmacokinetics of Drugs

Kinetic Effect	Diseases/Conditions
Absorption	
Delayed gastric emptying	Hypothyroidism, gastric ulcers, pyloric obstruction or stenosis, diabetic gastroparesis
Decreased gastric absorption	Gastritis, gastric ulcers, achlorhydria (for certain basic drugs)
Decreased intestinal absorbtion	Malabsorption syndromes
Distribution	
Altered volume of distribution	Dehydration, edema, congestive heart failure, amputations
Slowed delivery	Congestive heart failure
Reduced plasma protein binding	Hypoalbuminemia
Inactivation	
Reduced renal clearance	Glomerulotubular diseases, congestive heart failure, renal failure
Reduced hepatic metabolism	Viral hepatitis, toxic hepatitis, cirrhosis, obstructive jaundice, congestive heart failure (due to reduced hepatic blood flow)

tion, delaying and often lowering the peak plasma concentration. Total absorption from the gastrointestinal tract for certain drugs can be reduced by malabsorption syndrome. The ultimate concentration of absorbed drug in the distributive phase will depend on fluid volume effects of such disorders as essential hypertension or congestive heart failure. Older people have, on average, 10–15% less total body water, and this natural change can be intensified by dehydration. Changes in quantities of serum proteins may have important consequences on total blood levels of drugs that are usually significantly bound as well as the relative size of free to bound fractions. This is important because only the free fraction is pharmacologically active.

No doubt the most influential relationship between diseases common among the elderly and drug action are the diseases that affect the two main mechanisms of drug inactivation: metabolism by the liver and excretion in the urine by the kidneys. Some drugs are inactivated mainly by liver metabolism, some mainly by renal excretion, and some depend on both mechanisms. A very few drugs are inactivated by other mechanisms entirely. Elderly clients who have a degree of renal impairment will have much greater sensitivity to drugs inactivated primarily by renal excretion, but their response to drugs inactivated mainly by hepatic metabolism will be little affected. Conversely, those with a degree of liver failure can continue to receive drugs inactivated mainly by renal excretion at doses that would be appropriate for other elderly clients, but doses of drugs inactivated mainly by liver metabolism will have to be adjusted in proportion to the degree of liver failure. It is crucial, therefore, that prescribing physicians know the route of inactivation of drugs they prescribe and know the status of renal and hepatic function for each of their clients—particularly the elderly ones.

ALTERED PHARMACODYNAMICS IN OLDER PERSONS

Aging also influences the response of target tissues to local concentrations of drug (Table 4.1). One reason is that functional capacity of most major organ systems has declined, leaving less unused functional capacity in reserve. As a result, adverse effects impact more keenly on tissue systems already stretched to the limit.

In younger individuals, some actions of drugs are effectively counterbalanced by the vigorous physiological control mechanisms that maintain homeostasis. For example, when drugs increase blood pressure, the body often produces a compensatory decrease in heart rate, thereby decreasing cardiac output and partially canceling the drug-induced hypertension. This reflex, involving impulses along the vagus nerve to the heart, is less efficient for the elderly. Postural hypotension is likewise more common for elderly persons in response to drugs because the reflexive fine control over peripheral vascular beds, and thereby blood pressure, is not as responsive. Appetite control, a homeostatic activity of the hypothalamus, is likewise more fragile for an elderly person and more easily suppressed by anorexics such as amphetamine.

The brain of the elderly person is more sensitive to depressant influences of many drugs. For example, benzodiazepines impair motor function more in elderly people. Sedative-hypnotics cause more cognitive impairment, more depression, and more frequent episodes of paradoxical reactions among the elderly. Since older individuals often have poorer control of balance, they are more prone to ataxia and falls in response to depressant drugs. The brain is also more susceptible to intoxicating effects of digoxin even as the failing heart is likely to require increasing doses. Thus, the therapeutic index for digoxin declines and episodes of intoxication become frequent.

The elderly are more sensitive to many of the anticholinergic side effects of drugs with this property. Urinary retention and constipation are likely to be more severe, aggravation of glaucoma more frequent, as well as confusion and other central nervous system effects. Neuromuscular blockers will produce more muscle weakness in elderly individuals than younger patients.

The heart of the elderly person is more sensitive to some drugs, less sensitive to others. For example, responses to quinidine are usually less but increased with lidocaine. Older clients often develop resistance to insulin that they require for diabetes mellitus. Doses of insulin must sometimes be escalated many fold as a result.

REFERENCES AND RECOMMENDED READINGS

Adamson L: Drug treatment in the elderly. *Nurs. Times* 1978; 74:973–974.

Allen MD: Drug therapy in the elderly. *Am. J. Nurs.* 1980; 80(8):1474–1475.

Bishop T: Drugs and the elderly: A breeding ground for mishaps. *Nurs. Mirror* 1978; 147:49–50.

Dall CE et al.: Promoting effective drug-taking behaviors in the elderly. *Nurs. Clin. North Am.* 1982; 17(2):283–290.

Gibian T: Rational drug therapy in the elderly or how not to poison your elderly patients. *Aust. Fam. Physician* 1992; 21(12):1755–1760.

Goldberg PB: Why do older adults need different dosages? *Geriatr. Nurs.* 1980; 1:74.

Gotz BE, Gotz VP: Drugs and the elderly. *Am. J. Nurs.* 1978; 78:1347–1351.

Hayter J: The older adult and drug therapy. Why response to medication changes with age. *Geriatr. Nurs.* 1981; 2(6):411–416.

Hudson MF: Drugs and the older adult take special care. *Nursing* 1984; 14(8):46–51.

Lenhart DG: The use of medications in the elderly population. *Nurs. Clin. North Am.* 1976; 11:135–143.

Oppeneer C, Vervoren A: *Gerontological Pharmacology: a Resource for Health Practitioners.* St. Louis, C.V. Mosby Co., 1983.

Simons KJ et al.: Pharmacokinetics and pharmacodynamics of terfenadine and chlorpheniramine in the elderly. *J. Allergy Clin. Immunol.* 1990; 85(3): 540–547.

Sloan RW: Principles of drug therapy in geriatric patients. *Am. Fam. Physician* 1992; 45(6):2709–2718.

Stevenson IH, Hosie J: Pharmacokinetics in the elderly, in K. O'Malley and JL Waddington (eds): *Therapeutics in the elderly,* New York, Elsevier Sci. Publ., 1985, pp. 35–42.

CHAPTER 5

Adverse Reactions and Interactions in Geriatric Patients

It is difficult to obtain accurate data regarding the incidence of adverse reactions and interactions of drugs in the elderly because many of the most common kinds of adverse effects (Figure 5.1) resemble symptoms of disorders that are themselves common among the elderly. Common adverse effects such as falls (from drug-related orthostatic hypotension or ataxia); somnolence, confusion, cognitive impairment, or depression (from depressant medications); anticholinergic actions such as constipation or urinary retention, or dehydration from excess diuretic action may easily be mistaken for problems of aging. Even allergic reactions, such as skin rash, may not be recognized as drug-related. It is helpful in assessing whether an observed symptom is an adverse drug reaction to apply the following six tests.

1. Is the observed symptom one that is known to be a possible side effect of one or another drug that the client takes?
2. Did the observed symptom develop shortly after the addition of a new drug to the regimen or a dosage increase for an existing drug in the regimen?
3. Did the observed symptom subside when a drug was discontinued or the dosage reduced?
4. Did the symptoms reappear when a drug was reintroduced or the dosage increased?
5. What other factors might have led to or contributed to the observed symptom?
6. Has this client had a similar symptom in the past in response to this drug or another one?

Even if noxious symptoms are recognized as having a drug contribution, many times an adverse drug response involves predisposing variables as well, such as idiosyncratic (genetically determined) sensitivity, preexisting

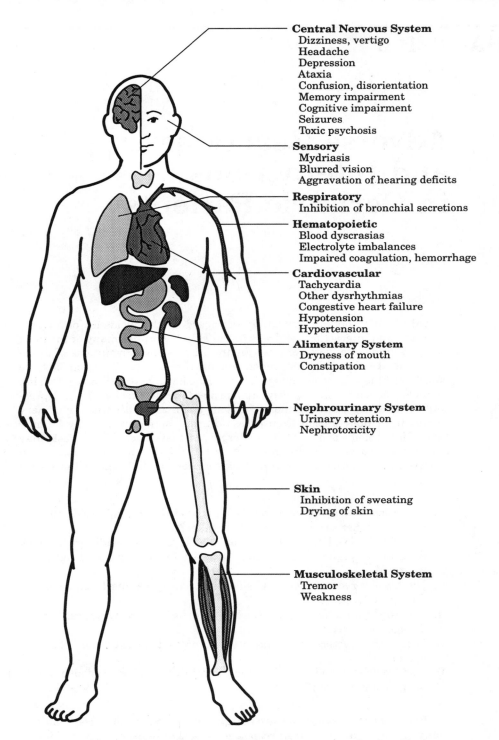

Central Nervous System
  Dizziness, vertigo
  Headache
  Depression
  Ataxia
  Confusion, disorientation
  Memory impairment
  Cognitive impairment
  Seizures
  Toxic psychosis

Sensory
  Mydriasis
  Blurred vision
  Aggravation of hearing deficits

Respiratory
  Inhibition of bronchial secretions

Hematopoietic
  Blood dyscrasias
  Electrolyte imbalances
  Impaired coagulation, hemorrhage

Cardiovascular
  Tachycardia
  Other dysrhythmias
  Congestive heart failure
  Hypotension
  Hypertension

Alimentary System
  Dryness of mouth
  Constipation

Nephrourinary System
  Urinary retention
  Nephrotoxicity

Skin
  Inhibition of sweating
  Drying of skin

Musculoskeletal System
  Tremor
  Weakness

Figure 5.1 Most common adverse drug reactions for the elderly.

disease states, or concurrent use of other drugs. The fact of nonadherence to regimens also complicates statistical analysis of the incidence of adverse drug effects, because clients who are not actually taking the prescribed medication will enlarge the apparent size of the group who do not experience a given adverse effect.

Nevertheless and in spite of these problems of analysis, it is well documented that the incidence of adverse effects of drugs increases with age. Among hospitalized elderly persons, an estimated 10–15% experience an adverse effect from their medication. Individuals over 70 comprise approximately 12% of hospital admissions, but experience about 16.5% of the adverse drug reactions. Adverse drugs reactions account for approximately 10–25% of admissions to geriatric hospitals. They account for 3% of *all* hospital admissions with 40% of those involving people over 60 years of age. One of the reasons for the higher incidence of medication-related problems in the elderly is the sheer number of drugs that they take on average (see Chapter 3). More drugs means more potential for more different side effects and more different drug interactions. Another reason is that most of the drugs most often responsible for adverse drugs reactions (e.g., aspirin and other antiarthritics, digoxin, warfarin, hydrochlorthiazide and other diuretics, antacids, and antihypertensives) are the drugs more widely used by elderly persons than by others.

Another contributing factor is the more frequent presence of preexisting disease which often leaves affected organ systems more vulnerable to drug effects. For example, some elderly people will be more susceptible to cardiovascular side effects because of preexisting hypertension, congestive heart disease, chronic renal failure, or angina pectoris. Some may be susceptible to psychiatric or neurologic side effects because they suffer depression, dementia, or sleep disturbances. Some may be more than typically prone to falls or fainting due to arthritis or gait disturbances. Or they might suffer greater impairments or nephrourinary function or gastrointestinal function because of preexisting incontinence or constipation. Sensory systems will be more affected by ototoxicity or ocular effects of drugs to the extent that hearing or visual impairments have developed. Also, homeostatic mechanisms are less effective in countering primary drug effects for the elderly. For example, the elderly are less able to regulate balance, body temperature, blood glucose, pulse rate, blood pressure, and bladder function.

Lastly, medical practice has still not yet come fully to grips with the need for dosage adjustment in the elderly because of the age-dependent pharmacokinetics (see Chapter 4). In other words, many elderly clients are receiving excessive doses of the medications that might otherwise be entirely appropriate medical interventions. Clients with impaired renal function—most usually an elderly person—are among those most likely to have adverse drug effects because of the higher plasma concentrations that occur with many drugs if renal clearance is diminished.

Elderly women have more adverse drug responses than elderly men, even adjusting for the larger number of elderly women. The main reason appears to be that elderly women use more drugs on average than elderly men. Drug interactions are likewise more common in older women than older men.

Adverse drug reactions can be classified according to two characteristics: (1) the most likely time of occurrence following initiation of drug therapy, and (2) whether they are predictable and dose-dependent or not. Many side effects appear soon after initiation of drug therapy and are termed *early* side effects. These side effects tend to subside with continued administration of the same drug dosage as tolerance develops. Most early side effects are dose-dependent, so that their likelihood is somewhat predictable based on the dosage of the drug that is required for the particular patient.

Two kinds of side effects that most often occur early are unpredictable, often exhibiting an intensity that bears little relationship to the dosage: **drug allergies** (also called hypersensitivity reactions) and idiosyncratic reactions. Drug allergies occur because drugs can serve as antigens or can combine with a component of the body and cause it to become antigenic. Either way, an immune response is triggered. Allergic reactions occur in a relatively small percentage of treated individuals with almost every class of drugs, the main exception being drugs that are the same as chemicals that also occur naturally in the body. Allergic reactions are a bit more common with antimicrobial drugs, local anesthetics, neuroleptics, and antidepressants than with most other drug classes. If a person is allergic to one drug, he or she will usually be allergic to any other drug of similar chemical structure, whether or not the drug belongs to the same or a different therapeutic classification. The main means of predicting potential allergic reactions in advance is the client's history of responses to the drug or ones of similar structure. Another technique used for drugs having a high risk of allergic responses is a sensitivity test, such as a skin patch test, in which a very small amount of drug is applied to test for unusual sensitivity. Allergic reactions can range from mild skin rash to life-threatening problems such as jaundice, anaphylaxis, anemia, or severe dermatologic eruptions.

Idiosyncratic reactions are usually intense reactions that occur because of the person's particular genetic make-up. Some people have, for example, a genetically based inability to metabolize certain drugs. This has been reported for succinylcholine, isoniazid, hydralazine, and phenytoin. Idiosyncratic reactions should be carefully recorded in the client's chart to guide subsequent health care providers.

Some categories of side effects occur only after long-term, chronic use of a drug. Tolerance and dependence are familiar examples. Tardive dyskinesias that stem from long-term use of neuroleptics is another. Drugs can cause so-called **iatrogenic diseases** that derive from tissue damage with long-term drug administration. The five most common examples of iatrogenic diseases are blood dyscrasias (a drop in white blood cell counts), liver damage, kidney damage, teratogenicity (damage to a fetus from maternal exposure), and skin eruptions. All but teratogenicity are more likely to occur in elderly than in younger patients.

COMMON ADVERSE DRUG REACTIONS IN THE ELDERLY

Although adverse effects in the elderly are qualitatively similar to those that occur in younger individuals, the incidence is higher, and the impact on the continuing health of the client is often greater. Older people are more susceptible to adverse drug effects on the brain, for example, including excess depression, toxic psychosis, and extrapyramidal reactions. Anticholinergic side effects, which include both central and peripheral examples, are more likely to occur not only because elderly clients are more likely to be taking two or more drugs with anticholinergic properties, but also because anticholinergic symptoms often add to preexisting health problems. Urinary retention, for example, might add to retention already present in a male client as a consequence of prostatic hypertrophy.

The cardiovascular system is likely to be more susceptible to adverse drug effects. Cardiac output, already reduced because of aging, can less afford the suppressant influence from the negative inotropic effect of beta-blockers. Dysrhythmias, orthostatic hypotension, and hypertensive responsives are also all more likely in older people because of less vigorous homeostatic control mechanisms and existing pathology.

Gastrointestinal motility, already diminished for elderly people, is more seriously impacted by drugs promoting constipation. The kidneys, after losing 1% of their filtration capacity each year for a number of years, are more susceptible to nephrotoxic effects of drugs. Electrolyte imbalances are more likely when diuretics are required.

Antibiotics, an often overused or irrationally used class of drugs especially in the elderly, are mostly excreted by the kidneys. Since renal function is usually less for elderly people, toxicity from antibiotics is more likely in theory and indeed more common in actual practice.

All professionals who work with elderly clients need to consider routinely that any newly developing symptoms might be an adverse drug reaction, especially if the symptom is one of those appearing in Table 5.1. The presumption that such symptoms are normal consequences of aging must be rigorously avoided until thorough evaluation rules out the possibility of a drug contribution.

COMMON DRUG–DRUG INTERACTIONS IN THE ELDERLY

Drug interactions are far more likely in the elderly, if for no other reason than because they take so many more medications. The elderly, who comprise 12% of the population currently, account for 32% of all prescriptions. This factor can hardly be overstated and its true import can be appreciated if one stops to consider that the number of possible two drug interactions increases almost geometrically as the number of drugs in the regimen increases. The number of possible two drug interactions for a regimen of n drugs can be calculated as $n \times (n-1)/2$. Thus, 2 drugs provide only 1 pairing for purposes of interaction, but 6 drugs provide 15 possible pairings, and 10 drugs 45. Moreover, some interactions develop from the combined effect of 3 or more of the drugs in the regimen, adding additional possibilities when regimens include large numbers of drugs. One large study found that the percentage of patients receiving drugs with potential for interaction was just 2.4% for 2 drug regimens, 8.8% for 3 drug regimens, 22.7% for 6 drug regimens, and 55.8% for 12 drug regimens. Of course, not all potential drug interactions manifest as clinically significant interactions.

Table 5.1 Most Common Adverse Drug Effects in Geriatric Patients

Adverse effect	Causative agents	
Central nervous system		
Excess depression: somnolence, fatigue, weakness, ataxia, confusion, disorientation, memory impairment, cognitive impairment	Antihistamines Antipsychotics Anxiolytics Cardiac glycosides Lithium Local anesthetics	Methyldopa Narcotics Phenytoin Reserpine Sedative-hypnotics
Seizures/coma	Penicillin G	
Psychiatric disturbances: psychosis	Cardiac glycosides Corticosteroids Levodopa	
Anticholinergic symptoms:		
Central: disorientation, poor attention, confusion, agitation, hallucinations, psychosis Peripheral: tachycardia, mydriasis, decreased salivary and bronchial secretions, inhibition of sweating, urinary retention, constipation	Antidepressants Antihistamines Antiparkinsonian drugs Antipsychotic drugs Quinidine	
Extrapyramidal symptoms	Antidepressants Lithium Neuroleptics	
Cardiovascular system		
Heart failure	Beta-blockers	
Dysrhythmias	Antidepressants Cardiac glycosides Phenytoin	
Hypotension: syncope, dizziness, headache, vertigo	Antidysrhythmics Antidepressants Antihistamines Antihypertensives Antipsychotics Benzodiazepines	Diuretics Levodopa Narcotics Phenytoin Vasodilators
Hypertension	Anorexics Nasal decongestants Stimulants	
Other		
Blood dyscrasias	Antineoplastics Antipsychotics Oxyphenbutazone Phenylbutazone	

Table 5.1 Continued

Adverse effect	Causative agents	
Other (cont.)		
Electrolyte imbalances	Corticosteroids Diuretics	
Gastrointestinal problems	Cardiac glycosides Clindamycin Colchicine Corticosteroids Diuretics	Hyperlipemic drugs Laxatives Narcotics Nonsteroidal anti- inflammatory drugs
Hemorrhage	Oral anticoagulants Heparin	
Nephrotoxicity	Aminoglycosides	
Ototoxicity	Aminoglycosides	

Moreover, there are other reasons that contribute to the higher frequency of drug interactions for the elderly—basically the same factors that serve to increase the likelihood of adverse reactions to individual drugs also operate to increase the likelihood of interactions: preexisting diseases, diminished tissue reserve, and less vigorous homeostatic compensations.

Although there are many possible drug interactions already known to occur, the task of predicting and preventing these can be a feasible one for physicians, pharmacists, and other healthcare providers because the collected set of all possible interactions is compiled in various computer programs and even in a portable chart format, called MEDISC. One of the keys to successful prevention of interactions is that at least one of the healthcare providers working with each individual has knowledge of the client's complete drug regimen, including all prescription, nonprescription, and recreational drugs being taken. Clients should be encouraged to consolidate their healthcare activities by, for example, filling all prescriptions and purchasing all nonprescription products from the same pharmacy and making sure that the pharmacy maintains a complete record of their drug requirements. Social service providers, visiting nurses, and physicians need to urge clients to discard out-of-date and unneeded drugs.

The drug interactions that occur most frequently in the elderly are summarized in Table 5.2. As research continues and new drugs are added each year to the existing pharmacopeia, undoubtedly additional examples of drug interactions will be identified. For the time-being, those listed in Table 5.2 represent the ones that most need to be anticipated by healthcare providers dealing with elderly persons. Caregivers must work together to simplify drug regimens for elderly clients and, in particular, to reduce the number of drugs whenever possible.

Table 5.2 Most Common Drug Interactions in Geriatric Patients

Drug or category	Interacting drug	Result
A vitamins	Mineral oil	Impaired absorption
Antiadrenergic antihypertensive drugs	Nasal decongestants	Hypertension
Anticholinergic drugs	Other anticholinergic drugs	Additive anticholinergic toxicity: urinary retention, constipation, drying, anxiety, poor attention, disorientation
Aspirin	Alkalinizing agents	More rapid excretion
	Acidifying agents	Slower excretion
	Corticosteroids	Lower plasma level and decreased effectiveness for aspirin
Cephalosporins (some) Chlorpropamide Griseofulvin Metronidazole Moxalactam Tolazamide Tolazoline Tolbutamide	Alcohol	Disulfiram-like interaction
CNS depressants	Sedative-hypnotics Anxiolytics Narcotics Neuroleptics Sedative antidepressants Antiepileptics Alcohol	Additive CNS depression: somnolence, ataxia, confusion, weakness, depression, cognitive impairments
Dexamethasone Methylprednisolone Other glucocorticoids Phenothiazines Quinidine Warfarin	Phenobarbital Phenytoin Secobarbital Other hypnotics Other antiepileptics Antihistamines	Faster metabolism of first drug after induction of liver enzymes by second drug
Digoxin	Quinidine	Increased plasma level of digoxin
	Diuretics	Digoxin toxicity from K^+ depletion
	Antidysrhythmics	Additive risk of block
Diuretics		
Thiazide & High ceiling	Glucocorticoids with mineralocorticoid activity	Increased potassium depletion
Potassium-sparing	Potassium salts ACE-inhibitors	Hyperkalemia
Guanethidine	Tricyclic antidepressants	Inhibition of benefit of guanethidine by blocking its uptake into neurons

Table 5.2 Continued

Drug or category	Interacting drug	Result
Insulin or sulfonylureas	Beta-2 blockers	Decreased benefit
Levodopa	Pyridoxine	Decreased entry of levodopa into brain
Phenytoin Tolbutamide	Chloramphenicol Methylphenidate Phenylbutazone Oxyphenylbutazone	Slowed metabolism of first drug
Tetracyclines Phenothiazines Isoniazid	Antacids	Decreased absorption
Sulfonylureas	Thiazide diuretics	Decreased benefit due to thiazide-induced glucose intolerance
Sympathomimetic amines	Tricyclic antidepressants	Potentiation of hypertensive effect
Warfarin Sulfonylureas Digoxin	Aspirin Other salicylates Phenylbutazone Phenytoin Other antiepileptics	Competition for plasma protein binding sites; mutual potentiation

REFERENCES AND RECOMMENDED READINGS

Blaschke TF, Cohen SN, Tatro DS, Rubin PC: Drug-drug interactions and aging, in Jarvik et al. (eds): *Clin. Pharmacol. and the Aged Patient.* New York, Raven, 1981, pp. 11–26.

McNamara TR: Adverse drug interactions in the elderly, in WG Wood, R. Strong (eds): *Geriatr. Clin. Pharmacol.* New York, Raven, 1987, pp. 141–147.

Roe DA: Drug-nutrient interactions in the elderly. *Geriatr.* 1982; 41(3):57–74.

Stewart RB: Adverse drug reactions, in Delafuente, Stewart: *Therapeutics in the Elderly.* Baltimore, Williams & Wilkins, 1988, pp. 121–131.

Vestal RE, Jue SG, Cusack BJ: Increased risk of adverse drug reactions in the elderly: Fact or myth?, in K. O'Malley and JL Waddington (eds): *Therapeutics in the elderly.* New York, Elsevier, 1985, pp. 97–104.

CHAPTER 6

Clinical and Outpatient Support for Drug Therapy

In order for drugs to be effective and serve their intended purpose, they must be appropriately prescribed, taken by the client as directed, and act as anticipated to produce the desired results. The first of these matters, appropriate prescription of drugs, is an issue that must be dealt with by physicians and other primary health care providers. Positive attitudes and education about pharmacokinetics and pharmacodynamics as related to special problems of the elderly is necessary for all who prescribe for elderly persons. Medical licensure helps ensure competent medical practice, and regulation agencies assist by ensuring that only approved drugs can be prescribed.

The second area, taking drugs as directed, is at present a primary concern. Nurses and other health care professionals who interact with clients provide an important service in this regard—by educating and guiding clients in accurate administration of drugs.

The third area, the effect of the drug once it enters the person's body, is often difficult to predict and control. Actions to minimize unexpected adverse drug reactions can only be accomplished if there have been careful assessment and follow-up of each person taking the medications. Client education, including any special instructions, restrictions, and precautions associated with the medications in use is critically important to ensure the intended effect of the drug.

Drug use and misuse, changes in how drugs are absorbed or inactivated in the body, and adverse effects of drugs among elderly persons were discussed in Chapters 3 and 4. With an understanding of these problems as a base, this chapter will focus on information that can assist nurses and other health care professionals in educating and supporting the elderly who require drugs. The problem of compliance and issues pertaining to self-care will be reviewed with an eye toward ways of assessing medication use and responses. Adverse effects of drugs can be minimized through well-designed interventions, including good communication skills, education, environmental modification, regimen simplification, and careful monitoring.

Problems with medications among the elderly can be client-centered or physician-centered (Figure 6.1). Interventions by nurses and other health

59

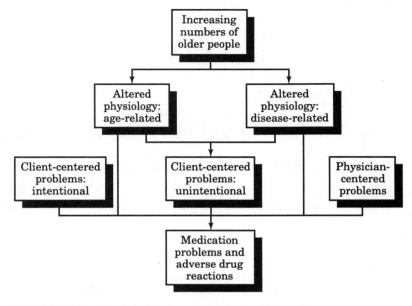

Figure 6.1 Factors contributing to problems with medications.

care professionals are best directed at the level of client-centered problems (both intentional and unintentional), whereas physician-centered problems are best handled through client advocacy.

COMPLIANCE

Use of the word *compliance* has sometimes been criticized because it suggests a power imbalance of weaker patients complying with more powerful physicians' "orders." In an effort to adopt a word without such negative connotations, some authors have used the word *adherence*, which refers to the client's adherence to the medical regimen. In this book, the words *compliance* and *adherence* are used interchangeably to mean the client's behavior of actively participating in and following the suggested plan of treatment, including directions for taking specified amounts (doses) of medications at specified times and particular ways/routes of administration.

Enloe has suggested that a participation model in which an older individual's power and control are acknowledged is a more productive model than compliance. "In reality, it is the older person who chooses and engages in the level of integration of health monitoring and treatment in [his or her] life" (Enloe, 1993, p. 21). Although a power imbalance is probably inherent within the patient-physician relationship, the assumption here is that the patient is a consumer who pays for a service. This service, to be fully effective, involves tasks to be accomplished by the consumer, who can then choose whether or not to continue with the follow-up tasks as directed. The greatest success results when consumers, or clients in the case of health care services, fully and actively participate in all aspects of their care—including appropriate follow-up of their physician's recommendations. Acceptance of an active participation model by health care professionals can help ensure that clients will be more successful in following the directions given to them regarding their drugs and medical regimen.

Patient compliance with prescribed medication regimens has been of great interest to researchers, but this is a difficult area to investigate because of problems with defining and measuring behavior. It is assumed that noncompliance leads to adverse drug reactions or increased problems from the disease for which the drug was prescribed; however, these outcomes also are difficult to measure. When deviations from compliance are extreme, such as overuse or abuse of a potent drug, adverse consequences are easily identified, but the relationship between smaller degrees of noncompliance and adverse drug effects is difficult to establish.

In general, the greater the number of medications and the greater the complexity of the drug-taking regimen, the higher the risk of adverse drug reactions and noncompliance. Interestingly, the elderly have not been found to have greater problems with noncompliance than younger people. Factors that have been identified as associated with noncompliance with prescribed medications include living alone, unpleasant side effects of drugs, financial problems, types of disease, relationship between patient and physician, complexity of medical regimen, cognitive and sensory deficits, and lack of understanding of the medication regimen (Simonson, 1984).

The most powerful motivation for compliance is a perception that the medication is alleviating existing symptoms quickly. On the other hand, a perception that not taking the medication will result in serious consequences is a strong motivator. Physician characteristics have also been found to influence compliance behaviors. Although personal characteristics such as age, sex, and ethnic group had no effect on compliance, clients were more likely to follow their doctors' advice if their doctors had busy practices, were happy in their work, and took time to answer questions and followed up with phone or office visits (DiMatteo et al., 1993).

Estimates of compliance with medication instructions among community living elderly have varied widely; however, a recent review reported a range from 52% to 65%, with only 5% of these errors likely to result in adverse drug reactions (German & Burton, 1989). One study of 50 older people found that 25% took medications differently than instructed on the label; however, most subjects stated that their physicians had given them verbal instructions to do so (Lundin, 1978). Verbal changes in instructions for medication regimen have not been adequately taken into account by most studies of compliance behaviors, thus limiting the value of the results.

Noncompliance with prescribed medication regimens can take several forms and result from **intentional decisions** or **unintentional errors.** Intentional decisions not to comply include not taking the drug or adjusting the dose because of unpleasant side effects, perceived improvement in condition, unacceptably high cost, fear of dependency on the drug, or lack of trust in the physician. A few older people purposefully do not take their drugs as prescribed in order to cause a decline in their health status because they experience positive effects from being sick. The older person who is suicidal may also misuse drugs to end his life.

Unintentional errors may result from a lack of understanding regarding the disease, drug dose, time or route of administration; from scheduling difficulties; from cognitive deficits resulting in memory problems; and from functional limitations making access to the drug difficult. Most of these errors result in underuse of prescription drugs. Overuse or abuse are rarely reported as problematic among elderly.

There are occasions when noncompliance with prescribed medications may result in fewer adverse drug reactions and improved health. Some older people have a very good understanding of their disease process and their medications, as well as a heightened sense of the internal physical state of their own bodies. For these people, self-regulation and management of their medication regimens based on their symptoms, which according to definition is noncompliance, may result in closer regulation of disease states and improved health outcomes.

COMMUNICATING WITH THE OLDER PERSON

Good communication skills are essential when delivering care to clients of any age. Although it is beyond the scope of this chapter to review basic communication skills, some information that may assist in fostering

Table 6.1 Barriers to Communication with Older Adults (Miller, 1990, p. 128)

Barriers in Older Adults
- Sensory impairments
- Physical discomfort (e.g., pain, thirst, hunger)
- Effects of medications or pathological conditions
- Impaired psychosocial functioning secondary to dementia or depression
- Diminished contact with reality

Barriers in the Interview Atmosphere
- Environmental noise and distractions
- Too much information at one time
- Too many people involved in the interview
- Cultural differences
- Language differences
- Prejudices and stereotypes

Barriers in the Inteviewer
- Insensitivity
- Poor listening skills
- Trite remarks
- False reassurance
- Judgmental attitudes
- Use of inappropriate or unacceptable names
- Inarticulate speech
- Obstructive mannerisms

Table 6.2 Techniques to Enhance Communication with Older Persons (Adapted from Miller, 1990, p. 133)

Verbal and Nonverbal Communication
- Begin interaction with an exchange of names and a handshake.
- Use touch sensitively and purposefully to reinforce verbal messages and as a primary method of nonverbal communication.
- Explain the purpose of the interaction in relation to identified goals.
- Begin with questions that are general in nature.
- Periodically clarify the messages using reflection (restating the message as you have understood it and asking for verification of meaning).
- Maintain good eye contact, use attentive listening, and encourage the person to elaborate on information.
- Remain nonjudgemental in responses, but show appropriate empathy.
- Sit in a face-to-face position.
- Ensure as much privacy as possible.
- Provide good lighting and avoid background glare.
- Eliminate as much background noise as possible.

understanding between the older person and the nurse or caregiver will be presented.

Barriers to communication with older persons may include hearing or vision impairment, overload from too much information, too many people talking, or too much background noise, internal distractions arising from physical discomfort, neurological disorders, or cognitive deficits. Other behaviors by health care providers that may create barriers include addressing older people in a manner considered disrespectful by them, giving false reassurance or avoiding sensitive issues, minimizing the person's feelings, communicating while performing other activities, or cultural differences (Table 6.1).

Health care providers can reduce or eliminate these barriers to communication. Techniques to enhance communication involve both verbal and nonverbal behaviors and special attention to the environment in which the interaction takes place (Table 6.2).

ASSESSMENT OF MEDICATION USE

Support of clients receiving drug therapy begins with a comprehensive assessment of the drugs they are taking, how they are taking them, and any problems they may be having related to the medication. A 24-hour drug history, similar to the widely used 24-hour nutrition history, has been found to be a useful way to begin assessing medication use. Doris Schwartz, the

Table 6.3 Guidelines and Questions for Medication Assessment

Begin with recording the 24-hour recall of drugs taken yesterday.

1. In addition to these drugs, do you take any other prescription pills, liquids, injections, eye drops, nasal sprays, skin preparations or patches, nonprescription pills or liquids that you buy yourself, vitamins and minerals, herbal or home remedies?
2. Are you allergic to any medications?
3. How much alcohol, caffeine, or tobacco do you use on a daily basis?
4. Are you taking medications prescribed for anyone else?
5. What do you do to help yourself remember to take your pills or keep track of those you have taken? What do you do when you forget a dose?
6. Do you have any problem getting your prescriptions filled? Any problem taking the medications? (Review the 24-hour recall list of drugs and ask questions specifically about each drug.)
7. What are you taking this medication for? What problems were you having when this medication was prescribed for you or when you purchased this drug (for OTC drugs)?
8. For drugs that are prescribed or the directions say to be taken as needed, how often do you usually take this drug? How do you decide when to take it?
9. What have you been told by the doctor or nurse about this medication?
10. Are there special instructions or things you should avoid when you take this drug, e.g., do not take with alcohol, or certain foods? Do you ever eat or drink these things while taking this drug?
11. How does this drug make you feel? Have you noticed any change in the way you feel since you began taking this drug? (If possible, ask to see the medications they are taking. Check bottles for drug names and instructions consistent with 24-hour recall. Look for discrepancies between directions on the labels and the way the client is taking the drugs.)
12. Has the doctor given you any verbal instructions that are different than those indicated on the bottle? (Note the name(s) of the prescribing physician(s).)
13. If more than one physician, are all these physicians caring for you aware of all the drugs being prescribed by each other? Ascertain if there are any medications being duplicated by different physicians.

If the dates on the bottles are different:

14. Were more recently prescribed medications added to the regimen or were they intended to replace older dated medications? (The client may not know the answer to this and the physician may need to be contacted if this seems to be likely.)

If problems with compliance are suspected and there is opportunity for home visiting and follow-up, monitoring the medication regimen by counting the pills remaining in the bottles week to week is a more accurate way of assessing adequacy of the medication regimen.

first nurse-researcher to look at problems of medication use among the elderly in the 1960's, suggested the following series of questions:

> Let's take yesterday. Starting with when you woke up in the morning, what was the first medicine that you took? How much? How many times a day do you take it? What are you taking that medicine for? What other medicines are you taking? (Anderson, et al., 1982, p. 195).

An analysis and verification of this 24-hour recall can elicit most essential drug information. Some additional questions and probing may be necessary to piece together the entire picture of when and how the older person is taking the drugs. An assessment of the older person's responses to the medications is also important to ascertain whether any possible drug reactions may be occurring. Some questions have proven their usefulness for obtaining complete information about medication regimens, how they are being taken, and the effect they are having (Table 6.3).

Assessment provides the basis for identifying problems, which in turn sets the stage for determining appropriate strategies for resolving or alleviating the problems. Nursing diagnoses have been developed and widely utilized within the nursing profession to identify and label client problems. For example, nursing diagnoses, such as noncompliance related to medication administration, knowledge deficit related to self-administration of medications, or health management deficit, may be relevant. Once problems have been accurately assessed and validated with the client, planning can occur, client-centered goals can be set, and interventions designed to meet these goals undertaken.

PLANNING

Planning is an essential step between assessment and intervention and one that is frequently overlooked. The key to successful planning is including the client in the planning process. Without the step of setting mutual goals with clients, client participation in their care is minimized and feelings of powerlessness may perpetuate noncompliance behaviors. Through active participation in the management of all aspects of their health care regimens including their drug regimens, feelings of competency and self-esteem of clients can be enhanced.

Goal setting that should be carried out jointly between health care professionals and clients includes both long-term goals and short-term objectives which, if met, will solve the problem. An example is a client who is directed to take 6 medications every day at different times. The assessment reveals that the client is only taking 4 of the drugs as prescribed, not taking 1 at all because she believes that it gives her a headache, and only taking half a dose of another to make it last longer because it is so expensive and she has noticed no ill effects. The problem, in this case, could be identified as knowledge deficit related to self-administration of medications. Clients may be more successful in following their prescribed regimens if they are aware of the necessity of taking all 6 of their medications as prescribed (even though they may be asymptomatic) and know the side effects, adverse reactions, and the possible ramifications of not taking all the medications.

The nurse or health care professional must further assess the nature of the knowledge deficit and whether or not this is the only problem. With drugs, the knowledge deficit usually centers around lack of knowledge about the relationship between the drug and the disease, side effects, and the possible consequences of lowering the dose on one's own initiative. Thus, two long-term goals, derived mutually by the health care professional and the client, might be

1. Client will demonstrate knowledge of her medication regimen.
2. Client will demonstrate the ability to self-administer her medications as directed.

Short-term objectives to meet this goal might be:

1. Client will be able to state the names and purposes of each of the prescribed drugs within one week.
2. Client will set up a daily schedule of administration of medications demonstrating correct dose and time for each.
3. Client will describe possible side effects and adverse reactions for each of the medications within two weeks.
4. Client will explore with the pharmacist and physician the possibility of medication assistance programs or changing medication to a less costly drug.
5. Client will evaluate ability to self-administer medications within one month.

It should be noted that all goals and objectives that are client-centered should begin with "client will." In addition, the verbs in the sentences are all action verbs such as "state," "set up," and "evaluate." Writing the plan in this way facilitates designing interventions and evaluations, so that at the end of a week or month, the client and the nurse can easily ascertain whether or not each objective has been met.

INTERVENTIONS

The major areas in which interventions can be focused are in providing education when there is a knowledge deficit, modifying the environment when this causes problems, simplifying the medication regimen, decreasing medication costs when possible, and promoting motivation to successfully manage the drug regimen. The most optimal setting for all of these is in the client's home. Because this is not possible in most instances, creative strategies for good assessment and education should be used within physicians offices, clinics, hospitals, senior citizens centers, and any other place where older people gather.

Education

Before discussing strategies for client education, it is important to review learning features of older adults. Healthy older adults show no declines in areas of intelligence affecting their ability to learn new material such as that necessary for understanding medication regimens. They may actually improve in their judgment, vocabulary, coordination of facts and ideas, and scope of knowledge and experience. Some slight declines have been noted in abstract thinking ability, verbal comprehension, word fluency, and spatial orientation among many older adults. Memory, both long-term and recent, probably both decline somewhat among older people, but memory is greatly affected by health status, sociocultural and educational background, personality, motivation, and expectations.

Older people learn new things as well as younger people, sometimes even better, if they are given adequate time and a comfortable environment without the imposition of time or performance stress. In general, older persons process information more slowly than younger people and are more cautious in their responses. Consideration must be given to the relevance of the material to be learned. Adults learn best when they can immediately apply the information in their lives. Also, differences in values might conflict with new knowledge. An older person may view taking pills as a drug addiction and be afraid to become "addicted." There may then be a negative response to learning about the necessity of taking a drug four times each day. Sensory deficits may also inhibit learning if the teacher has not made changes to ensure adequate communication and understanding of information.

Prior to beginning any client education, further assessment of the client's cognitive status, educational level, knowledge base, functional abilities, learning style, and resources is important. Management of the learning environment must include reducing background noise, maintenance of physical comfort, and promoting a relaxing atmosphere. The presenter must have a positive attitude toward older people, be knowledgeable about medications and their administration, and be flexible and creative in suggesting solutions to individual client problems. An informal approach similar to a dialogue rather than a presentation, in which the client feels free to ask questions and to share ideas, works best to accomplish mutual goals. Practical, easily applicable information is learned most readily and retained longest. Health care providers have found that certain factors need to be considered in the areas of assessment, environment, presenter, and the presentation when designing a teaching plan for the diagnosis of knowledge deficit related to medication administration (Figure 6.2).

Environmental Modification

Several common problems contribute to the inability of older persons to successfully manage their drug regimens. These include difficulty opening childproof containers, dividing pills or preparing medications because of functional or sensory limitations, poor memory, cognitive deficits, or busy schedules.

To ease medication administration for those with functional limitations, nonchildproof caps can be requested from the pharmacist. Although it is never a good idea to remove a medication from its own labeled container, over-the-counter drugs, which are always packaged in childproof bottles, may be transferred to containers that are easily opened as long as they are clearly labeled and essential drug information is attached to the container. If difficulties arise in dividing pills in half or in preparing correct amounts of medications (liquids, tablets, or medications for injections), family members

Environment
- Can client see and hear nurse?
- Is client physically comfortable?
- Is client free from anxiety and distractions?
- Is there privacy?

Assessment
- Cognitive status
  Able to manage medication schedule
  Able to learn and retain new information
- Educational level
  Current knowledge base
- Physical function
  Able to obtain and self-administer medications
- Learning style
  How client has learned and retained new information in the past
  Motivation for learning
- Resources
  Support persons available to assist with medications
  Primary case provider
  Finances

Presenter
- Positive attitude toward older persons
- Belief in promotion of self-care among older persons
- Flexibility when teaching
- Knowledge of age-related changes that may affect medication use by older individuals
- Knowledge of medications

Presentation
- Assess current knowledgebase.
- Build on client's current knowledge base.
- Pace the presentation by discussing small amounts of material at a time.
- Have the client describe and/or demonstrate self-administration of medications.
- Answer the client's questions and concerns as they arise.
- Monitor client's energy level/attention span.
- Provide cues (chart of administration schedule, pill box, timers).
- Focus on priorities.
  Administration and purpose of most important medications
  Emergency side effects

Figure 6.2 A sample teaching plan for nursing diagnosis of knowledge deficit. (From Dellasega et al., 1994, p. 35. Reprinted with permission.)

or neighbors can be taught to prepare medications in advance and carefully label them for the elderly person to take at later times. For isolated individuals who are unable to prepare their medications and who have no support, visiting nurses may prepare medications for a week or more in advance.

Medication lists and calendars can serve as important memory aids for the older person. Medication lists should include the name of the drug (including generic and trade names), description of the appearance of the tablet, the purpose of the drug, dose (including how many tablets equal that dose), times the drug is to be taken, and any special instructions. A medication calendar can be used to record when each dose is taken to prevent confusion as to whether the drug has been taken or not. Memory aids such as turning the medication bottle up-side down when the last dose has been taken may also help. These aids are only useful, however, to the degree the person refers to them or remembers to mark off the dose as taken. Placing medications in a visible place on the table or at the bedside may be used as a reminder to take the drug with meals or at bedtime.

Special containers which have separate compartments for pills for seven days or for multiple times each day for seven days are available. These can be very effective especially for persons who are confused about the drug regimen, but the containers must be accurately filled a week in advance. Some pill containers also require fine motor function to open, preventing their use by those with limited functional abilities. Simpler drug organizers can be creatively made for clients with such things as envelopes and a shoe box, with the day and time written on each envelope containing drugs to be taken at designated times. Monitoring how clients are taking their drugs is also easier with a system such as this.

Regimen Simplification

Complicated medication schedules, such as several medications that look alike and are to be taken at different times or frequently throughout the day, have been found to be associated with higher rates of noncompliance and drug errors. Efforts to simplify the regimen may be directed toward fitting medication times into the person's normal daily routine and existing schedules. Sometimes multiple ingredient tablets can be substituted for several single ingredient pills, so that the older person can take one medication instead of several. Caution should be used when recommending these multiple ingredient medications for older persons, however, because these also increase the incidence of adverse drug effects and drug interactions. The nurse or health care professional can act as an advocate for clients to alert physicians to problems caused by too many medications and can suggest changes that might improve the clients' ability to take their medications as directed.

Cost Reduction

Although the cost of medications is not within the scope of influence of clients or individual health care providers, programs are available in some states to assist older people with the cost of commonly used medications. Senior citizens centers or state departments of elderly affairs are good resources for information about such medication assistance programs. Older people also need to know the savings that can be incurred by taking a generic drug instead of a brand name drug. Cost concerns need to be discussed with prescribers who can then write prescriptions for generic drugs for pharmacists, if substitutions are allowed. Education regarding the differences between generic and brand name drugs needs to accompany any change, as the same drug in generic form may be a different size, color, and shape than the brand name drug. Also, a few generic drugs cause different responses for people than the same brand name drug and can thus contribute to adverse drug reactions. Pharmacists are excellent resources for drug information and monitoring.

EVALUATION

Careful attention to evaluation of older people taking medications is essential. The primary responsibility for this lies with the physician prescriber; however, any nurse or health care professional who has the opportunity to interact with older people on a regular basis can assist in this important task. Follow-up must occur if goals and objectives are to be evaluated.

Evaluation is done by repeating the assessment questions and comparing past medication-taking behaviors with current ones. Each objective needs to be evaluated individually as well. If progress in health status has not been made, or compliance continues to be a problem, a new approach may be needed.

Pharmacists can play an important role in monitoring and follow-up of clients taking multiple medications. To do this effectively, clients must obtain all their prescriptions from one pharmacy, which keeps a history of all prescriptions filled there. An astute pharmacist can then determine incompatible drugs, duplicate prescriptions from different doctors, and drugs that are contraindicated for certain conditions.

Finally, community-based programs, such as the "Brown Bag" program, initiated by the University of Rhode Island College of Pharmacy in 1982, have been very successful in assessing problems clients have taking their medications and providing education to alleviate the problems. In this program, elderly are encouraged to bring all their drugs into a central location, often a senior center, where they are reviewed by a pharmacist. The pharmacist is then able to check for any adverse effects, drug interactions, problems with drug administration, or misunderstandings about the drug regimen. The programs are available to provide much needed education about the drugs as well as answer any questions the older person may have.

CONCLUSION

Clinical and outpatient support for drug therapy necessitates knowledge of factors that inhibit older persons from taking their drugs as prescribed. The emphasis of this chapter has been on how drugs are taken by clients, because this is the area most amenable to intervention. Compliance, types and causes of noncompliance, and factors which promote compliance were described. The importance of using good communication techniques and assessing medication-taking behaviors of clients was discussed and an assessment guide was included. The process of mutual planning and goal setting with clients prior to intervening was outlined. Lastly, interventions including education, environmental modification, regimen simplification, and cost reduction were described. Follow-up and evaluation are critical for support of clients' medication therapy and change to more healthy drug-taking behaviors. Through comprehensive assessments, careful planning, well-designed interventions, and conscientious evaluations, adverse effects of drugs can be reduced.

REFERENCES AND RECOMMENDED READINGS

Anderson WF, Caird FI, Kennedy RD, & Schwartz D: *Gerontology and geriatric nursing.* New York, Arco, 1982.
Dellasega C, Clark D, McCreary D, et al.: Nursing process: Teaching elderly clients. *Journal of Gerontological Nursing,* 1994; 20(1):31–38.

DiMatteo MR, Sherbourne CD, Hays RD, et al.: Physicians' characteristics influence patient adherence to medical treatment: Results from the medical outcomes study. *Health Psychology,* 1993; 12(2):93–102.

Enloe C: Assessment in the elderly. In DL Carnevali & M Patrick (eds). *Nursing management for the elderly,* 3rd ed. Philadelphia: J. B. Lippincott, 1993, pp. 21–49.

German PS, & Burton LC: Medication and the elderly: Issues of prescription and use. *Journal of Aging and Health,* 1989; 1(1):4–34.

Lundin DV: Medication taking behavior of the elderly: A pilot study. *Drug Intelligence and Clinical Pharmacy,* 1978; 12:518.

Miller CA: *Nursing care of older adults: Theory and practice.* Glenview, IL; Scott, Foresman, 1990.

Simonson W: *Medications and the elderly.* Rockville, MD; Aspen Systems, 1984.

CHAPTER 7

Legal and Ethical Issues
in Health Care
for the Elderly

Both health care providers and their clients have rights and responsibilities regarding prescriptions, drug administration, and medication-taking behaviors. Some rights and responsibilities are controlled by law through legal restrictions that control practice or licensure requirements that regulate entry into professional practice. Other matters that are less strictly regulated may nevertheless be guided by standards of practice established by each profession. These accepted standards of practice, general and specific, are used as guides to determine responsibility of health care providers in cases of legal action where there are questions regarding the appropriateness of actions taken by health care professionals.

Ethics refers to the standards of acceptable conduct and individual moral judgments that must be made daily to assist in determining right and wrong courses of action. **Professional ethics** are codes of behavior reflecting values and standards or principles of behavior agreed upon by members of the profession that are viewed as necessary to protect the well-being of clients. They are often formulated as statements about how members of the profession *should* behave rather than how they *do* behave. Ethical standards are goals, not descriptions, to which members of the professional group have agreed they will aspire.

It is useful to consider legal and ethical issues together because they are related in the areas they address; both attempt to promote the health of clients and the rights and responsibilities of all involved in health care delivery. Different professionals may vary in the means used to accomplish these goals, which can result in conflicts. Legal mandates, for instance, may conflict with ethical decisions based on accepted standards and values. Sometimes, the concern to act in a way that can be defended legally takes precedence over the desire to act ethically. In a litigious society such as ours, legality frequently overrides the concern for ethical behavior. In the best circumstances, these two act in concert, but changes will need to be made before true synergism between ethics and legal controls can be viewed as anything close to universal.

Older people and their families face many ethical dilemmas and legal difficulties which are often a result of deteriorating health status. For purposes of this book, ethical and legal issues will be considered expressly as they relate to prescriptions, administration of medications, and self-care. This chapter begins by considering issues that could precipitate ethical and/or legal problems, based on rights and responsibilities of clients and health care professionals, and legal regulations that govern professional action and protect clients' rights. The chapter concludes with a portrayal of some of the kinds of dilemmas that clients, families, and health care professionals face in the care of older people, as a vehicle for examining ethical issues and decision making.

ETHICAL AND LEGAL DILEMMAS EXPERIENCED BY THE ELDERLY

Ethical and legal dilemmas are especially likely to occur in medical care for older people because of the nature of their diseases and associated changes in capabilities that accompany aging. At the same time, new developments in the health care system are adding additional ethical and legal challenges as well. One prime concern is the issue of autonomy in decision making when mental competency is in question. Because mental competency is more likely to be compromised for an elderly person than for those in the younger population, there may be evidence of memory lapses, poor judgment, or noncompliance with medical regimens. This may lead family caregivers to believe that the older person is at risk for making poor decisions. When this occurs, it is necessary to determine mental competency and possibly assign a legal guardian if the older person is deemed not mentally competent.

Medical technology, including artificial organs, laser treatments, ultrasound, and new drug therapies have presented new ethical dilemmas of safety as well as issues of access to these innovative technologies. Once a treatment is determined safe, cost and access issues determine who will be able to take advantage of the treatment.

Research activities can also raise important ethical or legal issues. Three concerns related to research are design and sample, protection of human subjects, and informed consent. Design and sample issues may result in invalid and unreliable data or data that are not relevant for the older population. On the other hand, when older persons are included in studies, they may not feel free to withdraw from participation or may experience discomfort such as tiring easily as a result of a long interview. Truly informed consent may be difficult to obtain if there are cognitive deficits that affect the client's ability to fully understand the study requirements.

A third area that presents ethical and legal dilemmas is the conflict between limited health care resources and growing numbers of older adults. As financial constraints become more obvious, decisions about who receives which treatments will have to be made more frequently. Discussions about rationing of health care have necessarily targeted older adults because they are consumers of health care resources. Callahan (1987) suggested that when an individual reaches the end of a natural life span, somewhere between the ages of 78–82 years of age, no life-extending measures should be used to attempt to avoid a natural death. Others have argued that age alone is a poor indicator of health potential and inappropriately places emphasis on material productivity as a measure of value of life.

A whole series of issues surrounds the end of life specifically, including rights to refuse treatment, right-to-die issues (including advanced directives and living will options), and the emotionally charged issue of euthanasia. Central to these dilemmas is a discussion of quality of life and the basic question of purpose and meaning in life. These are not easily answered questions and will remain ethical and legal dilemmas for many years.

RIGHTS AND RESPONSIBILITIES

Human beings have rights to life, liberty, and the pursuit of happiness awarded to them through the U.S. Constitution. In 1971 the White House Conference on Aging outlined nine basic human rights for older Americans. The first is as follows:

> The right to freedom, independence and the free exercise of individual initiative. This should encompass not only opportunities and resources for personal planning and managing one's lifestyle but support systems for maximum growth and contributions by older persons to their community.

Additional rights have been recognized as important for older adults. These include the right to refuse treatment or medication and the rights to informed consent; privacy; high quality, prompt medical care and treatment; freedom from procedures that are injurious to their health; and freedom to choose their own lifestyle.

Along with these rights come important responsibilities (Table 7.1). Clients have the responsibility to actively participate in their health care through reporting their symptoms to health care providers as accurately and completely as possible. If clients do this, they have the right to expect the best possible health care, including medications prescribed appropriately for their health and physical state. Older persons also have the responsibility to take steps to ensure that their wishes regarding their health care and their death will be carried out in the event that they are unable to make their wishes known at the time. Taking responsibility for designating a person to make health care decisions for them and communicating specific instructions regarding life-sustaining treatments in writing is important for older persons.

Health care professionals including physicians, nurse practitioners, nurses, pharmacists, social workers, and case workers have rights and responsibilities also (Table 7.1). They have the basic human rights afforded everyone in the United States, along with rights and responsibilities given to them by the mandates of their professions. Among these, for prescribers,

Table 7.1 Rights and Responsibilities

	Rights	Responsibilities
Client	1. To freedom, independence, and self determination 2. To informed consent, including to refuse treatment 3. To privacy 4. To competent care	1. To participate in their health care 2. Not to infringe on the rights of others
Nurse	1. To expect own rights to be respected 2. To safe and functional equipment and facilities 3. To compensation for services 4. To competent assistance	1. To act as a reasonable and prudent nurse 2. To render care commensurate with standards of care, updating knowledge regularly 3. To fulfill contract with employer
Physician	1. To expect own rights to be respected 2. To safe and functional equipment and facilities 3. To compensation for services 4. To competent assistance	1. To act as a reasonable and prudent physician 2. To render care commensurate with standards of care, updating knowledge
Hospital	1. To expect institution's rights will be respected 2. To competent service from employees 3. To compensation for services	1. To supply and supervise competent staff 2. To provide safe and functional equipment and facilities

Adapted from Fenner KM: *Ethics and nursing law*. New York, Van Nostrand Reinhold, 1980, p. 90.

is the responsibility to prescribe the drug with the highest probability of success in treating a particular medical problem. To do this, they must carry out high quality assessments of their clients and be current in their knowledge of new developments in their fields, including new information about drugs.

Nurses and other health care professionals in whatever settings they may encounter older people have responsibility for assessment and follow-up of difficulties that older persons report having with their health, particularly their medications. Health care professionals also have responsibility for educating older clients about their medications. This helps clients to become informed consumers who can actively participate in their health care.

In our society, institutions such as hospitals and nursing homes accept responsibility for the environments they provide and the people they employ to deliver care within specified job descriptions. Institutions also have rights that enable them to operate under contractual arrangements and to receive reimbursement for the services they provide. Institutions have responsibility to state their purposes, make clear the limits of their services, and ensure that measures are taken to monitor the quality of the services they offer.

LEGAL ISSUES

Legal responses to issues arise in two ways in the United States: through local, state, and federal legislation and through judicial decisions that result from rulings made by a court in a lawsuit. These rulings become part of common law and serve as precedents for lower courts in the same jurisdiction. Precedents for all lower courts in the United States are set by the Supreme Court's rulings. Laws that affect health care of older adults include laws that guarantee individual autonomy and rights such as the Patient Self-Determination Act (Living Will and Durable Power of Attorney documents, Do Not Resuscitate orders) and laws that specify how mental competence is to be determined and how guardianship is to be awarded.

Laws about patients' rights and autonomy are well-established. In an early case in 1914, the judge ruled that all adults who are of sound mind have a right to determine what should be done with their bodies (Jonsen, et al., 1982). These rights include the notion of informed consent or refusal of consent for treatment of competent adult clients. Clients must be assumed to be mentally competent unless there is good reason to suspect otherwise. Mental incompetency is a legal determination requiring a psychiatric evaluation and a competency hearing by a court. If the judge rules the person incompetent, a guardian is appointed to be a surrogate decision maker on behalf of the client.

The Patient Self-Determination Act is federal legislation that was passed in 1990. It directs personnel in health care institutions to explain to all patients on admission that patients have a right to make decisions about their medical care, including decisions to accept or refuse treatment and the right to specify advanced directives. Advanced directives are documents such as Living Wills and Durable Power of Attorney documents that give directions regarding peoples' wishes about aggressive treatment in the face of terminal illness and designate another to make health care decisions for them.

Nurses and other providers of care are greatly impacted by our legal system. The professional practices of physicians, nurses, and pharmacists are all regulated by licensure, ensuring that only those who are able to meet minimum standards by passing a professional licensure examination are given the credentials to practice. State practice acts specify the care that is to be given by each profession. In many states, evidence of continuing education for relicensure is necessary, ensuring the maintenance of current knowledge and practice. In addition, professional organizations, such as the American Nurses Association, have established standards of practice, both general and specific, for individual specialty areas, which serve as guidelines for quality practice. Although not enacted into law, these standards are used as criteria to determine what might be considered competent practice.

The major criterion by which the competency of service is evaluated is that of **reasonableness and prudence.** The standard of care for the health care provider becomes that which would have been done by a reasonable and prudent professional, with similar preparation and education, and under similar circumstances (Fenner, 1980). Liability refers to one's responsibility for one's own actions and the actions of those whom one supervises. Legal determinations of competency and liability have been made through court rulings and have become part of common law.

Licensure exams for physicians and nurses contain questions about general drug information as well as questions concerning drug administration, assessment, education, and follow-up. This ensures that professional providers have a beginning level of knowledge for entry into professional practice. It is the professional persons' responsibility to use this knowledge and to practice safely.

Laws pertaining to drug standards help safeguard the public from substandard or defective medications. According to the American Products Liability Doctrine, manufacturers are required to warn consumers of potential dangers that may be incurred by taking medications. Information about the drug must also be provided to the prescriber who is responsible for acting as the "learned intermediary" between the consumer and the drug manufacturer. Persons prescribing medications must exercise judgment in determining what information regarding risks of the drug is to be shared with the client. There are special laws that regulate the administration and monitoring of narcotic drugs. For over-the-counter drugs, proper labeling must include adequate directions for use, written in terms understandable to the consumer (Inman, 1986).

ETHICAL ISSUES

Ethics refers to a systematic process of determining right and wrong courses of action. Professional ethics are codes of behavior, open to public scrutiny, reflecting values and standards of conduct or principles of behavior agreed upon by members of the profession that are viewed as necessary to protect the well-being of clients. Personal ethics is also an element of professional practice as most people enter the health care professions with the intent to help others. How "helping others" is accomplished, however, can vary from individual to individual, depending on one's personal code of ethics. For instance, preserving life no matter what the circumstances may be one person's priority, while another may believe that preserving life is not in the best interest of the patient if it significantly prolongs suffering.

Codes of ethics have been developed by professional organizations to provide a standard of conduct. These often exceed the legal standards specified in the practice acts and violation of the code of ethics is not punishable by law. Instead, violations may result in sanctions such as reprimands or suspension. An example is the Code of Ethics for Nurses (Table 7.2).

Although there are various philosophical positions for making ethical decisions presented in the literature, three of the most common are described by Aroskar (1980): utilitarianism, egoism, and formalism (or deontological method).

Table 7.2 Code for Nurses (Reprinted with permission from Code for Nurses with Interpretive Statements, © 1985, American Nurses Association, Washington, DC.)

Preamble

The *Code for Nurses* is based on belief about the nature of individuals, nursing, health, and society. Recipients and providers of nursing services are viewed as individuals and groups who possess basic rights and responsibilities and whose values and circumstances command respect at all times. Nursing encompasses the promotion and restoration of health, the prevention of illness, and the alleviation of suffering. The statements of the *Code* and their interpretation provide guidance for conduct and relationships in carrying out nursing responsibilities consistent with the ethical obligations of the profession and quality in nursing care.

1. The nurse provides services with respect for human dignity and the uniqueness of the client unrestricted by considerations of social or economic status, personal attributes, or the nature of health problems.
2. The nurse safeguards the client's right to privacy by judiciously protecting information of a confidential nature.
3. The nurse acts to safeguard the client and the public when health care and safety are affected by the incompetent, unethical, or illegal practice of any person.
4. The nurse assumes responsibility and accountability for individual nursing judgments and actions.
5. The nurse maintains competence in nursing.
6. The nurse exercises informed judgment and uses individual competence and qualifications as criteria in seeking consultation, accepting responsibilities, and delegating nursing activities to others.
7. The nurse participates in activities that contribute to the ongoing development of the profession's body of knowledge.
8. The nurse participates in the profession's efforts to implement and improve standards of nursing.
9. The nurse participates in the profession's efforts to establish and maintain conditions of employment conducive to high quality nursing care.
10. The nurse participates in the profession's effort to protect the public from misinformation and misrepresentation and to maintain the integrity of nursing.
11. The nurse collaborates with members of the health professions and other citizens in promoting community and national efforts to meet the health needs of the public.

Utilitarianism emphasizes calculating the consequences that will result in the greatest good for the greatest number of people. The focus is on the community rather than the individual, and may be in conflict with the traditional medical ethic of doing everything possible for the benefit of a single individual. This has important implications for making decisions regarding rationing of scarce health care resources.

Egoism views the best solution to an ethical dilemma as one which is best for the health care professional. There is no reason to act to benefit others unless it also brings personal benefit. The health care provider must feel comfortable with the decision regardless of how the client feels about it.

Formalism is also called the **deontological approach** and is founded on the discovery and confirmation of rules and principles that govern the ethical dilemma to be solved. These principles are applied to all cases regardless of the circumstances and without regard to the consequences of the decision or the personal position of the health care provider.

A fourth position, **relativism,** can also be called situational ethics. Within relativism, right and wrong are viewed as relative to the situation. The most extreme relativist belief holds that individual variation is acceptable regarding ethical correctness. Others believe that individual beliefs should conform to the general beliefs of society (Eliopolous, 1993). The latter belief is more similar to the formalist view.

Basic moral principles that are generally accepted guides to ethical decision-making in health care professions include the following:

- Beneficence—doing the highest good for the client
- Nonmaleficence—doing no harm to the client
- Justice—acting in fairness and equitably giving clients the services they need
- Fidelity—respecting one's words and responsibility to clients as a health care professional
- Autonomy—respecting client's worth, rights and freedoms

Delivering health care to clients often presents providers with complex problems in which one or more of these ethical principles is compromised. Conflicts can arise between the nurse's own values, standards of care defined by the hospital or legal system, and the rights of the client. In difficult dilemmas such as these, ethical theories and principles are called into use. For example, ethical issues arise related to the decision to administer pain medication to a terminally ill elderly person or the use of chemical restraints for an agitated older adult. The following specific case may serve to illustrate the use of ethical principles in a nursing practice situation.

> Mrs. M. is a 79-year-old patient on the medical unit where Nurse R. is working as staff nurse on the evening shift. Mrs. M. is terminally ill, in the last stages of metastatic cancer, and is complaining of a great deal of pain. She also has ascites and labored respirations, but is mentally alert and able to communicate from time to time with her daughter, who remains at her bedside. She has an order for morphine for pain as needed which Nurse R. must make the decision to administer. Mrs. M. has also given instructions for comfort measures only—for no life-prolonging treatments to be carried out.

Two nursing goals are important here: to protect the life of the patient and to alleviate the patient's suffering and pain. Other considerations are the patient's own wishes and her continued but limited ability to communicate with her daughter. Ms. R. believes that giving the pain medication may relieve Mrs. M's pain but may also hasten death by suppressing respirations—the essence of an ethical dilemma. In this example, legal issues do not seem to be complicating the situation because of the advanced directive. Nurse R. must decide whether it is better to relieve the patient's pain and risk contributing to her death or to prolong her life without relieving her suffering. Ordinarily, when the patient is terminally ill, relieving pain and suffering takes highest priority and prolonging life becomes second in importance. Administration of the pain medication in this instance is ethically justifiable.

A useful framework for analyzing ethical problems has been described by Thompson and Thompson (1981) and modified by Matteson and McConnell (1988). These guidelines are as follows:

1. Review the situation.
   a. What health problems exist?
   b. What decisions need to be made?
   c. Which are ethical components and which are based on scientific knowledge?
   d. Who are the individuals or groups affected by the decision?
2. Gather additional information necessary to make the decision.
3. What are relevant ethical principles?
   a. What are the historical, philosophical, and religious bases for each of the principles?
4. What are your own values and beliefs?
   a. from your family and other personal experience?
   b. from the Code for Nurses?
5. What are the values and beliefs of others involved in the situation?
6. What are the value conflicts in the situation?
7. Who is best able to make the decisions?
8. What is the fullest range of possible decisions and actions?
   a. What are implications/consequences of the possible decisions and actions?
   b. What is the congruence between possible decisions and actions, and the Code for Nurses?
9. Decide on a course of action and take steps to implement.
10. Evaluate the outcomes of the decision and use this information for future decision making.

Ethical decisions should not be made in isolation. Many institutions have ethics review boards whose task is to assist health care professionals in resolving ethical dilemmas in the best way possible. It is helpful to have other professionals to discuss and assist with the steps of the decision making process, although issues of confidentiality must always be considered.

CONCLUSION

Ethical and legal problems related to medication usage by older persons were presented in this chapter along with related issues for health care professionals. The legal and ethical standards governing professional practice ensure the protection of individual client's rights, autonomy, and informed participation in all aspects of their care. Although most ethical dilemmas pertaining to older clients are not related to prescribing or administrating medications, thoughtful decision making for successful resolution is required when these issues do arise. Issues relating to fundamental human rights and responsibilities frequently impact on the health status of clients, their treatment with medications, and even, at times, on their very survival.

REFERENCES AND RECOMMENDED READINGS

American Nurses' Association. *Code for nurses with interpretive statements.* Kansas City, MO, American Nurses' Association, 1976.

Callahan D: *Setting limits and medical goals in an aging society.* New York, Simon & Schuster, 1987.

Eliopolous C: (1993). *Gerontological nursing,* 3rd ed. Philadelphia, J. B. Lippincott, 1987.

Fenner KM: *Ethics and law in nursing: Professional perspectives.* New York, Van Nostrand Reinhold, 1980.

Inman WHW Ed: *Monitoring for drug safety,* 2nd ed. Hingham, MA, MTP Press, 1986.

Jonsen AB, Stegler M, & Winslade WJ: *Clinical ethics.* New York, Macmillan, 1982.

Matteson MA, & McConnell ES: (1984). *Gerontological nursing: Concepts and practice.* Philadelphia, W. B. Saunders, 1984.

Omnibus Budget Reconciliation Act of 1990. *The Patient Self-determination Act,* 123:776.

Thompson JB., & Thompson HO: *Ethics in nursing.* New York, Macmillan, 1981.

White House Conference on Aging, 1971.

CHAPTER 8

Drug Therapy and Organic Brain Syndrome

Organic brain syndromes are disorders of cognitive or psychological functioning caused by neuronal loss or damage. Over time, the brain gradually suffers from the accumulated effects of aging, stress, chronic diseases, and nutritional or metabolic deficiencies resulting in impaired function for neurons, some more than others. The term **organic brain syndrome (OBS)** describes a category of problems that have many different possible etiologies, but which have in common an organic basis and a constellation of clinical manifestations. The six characteristic manifestations of OBS are

1. impairments of memory, recent or remote;
2. impaired arousal or attention, with possible disorientation or diminished motivation;
3. impaired cognition or intellectual function;
4. distortions of sensory perception or ideation;
5. psychological disturbances, ranging from anxiety or personality disturbances to depression or psychosis;
6. neurologic symptoms including such possibilities as fainting, dizziness, anorexia, or headaches.

Several, but not all, of the causes of organic brain syndrome are age-related; that is, they occur more frequently in older people than younger ones. Moreover, any damage to neurons that occurs from a specific etiology will be superimposed, in the older person, on a degree of deterioration in brain and neural functioning that occurs as a natural consequence of aging (see Chapter 1). The incidence of organic brain syndromes, taken collectively, increases dramatically with aging. Approximately 5% of those over age 65 suffer from severe dementia and about 10–18% from any degree. After age 80, the incidence of severe dementia rises to 20–25%.

The terminology used by neuroscientists and healthcare practitioners relating to organic brain syndromes, terms like *Alzheimer's disease, senility, dementia,* etc., sometimes imply a greater level of understanding and a greater specificity of etiology than actually exists. In spite of a tremendous surge of research activity in neuropathology, little is known about the cause of most cases of organic brain syndrome and still less about effective treatment. Nevertheless, those who work with elderly individuals to provide support or clinical services can expect important advances in this field in the years ahead. On the other hand, one needs to add the *caveat* that the reporting in the public media of research in this area is notoriously inaccurate. The need to attract interest in their stories often leads the media to describe, with hyperbole, the many relatively small advances in our knowledge of organic brain syndrome as major breakthroughs. Odds are that progress in this area will come, ultimately, as the result of many contributions, individually insignificant, as the puzzle is gradually pieced together.

If, like other major organ systems, the brain deteriorates as a natural part of aging, it may be unrealistic to expect that medical advances can eliminate organic brain syndromes entirely. Two more likely contributions that research might make would be to advance the average age at which organic brain syndrome becomes evident by, say, a decade and to determine and address the factors that cause the condition to manifest early in some individuals. With the continuing advance of average life expectancy, such research may go a long way in determining whether we simply live longer or whether we live better during the late years of life.

Organic brain syndromes need to be viewed as a multidimensional problem by those who provide services to such clients and their families. Besides the illness itself, those afflicted must often cope with job pressures or loss, financial problems, changes in family roles, isolation, loss of self-esteem, and depression. In those cases that are progressive, families will be strained to the limit by the need to continuously adjust coping strategies to ever-increasing levels of deficit. Feelings of guilt, depression, anxiety, and frustration may consume family resources without effective help from counseling and support services. Family members are unsettled by the changes they observe in their loved one and may be overcome by guilt or anger in being unable to do more to help. A particularly critical point in the progression comes when the family must confront the issue of placement when the deterioration has progressed beyond what they can effectively manage in the household. Feelings of guilt, anger, depression, and most of all, uncertainty, will inevitably surround this decision.

DIAGNOSIS OF ORGANIC BRAIN SYNDROME

Diagnosis of organic brain syndrome and, in particular, its differentiation from functional psychiatric disorders (see Chapter 9), is of utmost importance for a number of reasons. It is also of utmost difficulty in some cases. The psychiatric symptoms of OBS can mimic many of the functional disorders, including major depression, schizophrenia, paraphrenia, generalized anxiety disorder, or personality disorders. Sometimes, clients thought throughout the end stage of their lives to have a functional disorder are found to have suffered from OBS only after autopsy of their brains reveals the characteristic changes of OBS. Thus, even when the best effort at differential diagnosis is made, some individual cases will be misdiagnosed.

Nevertheless, the effort is an important one because the diagnosis directs the treatment effort, including the drug selections that might be made and the therapeutic outcomes that can be expected. The psychiatric symptoms of OBS are managed with the same kinds of drugs used for functional disorders of similar expression (for example, anxiolytics for anxiety of OBS, antidepressants for the depression), but, on average, psychiatric symptoms secondary to OBS respond less well to medication than do the true functional disorders, and remissions after a short course of drug therapy are virtually out of the question. Therapeutic objectives must be adjusted accordingly.

Although the more common diagnostic error is the assumption of a functional disorder when the problem is in fact OBS, the opposite error can be equally disadvantageous to the client. Some individuals present with dementia that is, in reality, secondary to severe depression. This circumstance is termed **pseudodementia** or **pseudodementing depression.** When dementia is not recognized as secondary to functional depression, the client is likely to receive less aggressive intervention than would be usual for major depression. The evidence suggests, however, that the dementia of pseudodementia responds when the depression responds and that depression with secondary dementia is as responsive to antidepressants as is depression without dementia.

In weighing whether psychiatric problems are functional or secondary to OBS, differential diagnosis is based on psychiatric appraisal, a review of the premorbid history, and neurological testing. Theoretically, OBS is indicated when (1) the degree of cognitive or memory impairment is great relative to the degree of psychiatric disturbance; or (2) when neurologic tests reveal presence of abnormality. Individuals with dementia typically exhibit diffuse, symmetrical, and progressive slowing of the EEG, reduced cerebrovascular bloodflow, and diminished glucose utilization by cortical cells.

When organic brain syndrome is evident, four further matters of characterization can be considered.

1. Is the deficit global or selective?
2. Is the condition acute or chronic?
3. Does the age of onset indicate a presenile or senile condition?
4. What is the etiology?

Delirium

Most often, OBS presents as one of the two global forms: delirium or dementia (see Table 8.1). **Delirium,** a disturbance of consciousness that impairs attention, orientation, perception, memory, motor activity, and sleep patterns, is always acute in onset and suggests some specific physiologic disturbance.

Typical causes include infections of the central nervous system, metabolic imbalances such as acidosis, irregular blood glucose levels, electrolyte disturbances (hypercalcemia, hypernatremia, hyponatremia), unusual

Table 8.1 Organic Brain Syndromes and Their Etiologies

Type	Typical etiologies
Global impairments	
A. Delirium	CNS infections; imbalances of blood gases, blood glucose levels, electrolytes or pH; hepatic or renal disease; postoperative or postictal states; drug intoxication or withdrawal syndromes; head trauma or masses; poisonings
B. Dementias	
1. Primary degenerative	
a. Presenile	Alzheimer's disease, Pick's disease
b. Senile	Senile dementia of the Alzheimer's type
2. Multi-infarct	Cerebral arteriosclerosis
3. Pseudodementia	Severe depression
4. Nutritional deficits	Vitamin B_{12}, B_6, or B_3 deficiency
5. Other	Anemias, normal pressure hydrocephalus, CNS infections (e.g., Creutzfeldt-Jakob disease), head trauma (e.g., blows from boxing), degenerative diseases (e.g., supranuclear palsy), hypothyroidism, chronic poisonings, anoxia, or hypoglycemia, brain masses, dyalysis, chronic renal or hepatic disease
Selective impairments	
A. Amnestic syndrome	Wernicke's-Korsakoff syndrome or incomplete recovery from head trauma, hypoxia, cranial infarcts, or encephalitis
B. Organic hallucinosis	Alcohol, hallucinogens, sensory deprivation, seizure auras
C. Organic delusional syndrome	Amphetamines, cannabis, psychedelics, Huntington's disease, temporal lobe epilepsy
D. Organic affective syndrome	Depressant drugs, thyroid or adrenal gland disorders, CNS infections
E. Organic personality syndrome	Head trauma or neoplasms, temporal lobe epilepsy, cerebrovascular disorders, Huntington's disease, multiple sclerosis

blood oxygen levels, elevated intracranial pressure, hepatic or renal failure, postseizure or postoperative states, substance intoxication, or drug withdrawal syndromes.

Common drug contributions to delirium include alcohol, barbiturates, benzodiazepines, narcotics, levodopa, anticholinergic drugs, phenothiazines, stimulants, digoxin, diuretics (due to hypokalemia or dehydration), antidiabetics (due to hypoglycemia), and antihypertensives (due to excess hypotension).

The level of severity of delirium may fluctuate with severe disorientation alternating with unpredictable periods of lucidness. The individual may be agitated, even uncontrollably so, or quiet. Since delirium indicates a physiological disturbance of abrupt onset, treatment focuses on identification and treatment of the underlying problem.

Dementia

Dementia is a loss of intellectual abilities to an extent that there are interferences with normal social and occupational activities. Memory is also impaired in at least some component, but consciousness is not clouded, which distinguishes dementia from delirium. Dementias are usually chronic, that is, irreversible, and often progressive, but 15–20% of cases are acute and reversible with appropriate intervention. Alzheimer's disease and multi-infarct dementia (MID), or combinations of the two, account for approximately 75–80% of the chronic dementias, while a large number of relatively infrequent conditions account for the remainder of instances (see Table 8.1). Reversible dementias can derive from endocrine problems, nutritional deficiencies, brain masses (e.g., tumors, hematomas), or drug or chemical poisonings. However, the most frequent cause of reversible dementia is **pseudodementia**—dementia secondary to severe depression.

Selective Varieties of OBS

Selective varieties of OBS are less common than the global types. They include amnestic syndrome, organic hallucinosis, organic delusional disorder, organic affective disorder, and organic personality syndrome (see Table 8.1). Most of these conditions are toxic disorders triggered by high doses of alcohol, cocaine, psychedelics, or other drugs of abuse. Thiamine deficiency associated with alcoholism can produce an amnestic syndrome. The neurologic damage that occurs in this event is called **Wernicke's encephalopathy** and the behavioral syndrome is known as **Korsakoff's syndrome.**

Presenile and Senile Dementias

Somewhat arbitrarily, dementias that arise prior to age 65 are termed **presenile dementias,** while those developing after age 65 are called **senile dementias.** If there is value in this distinction, it is in reminding us that there may well be two components in the overall occurrence of organic brain syndrome: a "disease" component causing some people to develop dementia at an unusually early age and a "natural" component that reflects the wear and tear that a long life inevitably exerts on neural function. Research has already indicated that the genetic component in the occurrence of dementias is much stronger for the early onset cases than for those developing late in life. Some specific types of dementia have a characteristic presenile onset, including notably Huntington's disease and Pick's disease— both conditions carried by a single dominant gene. The two most prevalent examples of primary degenerative dementia, Alzheimer's disease and multi-infarct dementia, deserve some additional consideration and are further discussed in the following two sections.

Onset of dementia is usually insidious. Earliest signs often consist of inability to recall events or details, perception errors, and depression. Activities become more self-centered and less varied. New activities become difficult to acquire, much less master. As dementia progresses, intellectual impairments become more profound and the activities of which the person remains capable become fewer and fewer. Personality changes become more pronounced.

Alzheimer's Dementia

It is likely that the societal significance of dementias will escalate in the immediate future in the United States as the demographic shift toward increasing numbers of elderly people continues. Medical advances in control of cancer and heart disease, if they occur, will increase the percentage of the population that survives into the years when dementia takes its greatest toll.

Alzheimer's dementia is the most commonly diagnosed type of dementia, although the diagnostic category may currently subsume more than one etiology. A diagnosis of Alzheimer's disease is usually arrived at by exclusion—ruling out all of the known specific etiologies for dementia. (A small percentage of early onset cases can be diagnosed by a genetic marker technique.) Thus, this diagnostic category is a kind of diagnosis of last resort that indicates, in effect, etiology unknown. One of the major controversies, at present, is the extent to which Alzheimer's disease represents the inevitable consequences of aging and to what extent a disease. Most likely, it involves both of these elements. The situation might well be like that for automobiles. We expect that every car will break down sooner or later, but some models have the troublesome habit of breaking down prematurely. We are perhaps closer to being able to explain and prevent the defects that result in earlier than average breakdown than in building a vehicle that can be maintained indefinitely. The observation that the genetic contribution is greater for early onset cases than for late onset cases is consistent with an interpretation that postulates both a disease component and a contribution from the aging process. Nevertheless, even the part of the problem that comes from aging may be delayed, though probably not "curable," if we succeed in identifying which factors of lifestyle and which health practices are most influential.

Two of the characteristic changes that occur in the brain of individual's with Alzheimer's disease are **Alzheimer's tangles** and **senile plaques.** The tangles are thought to be residues formed from the disorganization of the neurotubular transport system of degenerating axons. The plaques are amyloid-rich deposits formed from degenerated nerve terminals. The cholinergic neurons of the brain, especially those with cell bodies in the basal nucleus of the forebrain with axons extending into the cerebrum, are likely to be the first to undergo deterioration as Alzheimer's disease develops.

Another neuron group often affected early on is the catecholamine pathways. Parts of the temporal lobe (the subiculum and entorhinal cortex) that lie immediately adjacent to the hippocampus exhibit cell level pathology, as well, in patients with Alzheimer's disease. These areas contain the pathways that enter and exit from the hippocampus. This is an important finding because the hippocampus plays a major role in memory, and memory loss is a nearly universal symptom of Alzheimer's disease. Many of the afferent neurons to the hippocampus are cholinergic ones.

There are several theories currently being tested regarding causes of Alzheimer's disease. One study suggested a possible infectious origin possibly involving a slow-virus, or prion, similar to pathogens responsible for scrapie, kuru, and Creutzfeldt-Jakob disease. There are other examples, in medicine, of viruses that associate with and replicate in nerve cells. Diseases like kuru and Creutzfeldt-Jakob disease that have already been linked to prions are also associated with amyloid plaques. One study has suggested that prions may in fact be a constituent of the plaques of Alzheimer's disease. This area of research continues to be hotly pursued.

Some suggest that autoimmunity may play a role because the amyloid that prevails in the senile plaques could derive from immunoglobulins. Antibodies that have been produced against neurofilament preparations have been reported to be reactive against Alzheimer's tangles. Other researchers are working to identify the exact structure of the proteins that make up the tangles, which appear to consist of paired helical filaments.

Aluminum toxicity has sometimes been advanced as a cause of Alzheimer's disease. No doubt, when aluminum intake for a person is such as to allow significant accumulation, an Alzheimer's-like dementia does occur. Some studies have reported as much as three-fold higher levels of aluminum in the brain of Alzheimer's patients, but other studies have not. Aluminum content in the water supply may be higher in some locales than others, but data are lacking on whether geographic location or employment in industries that expose workers to aluminum are correlated with incidence of dementia. Little is known about the quantitative relationship between aluminum levels and toxicity. An aluminum chelator (a drug that forms a complex with aluminum to facilitate its excretion from the body), deferoxamine, is being tested currently.

Although a genetic contribution has been established for early onset cases, genetics play much less of a role in senile dementias. If late onset cases entail, as we suggested, specific disease contributions superimposed on the aging process, the genetic contribution and its mode of inheritance will be more difficult to determine. Some cases of Alzheimer's disease occur in association with Down's syndrome. Correlation of Alzheimer's disease has also been suggested with certain autoimmune disorders, lymphoma, and leukemia, but further documentation of these relationships will be required. Hypothyroidism, which is more common in women than men, has been suggested as a factor in the greater incidence of dementia in elderly women than elderly men.

Lastly, head trauma may contribute. The relationship between trauma to the head and dementia is most obvious in the type called **dementia pugilistica** that is described in boxers who have "taken too many punches." The principle may apply in a less obvious way to dementias in general. One study reported that instances of prior head injury were greater among those suffering senile dementia than for matched controls.

Multi-Infarct Dementia

Cerebral arteriosclerosis is evident in perhaps as many as one-third of individuals with organic brain syndrome. Cerebral arteriosclerosis is a disorder of the blood vessels brought about by accumulations of lipids that thicken the blood vessel wall and narrow the diameter of the vessel, thereby restricting blood flow. Pressure in the cerebral blood vessel bed rises, but exchange of nutrients, oxygen, and waste materials between the blood and brain is hindered. Cerebral arteriosclerosis can be generalized causing diffuse changes in brain function with reductions in awareness and mental activity.

Othertimes, the loss of perfusion is localized resulting in specific deficits of sensory or motor function. Arteriosclerosis also establishes the conditions for small infarctions. **Multi-infarct dementia (MID)** is the name given to the deficits of intellect that may follow from multiple infarcts often developing over a period of years. Autopsy ultimately reveals the presence of many local infarctions. In multi-infarct dementia, the deterioration tends to occur in many small steps, rather than as a continuous, linear process. Steps typically occur at about 5-year intervals. Some intellectual functions may be relatively spared. Neurological deficits will often be asymmetrical. Personality and insight may be little altered.

Arteriosclerosis most often develops in men and usually after age 65. Hypertension is likely to be present. Ischemic heart disease is likely to occur in conjunction with MID because cerebral arteriosclerosis is the major predisposing factor for both conditions. Myocardial infarction is likely to be the ultimate cause of death. Vascular causes of dementia can often be differentiated from primary degenerative dementias (such as Alzheimer's disease) by studies of cerebral blood flow and blood levels of glucose and oxygen entering and leaving the brain. When blood flow is impaired, the brain extracts a higher fraction of the oxygen and glucose available to compensate for the reduction in blood flow. Thus, the difference in arterial and venous levels of these crucial substances will be greater when dementia has a primarily vascular basis.

Although dementias with a primarily vascular origin are irreversible, they are also the current best example of a dementia that is at least somewhat preventable, since many of the risk factors for cerebral arteriosclerosis are matters of lifestyle. Thus, diets high in cholesterol and saturated fats, lack of exercise, obesity, smoking tobacco, drinking alcohol, stress, and inappropriate use of androgens all contribute adversely to the risk of dementia of vascular origin. Diets rich in polyunsaturated fats, exercise, and estrogens reduce liability. Factors over which there is little or no control that also contribute adversely are aging and presence of diabetes or hypotension.

DRUG THERAPIES FOR ORGANIC BRAIN SYNDROME

Nondrug components of the therapeutic plan for chronic OBS are often the more important part of intervention. Specific objectives might include provision of support services; helping the client and family members cope with changing family roles, feelings of guilt, depression, or anxiety; improving the reality orientation of the client; or modification of detrimental behaviors.

Drug therapy for chronic organic brain syndromes centers on two objectives: (1) to relieve the psychiatric symptoms that are secondary to the disturbance; and (2) to improve cognitive functioning to the extent possible. The first objective is accomplished reasonably well with the use of neuroleptics (most often, thioridazine) for thought disorders or agitation, anxiolytics for anxiety, and tricyclic or second-generation antidepressants for depression. Benzodiazepines can be useful for anxiety, but cause more frequent paradoxical reactions in the elderly than in younger adults.

Sleep disturbances are common among the elderly with organic brain syndrome. Some even develop a reversal of sleep pattern, napping frequently throughout the day and becoming restless at night. This pattern has been dubbed "sundown syndrome." Taking measures to keep the client awake during the day can sometimes help in correcting this problem. Otherwise, administration of a short-acting hypnotic at bedtime might be considered. Sleep disorders secondary to OBS present a special therapeutic problem because conventional sedative-hypnotics have limited periods of effectiveness and also tend to worsen whatever degree of cognitive impairment is already evident. Sedative antidepressants, such as imipramine, might be used for double duty: to alleviate depression and, by giving the major part of the daily dose at bedtime, to facilitate sleep. However, tricyclic antidepressants with anticholinergic properties may aggravate mental confusion, particularly if other drugs with anticholinergic activity are included in the regimen.

Neuroleptics, though useful for controlling agitation, can further diminish alertness and aggravate motor deficits if extrapyramidal side effects develop. Moreover, pointed criticism has been levied against healthcare facilities that cater to the elderly for excessive use of neuroleptics for the apparent main purpose of rendering the client manageable. Some critics have estimated that as much as 80% of neuroleptic use in the institutionalized elderly is for this purpose. Whenever possible, tractability should be achieved by provision of a warm, supportive, conducive environment rather than by tranquilization. Thioridazine is sometimes projected as the drug of choice for use in elderly demented clients. It is unlikely to cause extrapyramidal side effects and contributes less to depression and sedation than does chlorpromazine.

The second objective of drug therapy, improving cognitive impairment, is one that is only marginally achievable at present. A large variety of approaches have been examined thus far and many experimental drugs are currently undergoing testing. The various approaches can be grouped into the following general categories:

1. Nootropics, or stimulators of cerebral metabolism
2. Drugs that elevate neurotransmitter levels
3. Cerebral vasodilators
4. Carbonic anhydrase inhibitors
5. Stimulants
6. Anticoagulants
7. Hyperbaric oxygen

8. Yeast ribonucleic acid
9. Drugs to reduce lipofuscin pigments in the brain
10. Vitamins
11. Procaine

Only the first three approaches have any identifiable claim of even marginal efficacy based on current evidence.

Nootropics

Nootropics is the term recently coined for drugs that act by stimulating metabolism of neurons. Investigation of nootropics is one of the most active areas of research for treatment of OBS. More than a half-dozen such drugs are currently in various stages of testing: piracetam, pramiracetam, oxiracetam, vincamine, bromvincamine, pebonin, naftidrofuryl, and suloctidil. At present there is just one nootropic approved for use in the United States—dihydrogenated ergot alkaloids (DHEA), sometimes also called dihydroergotoxine or ergoloid mesylates. Brandnames include Hydergine, Circanol, Deapril-ST, Gerimal, and Niloric. DHEA is a combination of three closely related ergot compounds (dihydroergocornine, dihydroergocristine, and dihydroergocryptine).

The precise mechanism by which DHEA works has not yet been elucidated. DHEA has weak dopaminergic activity, inhibits phosphodiesterase (the enzyme that breaks down an important cell regulator, cyclic-adenosine monophosphate), stimulates cerebral metabolism, and modestly increases cerebral blood flow. Which of these actions, if any, contributes significantly to its benefit has yet to be determined. Neurons in the brain that are deprived of adequate blood flow and oxygenation are forced to switch over part of their cellular effort from normal aerobic metabolism to a less natural anaerobic metabolism, as indicated by the kind of metabolites that pass out of the brain. DHEA promotes a return to the healthier aerobic metabolism, but it is unclear how much of this effect comes from improving "cellular efficiency" and how much comes from improvements in blood flow.

Clinical Indications in the Elderly.   Regardless of the weaknesses in the theoretical explanation, what we know from empirical clinical studies is that clients with dementia show modest improvements in cognitive function, regardless of whether assessment of improvements is based on the client's own perception or objective, external assessment by clinical personnel. Cognitive measures improve, but measures of physical health or daily functioning do not. Symptoms of anorexia and headaches may improve. Benefits are typically evident after 3 to 6 weeks of DHEA treatment and typically outlast benefits observed with cerebral vasodilators. Clients with measurable deficits in cerebral blood flow rates are more likely to benefit than others. Those with mild to moderate dementia are more likely to respond than those who have already progressed to severe dementia.

Pharmacokinetics or Pharmacodynamics in the Elderly.   After oral administration, less than 50% of a DHEA dose is absorbed in the systemic circulation. The half-life for DHEA is approximately 3.5 hours.

Adverse Effects and Contraindications in the Elderly.   No serious adverse effects have been identified for DHEA, which is one reason that its use is acceptable in spite of marginal benefits. Nausea or heartburn have been reported occasionally. Mild hypotension and/or bradycardia have occurred. Baseline measurement of blood pressure and pulse rate should be conducted before administration of DHEA and periodically thereafter. DHEA is contraindicated for use in functional psychoses.

Interactions in the Elderly.   None reported.

Administration in the Elderly.   Clients need to hold the tablets under the tongue until completely dissolved and not eat, drink, or smoke until the dissolution is complete. Sublingual irritation occurs occasionally. A liquid for oral administration is also available.

DIHYDROGENATED ERGOT ALKALOIDS   (Hydergine, Gerimal, Niloric, generic)

Recommended initial oral dose: 1 mg 3 times daily.

Young Adult initial dosage for comparison: not applicable.

Maximum doses: 4.5–12 mg/day.

All of the following drugs are experimental:

Bromvincamine
Naftidrofuryl
Oxiracetam
Pebonin
Piracetam
Pramiracetam
Vincamine

Drugs That Elevate Neurotransmitter Levels

It has been thought that drugs that increase levels of one or another of the major neurotransmitters might possibly alleviate some of the cognitive impairment that occurs in dementia. Attention has been especially focused on those transmitters associated with systems that show signs of degeneration in the earliest stages of Alzheimer's disease—the cholinergic and catecholamine systems. Experimental interventions have utilized either precursors, which potentially augment synthesis of the transmitter, or inhibitors of the degratory enzymes, which might help to preserve the existing transmitter molecules.

Choline, the precursor of acetylcholine, has been given to elderly clients with dementia. So too has lecithin, a dietary substance that breaks down into choline in the gastrointestinal tract. Quantities sufficient to double plasma choline concentrations have been without effect, an observation consistent with studies in laboratory animals that indicate that rates of synthesis of acetylcholine in the brain are not particularly responsive to precursor loading. Inhibitors of the enzyme cholinesterase hold out greater promise of ultimate usefulness. For many years, progress in testing the viability of inhibiting cholinesterase in the brain were hindered by the fact that most of the several anticholinesterase inhibitors already available for medical use do not penetrate the brain very well. That property is a distinct advantage when the medical intent is treatment of disorder at a peripheral site of action, such as myasthenia gravis or glaucoma, when the desire is to minimize central nervous system side effects. The same property limits usefulness of such agents for treatment of dementia. Of the traditional cholinesterase inhibitors, only physostigmine possesses significant central activity; its problem is a rather short half-life and duration of action necessitating administration many times per day for sustained inhibition of brain acetylcholinesterase. Clinical trials using a sustained release formulation of physostigmine are currently underway.

A centrally active cholinesterase inhibitor, tacrine (THA, tetrahydroaminoacridine, Cognex) began clinical testing in 1990 and received approval by the Food and Drug Administration in 1993. This drug is well-absorbed after oral administration and has a half-life of approximately 3 hours. Tacrine clearance is not influenced by age to a clinically significant extent. Side effects of tacrine are expected peripheral cholinergic actions: increased sweating, diarrhea, increased urinary frequency, nausea, and abdominal discomfort. More serious problems of hepatotoxicity, neurological toxicity, or hematological disturbances are also a potential with this drug. Velnacrine (Mentane), a derivative of tacrine, began testing in 1992. During the initial protocol trial, side effects with velnacrine resembled those of tacrine—peripheral cholinergic effects and hepatotoxicity. Seventy-eight percent of treated clients developed elevated liver enzymes in the plasma (a standard medical indicator of liver toxicity) severe enough to necessitate discontinuation. As a result, the FDA has not recommended approval of this drug even for further clinical trials.

Drugs that influence dopamine levels in the brain are also being tested. Dementia sometimes occurs in the late stages of Parkinson's disease, a condition long linked to dopamine depletion, and the cognitive deficits may either improve or get worse when treatment with levodopa, a precursor of dopamine, is undertaken. Like the motor deficits of Parkinson's disease, the cognitive deficits apparently improve in response to levodopa only if there are at least some remaining intact dopamine neurons to provide conversion of levodopa into dopamine. Treatment of clients with Alzheimer's disease with either levodopa or another precursor of catecholamines, tyrosine, failed to provide any improvement. Selegiline (Endepryl), a newly introduced selective inhibitor of type-B monoamine oxidase, an enzyme that breaks down catecholamine transmitters, has provided some promising preliminary results in clients with dementia.

Tryptophan, 5-hydroxytryptophan, and 1,5-hydroxytryptamine, all precursors of serotonin, have also been tested preliminarily, but have failed to increase serotonin levels or turnover in serotonergic neurons of the brain—neurons of the raphe system. There has been no evidence of beneficial results in dementia.

TACRINE   (tetrahydroaminoacridine, Cognex)

Recommended initial oral dose in the elderly: No adjustments required in relation to age.

Initiation of treatment: 40 mg/day given as 10 mg 4 times daily. Maintain this dosage for a minimum of 6 weeks while monitoring transaminase levels weekly.

Dose titration: After the six-week initiation period and provided that there is no elevation in transaminase levels or unusual adverse reaction, increase the dose to 80 mg/day given as 20 mg 4 times daily. The dosage level may be further increased by increments of 40 mg/day at intervals of no less than 6 weeks, to 120 mg/day and then 160 mg/day, with the daily dose divided evenly among four daily administrations. The rate of dosage escalation may be slower than six-week intervals but should not be faster.

Cerebral Vasodilators

The logic behind the use of cerebral vasodilators is that many older people, particularly those with dementia, have decreased cerebral blood flow and resultant cerebral hypoxia. Deficient oxygen supply then forces neurons to decrease their metabolic rate and shift toward abnormal anaerobic metabolic pathways. The EEG reflects the slowing of cellular activity on a global level. Decreased cerebral blood flow may be, in part, a consequence of developing cerebral arteriosclerosis or it may be, in part, a consequence rather than a cause of reduced cellular metabolism.

One of the major determinants of local patterns of cerebral blood flow is the metabolic demand of cells in that part of the brain. If diminished blood flow is a consequence of the problems of dementia rather than a cause, vasodilators cannot be expected to provide benefit. Even in the circumstance where arteriosclerosis was the cause of poor perfusion of otherwise healthy brain cells, vasodilators might fail to work, theoretically, because sclerotic blood vessels are less flexible in responding to dilating influences than healthy vessels. One can imagine that blood flow might actually be shunted away from areas of poor perfusion by the action of a cerebral vasodilator if the healthiest vessels dilate more than the most sclerotic ones. Moreover, drugs given the designation of cerebral vasodilators are actually not as specific as the term implies. All such drugs also dilate blood vessels elsewhere in the body, even if to a lesser extent, an action that might further shunt blood away from the cerebral vasculature.

Lastly, sclerotic vessels are not only thinner in diameter, but also provide poorer transfer of materials between the blood and tissue cells. This might even be the major deficiency in sclerotic vessels. Even if the cerebral vasodilator increases flow through a sclerotic vessel, there is no guarantee that higher flow will translate into greater provision of oxygen and nutrients to the tissue cells.

Clinical Indications in the Elderly. Theory aside, numerous trials have been conducted with cerebral vasodilators (such as papaverine and cyclandelate) with distinctly mixed reviews. The studies divide almost half and half between reporting benefit and not. One large study with 1772 clients having neurological symptoms attributable to cerebrovascular insufficiency specifically reported good to excellent responses in 81% of clients based on physician ratings or 75% based on client ratings. Those with minor cerebrovascular problems appear to benefit the most. Results from studies involving clients with dementia not specifically linked to cerebrovascular deficits have been much less supportive of value for these drugs. Thus, given the severity of adverse effects for these drugs, a reasonable case could be made for limiting the use of cerebral vasodilators to those clients with neurological problems, such as confusion, depression, dizziness, or social isolation, deriving specifically from cerebrovascular insufficiency.

Altered Pharmacokinetics or Pharmacodynamics in the Elderly. Age-dependent pharmacokinetics have not been established for papaverine. Approximately 54% is absorbed after oral administration and is 90% bound to plasma proteins in the blood. The half-life has not been definitively determined, but an administration interval of 6 hours provides reasonably consistent plasma concentrations.

Adverse Effects and Contraindications in the Elderly. Cerebral vasodilators may cause serious cardiovascular problems. Hypotension is virtually inevitable when these drugs are used and clients need to be warned to avoid rapid changes in position, particularly standing rapidly from a prone position. Heart rate may increase and cardiac dysrhythmias may develop from ectopic beats or block. Gastrointestinal problems, such as nausea, cramps, diarrhea, or constipation, are common. Neurologic side effects can include sedation or drowsiness. Vascular headaches are a possibility, as well. Papaverine has caused episodes of hepatic toxicity and hepatic function tests need to be conducted whenever it is employed.

Interactions in the Elderly. Papaverine has been reported to decrease the benefit of levodopa as an antiparkinsonian agent.

Administration in the Elderly. Papaverine can be administered orally or by injection. Sustained release preparations are available, but they are erratic and not recommended. Papaverine or cyclandelate is best given before, with, or shortly after meals, with milk or an antacid to minimize gastrointestinal side effects.

CINNARIZINE

Experimental.

CYCLANDELATE   (Cyclan, Cyclospasmol, generic)

Recommended initial oral dose in the elderly: No specific recommendation.

Adult initial dosage for comparison   1.2–1.6 g/day in divided doses before meals and at bedtime.

PAPAVERINE   (Pavabid, Cerespan, Genabid, and generic)

Recommended initial oral dose in the elderly: No specific recommendation.

Adult initial oral dosage   100–300 mg 3–5 times daily or 150 mg every 12 hrs for the timed release formulation.

Carbonic Anhydrase Inhibitors

This is a variation on the theme of cerebral vasodilators. Carbonic anhydrase inhibitors lower extracellular pH, which then causes vasodilation. One study using a centrally active carbonic anhydrase inhibitor in geriatric patients with dementia reported an increase in cerebral blood flow, but without mental improvement.

Stimulants

In one respect, these drugs are the most tested of all drugs for the neural consequences of aging, but that testing has been the informal, uncontrolled experience of millions of people who have used stimulants over the centuries for social and pseudomedical purposes. Stimulants have indisputable capacity to increase mental and physical energy, improve memory and learning (at least for simple tasks), enhance attention, and increase motivation. The well-documented drawback is that the benefits are short-lived and come at the cost of rebound deficits in these same parameters. Moreover, stimulants have abuse liability and can cause anxiety, irritability, restlessness, insomnia, poor appetite, and hypertension. Nevertheless, depression in the elderly is an unlabeled use of methylphenidate (Ritalin), a stimulant of intermediate potency.

If there is a rational place for stimulants in treatment of dementia, that place probably belongs to caffeine, the relatively weak, widely used stimulant found in coffee, tea, cola, and other sources. Caffeine consumed in the form of coffee or tea can provide modest improvements in attention and alertness, while simultaneously raising spirits merely by the provision of a warm, tasty treat. Provision of caffeine at selected times of day can also help to stabilize irregular sleep patterns by inhibiting daytime napping that might otherwise interfere with nighttime sleep. Excessive daily intake of caffeine is, however, linked to such health risks as ulcers, heart attacks, and anxiety.

Anticoagulants

A rationale for using anticoagulants would be most evident for those cases of dementia associated with arteriosclerosis and multiple infarcts. In these cases, anticoagulant therapy could help prevent further infarcts, or ministrokes, thus preventing further deterioration. Anticoagulant therapy has already been demonstrated to improve mental functioning for clients who suffer recurrent strokes or transient ischemic attacks in the cerebral vasculature. One test of the anticoagulant warfarin in clients with dementia failed to demonstrate improvement, but did report no further deterioration while a control group exhibited further decline. Since anticoagulants do not break up existing clots or infarcts but inhibit formation of new clots, the observed results are consistent with the experience with anticoagulants in other areas of medicine.

The potential for adverse effects is great with anticoagulants and this will undoubtedly hinder their acceptance as a standard therapy for dementia. Serious episodes of bleeding were reported, for example, in approximately 25% of individuals receiving the anticoagulant in the one study conducted so far in clients with dementia. Moreover, discontinuation of anticoagulant therapy brings with it an elevated likelihood of thromboembolic events. The potential risks may therefore very well outweigh the potential benefits for this approach. At the least, very careful client selection procedures would need to be implemented.

Hyperbaric Oxygen

The theory here is that better oxygenation of the blood might compensate for poor cerebral perfusion and resultant cellular hypoxia. Intermittent oxygenation by this method has produced good results in those individuals having dementia specifically related to cerebral vascular insufficiency. In studies using this procedure in clients with dementia of unspecified origin, results have been distinctly mixed, with positive outcomes reported in about half the studies for a few patients.

Yeast Ribonucleic Acid (RNA)

There are only very preliminary reports of benefit from administration of yeast in clients with memory loss stemming from arteriosclerosis. The study was not sufficiently controlled to rule out nonspecific improvements from increased attention that comes inevitably with any clinical study.

Drugs to Reduce Lipofuscin Pigments in the Brain

Lipofuscins are the pigments that accumulate in the brain over time and they produce the deeper coloration of the brains of elderly persons. Investigators have been intrigued by the possibility that these substances might contribute to impairments of cognitive function with aging. Centrophenoxine (Meclofenoxate), an experimental agent, facilitates removal of lipofuscins from the brain, reducing the residual levels. Studies to date have been too poorly designed to permit conclusions regarding the potential of this approach.

Vitamins

Various vitamins and minerals have been tested preliminarily for potential benefits. Occasional reports pertaining to benefit in individual cases surface from time to time because some cases of dementia are caused by deficiencies in vitamin B_1 (Wernicke's-Korsakoff syndrome), B_3 (pellegra), B_6, or B_{12}. At least one case of dementia has also been attributed to folate deficiency with subsequent positive response to folic acid administration. There is no adequate evidence that vitamins provide benefit in dementias not specifically attributable to vitamin deficiency.

Procaine Hydrochloride

Although there have been anecdotal reports of the rejuvenating potential of procaine hydrochloride, particularly from Romania, controlled studies in the United States have not supported the claims.

REFERENCES AND RECOMMENDED READINGS

Abraham IL, Neundorfer MM: Alzheimer's: A decade of progress, a future of nursing challenges. *Geriatr. Nurs.*, 1990; 11(3):116–119.

Cohan SL: *Neurologic diseases in the elderly*, in Reichel: *Clinical Aspects of Aging*, 3rd ed. Baltimore, Williams & Wilkins, 1989, pp. 163–176.

Cook P, James I: Cerebral vasodilators. *N. Engl. J. Med.*, 1981; 305:1508–1513, 1560–1564.

Coyle JT, et al.: Alzheimer's disease: A disorder of cortical cholinergic innervation. *Science*, 1983; 219:1184–1190.

Fisman M: Clinical pharmacology of senile dementia. *Prog. Neuropsychopharmacol.*, 1981; 5(5–6):447–457.

Katzman R (ed): *Biological Aspects of Alzheimer's Disease, Banbury Report 15.* USA, Cold Spring Harbor Laboratories, 1983.

Pepeu G et al.: Aging of brain cholinergic neurons: pharmacological interventions. *Clin. Neuropharmacol.* 1992; 15 (Suppl. 1, Pt. A):31A-32A.

Pricee DL: New perspectives on Alzheimer's disease. *Annu. Rev. Neurosci.*, 1986; 9:489–512.

Rabins RV, Mace NL, Lucas MJ: The impact of dementia on the family. *JAMA*, 1982; 248:333–335.

Shapiro J: Research trends in Alzheimer's Disease. *Gerontol. Nurs.* 1994; 20(4):4–9.

Yesavage JA: Pharmacology of the aged central nervous system. *Clin. Neuropharmacol.*, 1979; 4:199–220.

CHAPTER 9

Psychiatric Problems in the Elderly and Related Drug Therapies

Although it is generally conceded that estimates of the incidence of psychiatric problems among the elderly are less accurate than for younger populations, it is nevertheless clear that the prevalence of such disorders indeed increases with aging. The main question left unresolved, at present, is how large is the increase? One of the principal reasons for the lack of accurate data regarding psychiatric disorders in the elderly is that, as a society, we are likely to overlook incidents of deviant behavior or psychiatric symptoms in the elderly that we would less likely take for granted in younger adults or children. The natural but sometimes detrimental and often erroneous tendency is for family members to attribute all but the most obvious and severe alterations in mental functioning to aging. This tendency to overlook "odd behavior" in an older person may indeed have a quality of mercy when the behaviors are either minimally impairing or untreatable, but in other circumstances serves only to deprive the older person of timely interventions that might enhance or sustain quality of life.

Even when differential diagnosis is undertaken by competent medical personnel, it is often difficult, and sometimes even impossible, to determine when developing psychiatric symptoms are secondary to neurological changes of organic brain syndrome and when, in other cases, such symptoms constitute a functional psychiatric disorder. While it is true that organic brain syndromes, especially Alzheimer's disease, occur with ever increasing frequency as age increases, it is also true that the incidence of functional psychiatric disorders in the elderly is not insignificant. For example, an estimated 15–20% of those over 65 suffer from depression. Anxiety disorders are likewise commonplace.

To some extent, the distinction between organic and functional disorders of the nervous system may be an artificial one. The intent of the designation *organic* is to characterize the disorder as one with a strictly biological basis. Yet, clearly any significant change in the biological integrity of the neural tissue is bound to result in changes in personality or behavior which will in turn alter interpersonal relationships and the individual's ability to function in a social context. The label *functional* implies, on the other hand, that the disorder originates in the way that the neural network has been organized (or "programmed", to borrow a term from the computer age) in response to experience without actual biological damage to specific neurons. But, any such error of neural organization must be reflected in altered events at the neurochemical and electrophysiological levels. Even the "healthy" aging brain undergoes characteristic biological changes as it ages (as detailed in Chapter 1). Therefore, among the elderly especially, behavioral or emotional problems may frequently involve both kinds of elements, constituting impairments that truly justify the qualifier *neuropsychiatric*. Ultimately, whether a problem is organic in origin, functional, or mixed, there is only a limited variety of behavioral or subjective manifestations available through which the disorder can be expressed. As a result, a given set of neuropsychiatric symptoms could represent any of several combinations of organic and/or functional alterations. Nevertheless, the focus of this chapter will be those disorders currently classified as **functional;** those designated **organic** were considered in the preceding chapter.

THE INTERRELATEDNESS OF PSYCHOLOGICAL AND PHYSICAL HEALTH

The interrelatedness of biological changes in the brain and psychosocial stresses may indeed be even stronger among the elderly than for younger adults. Stresses such as loss of loved ones, restrictions on independence, fear of death, financial difficulties, loss of sexual function, chronic fatigue, or loss of professional status are more likely to bring on or exacerbate health problems for older persons than for their younger counterparts. This is most obviously the case for those disorders recognized as **psychosomatic**—tension or migraine headaches, certain instances of lower back pain, or peptic ulcers—but may also apply in less well-defined ways to a wide range of health problems. Less often recognized is the interrelatedness of psychological health and physical health as it applies in the opposite direction—the effect of physical health status on psychological well-being.

The advent of diminished organ system capacities, chronic debilitating diseases, and sensory system impairments (e.g., decreased visual acuity, diminished depth perception, loss of high frequency auditory acuity) can serve as added stresses that cause or exacerbate anxiety, depression, or even psychosis. One manifestation of the added strains imposed on psychological health by deteriorating physical health is the increase in suicide rates among elderly individuals—most often of all, white males who are widowed or divorced.

While younger people generally recognize that aging brings new burdens to life, few younger people can be expected to truly appreciate the full range of new stresses that accompany aging—until, of course, they, in turn, experience that phase of life. The unique stresses that accompany aging can

Table 9.1 Stresses of Aging

Added Physiological Stresses
- Declining functional capacity of major physiological systems (pulmonary, renal, cardiovascular)
- One or more chronic diseases
- Less vigorous homeostatic control mechanisms for blood pressure, heart rate, blood sugar levels, balance, appetite, and body temperature
- Increased incidence of gastrointestinal disorders/nutritional deficiencies
- Increased incidence of genitourinary disorders
- Degenerative events of the nervous system
- Impaired function of sensory systems (sight, hearing, etc.)
- Increased incidence of sleep disorders
- Neuromuscular problems with impaired mobility
- Increased risk of falls and other accidental injury

Added Psychosocial Stresses
- Loss of loved ones
- Loneliness, isolation
- Increased conflicts with family or friends
- Loss of status or self-esteem in relation to occupation
- Inadequate retirement income
- Loss of independence due to debilitating diseases
- Chronic fatigue
- Loss of sexual function or opportunities
- Poor nutrition due to substandard resources or disinterest in meal preparation

be loosely divided into two broad categories: physiological and psychosocial (see Table 9.1).

PSYCHOSIS AMONG THE ELDERLY

Schizophrenia is the most commonly occurring type of psychosis found among the elderly. The criteria set forth in the Diagnostic and Statistical Manual of the American Psychiatric Association, 3rd edition revised (DSM-IIIR) include one that specifies that the condition has been evident at least 6 months, including any prodromal phase. This duration criterion has an important inference because there is a fairly good chance that a psychosis may remit during the first 6 months (especially if it developed abruptly and previous level of functioning was good). Likelihood of recovery is much lower, however, if the psychosis has been continuously evident for more than 6 months. Thus, the diagnosis of schizophrenia as it is applied today suggests a disorder that is likely to be chronic—probably lifelong. Most older persons who are psychotic developed schizophrenia in their late teens or as a young adult, carrying the condition with them into later life.

Some elderly clients will have had one or more episodes of schizophreniform disorder, either in earlier years or more recently. *Schizophreniform disorder* is the designation used for a schizophrenic-like condition that does not meet the duration criterion of six months, hence, it is not chronic. Nevertheless, such **acute episodes** may be recurrent.

There are, however, two additional circumstances that may be the basis for psychosis in later life, both of later onset than schizophrenia. Frequently late onset psychosis is secondary to organic brain syndromes (see previous chapter), such as Alzheimer's disease. In this event, the thought disorders which are the hallmark of psychosis will be accompanied by some degree of cognitive impairments, memory impairments, and clouding of the sensorium. The second possibility is a late-onset schizophrenic-like condition, called **paraphrenia.** This designation indicates a late-onset psychosis that generally meets the criteria for schizophrenia except for onset prior to age 45. The condition is likely to include delusions and/or hallucinations, mood changes, and impairments of volition, but the sensorium remains clear. Paranoid thinking is more often evident in paraphrenia than in schizophrenia and may relate to the increasing loss of control and uncontrollable losses that frequently accompany aging. Paraphrenia occurs most often in elderly females, especially those who are disengaged from society and isolated from family contacts.

Antipsychotic Drug Use in the Elderly

Antipsychotic drugs are often effective in suppressing paranoid symptoms, delusions, hallucinations, and other florid symptoms of psychosis in the elderly. There is little difference in effectiveness of the various available drugs, but there are important differences in the severity of different categories of adverse effects.

Clinical Indications in the Elderly.   Antipsychotic drugs are indicated for elderly clients with a diagnosis of schizophrenia, delusional disorder, or paraphrenia. These drugs are also useful for suppression of psychotic symptoms secondary to organic brain syndrome. Neuroleptics also provide the main basis for short-term management of mania of bipolar disorder. They are sometimes used in small doses in elderly clients for nocturnal delirium (Sundowner's syndrome) characterized by frightening auditory and visual hallucinations. Antipsychotic drugs provide the main basis for symptomatic control of agitation but, because of the hazards these drugs present, they should no longer be considered appropriate selections for general sedative purposes.

Perhaps the single, greatest benefit afforded by antipsychotic drug therapy is the control of florid symptoms in the milder cases of psychosis, which would otherwise stand as a roadblock to continued involvement of the person in the community setting. The average family cannot cope well with an unmedicated psychotic family member. Proper medication may therefore mean the difference between continued presence with the family and institutionalization. This difference is not only often an important contribution to the continued happiness of the psychotic person, but also impacts more strongly on prognosis than any other single variable.

Chronic psychosis may entail episodic exacerbations and intervening periods of relative remittance. Drug doses may need to be adjusted in relation to such fluctuations. Dosage increases should not necessarily be considered permanent if the client's condition has previously shown evidence of fluctuations in severity. Some elderly clients who have had multiple instances of schizophreniform disorder will be on maintenance doses of an antipsychotic drug, but normally not until after the third or fourth such episode. Maintenance doses are typically just one-fifth to one-third the doses that would be used for chronic forms of psychosis.

Antipsychotic drugs occasionally find use for nonpsychiatric applications in the elderly. Prochlorperazine (Compazine), for example, might be used for suppressing the nausea and vomiting that often accompanies cancer chemotherapy or for minimizing preanesthetic apprehensiveness. Doses for these purposes are at the low end of the dosage range but may nevertheless result in significant adverse reactions for the elderly, who are more sensitive to such problems.

Altered Pharmacokinetics or Pharmacodynamics in the Elderly. Neuroleptic doses need to be substantially lower in older individuals. There is evidence that older people are more susceptible to the adverse effects when conventional doses are employed. Efficacy can also be achieved usually at lower doses. Neuroleptics are 99% metabolized prior to excretion and this process proceeds more slowly in elderly persons. It is not clear at this point whether pharmacodynamic factors (i.e., an increased response in the brain to a given plasma concentration) also contribute to the greater sensitivity of elderly people to neuroleptics.

Adverse Effects and Contraindications in the Elderly. Neuroleptics as a group have one of the worst sets of adverse effects for drugs in the psychotropic drug category. In fact, the adverse effects are severe enough to be given considerable weight in any risk/benefit analysis, and there will be times when the decision most in the client's interests will be to withhold antipsychotic drug treatment. Since elderly clients are more than typically susceptible to many of these potential problems, a thorough physical examination, including complete blood cell counts, and electroencephalogram, visual examination, urinalysis, and liver function tests, should be conducted before initiating neuroleptic therapy in an elderly person.

Adverse effects of antipsychotic drugs can be grouped into

1. **early side effects,** which are most intense shortly after therapy is initiated but subside;
2. **continuing side effects,** which remain at roughly the same level of intensity throughout the period of drug therapy; and
3. **extrapyramidal side effects,** which include both early and late varieties and which may pose a significant liability for the client.

Although the various neuroleptics resemble one another with respect to the overall set of potential side effects that may occur, the frequency and severity of side effects in various categories varies substantially from drug to drug (see Table 9.2).

Table 9.2 Side Effects of Various Neuroleptics

Drug	Early Side Effects				Continuing Side Effects		
	Anticho-linergic	Sedation	Orthostatic hypotension	Blood cell disorders	Lowered seizure threshold	Hypo-thalamic	Extra-pyramidal
Phenothiazines, Aliphatic							
Chlorpromazine	++	+++	+++	++	+++	++	++
Promazine	+++	++	++	++	+++	++	++
Triflupromazine	+++	+++	++	++	+++	++	++
Phenothiazines, Piperidine							
Thioridazine	+++	+++	+++	+	+	++	+
Mesoridazine	++	+++	++	+	+	++	+
Phenothiazines, Piperazine							
Prochlorperazine	+	++	+	++	+	++	+++
Perphenazine	++	+	+	++	+	++	+++
Fluphenazine	+	+	+	++	+	++	+++
Trifluoperazine	+	+	+	++	+	++	+++
Acetophenazine	++	++	+	++	+	++	+++
Butyrophenone							
Haloperidol	0	+	+	+	++	+++	+++
Thioxanthenes							
Chlorprothixene	++	+++	+++	++	+++	++	++
Thiothixene	+	+	+	++	++	++	+++
Dihydroindolone							
Molindone	++	++	+	+	0/+	+	++
Dibenzoxazepine							
Loxapine	+	++	+	++	++	+	+++
Dibenzodiazepines							
Clozapine	+++	++	+++	++	+	0/+	0
Benzisoxazoles							
Risperidone	+	+	+	+	+	+	0/+

+++ high degree; ++ moderate degree; + slight degree; 0/+ slight or not at all; 0 not at all.

All of the major examples of early side effects of antipsychotic drugs pose a greater threat to elderly individuals than to younger clients. **Agranulocytosis** and **allergic reactions,** such as urticaria, photosensitivity, and cholestatic jaundice, occur more often in older clients. The drug history of the client is the best advanced indication of potential allergic reactions, so the client's previous drug responses should be thoroughly evaluated before initiating neuroleptic therapy. Photosensitivity can be a particularly injurious side effect. One manifestation, retinopathy, can culminate in blindness if not recognized and addressed. Clients receiving neuroleptics should receive periodic visual examinations and should be taught to employ UV-blocking sunglasses when in bright sunlight.

The sedative action of neuroleptics, though less than that produced by sedative-hypnotics, can be troublesome for older clients by worsening intellectual impairments for those who are already suffering from some degree of organic brain syndrome. Geriatric clients living in the community need to be warned that the sedative action of neuroleptics may impair ability to drive or perform other tasks requiring alertness.

Orthostatic hypotension and **cardiotoxicity** are likely to be of greater consequence for elderly individuals. Even in the absence of specific ailments, aging entails a diminished sensitivity for various homeostatic mechanisms. One such example is a slower response time for vascular adjustments in relation to changes in bodily position. Balance is also impaired. So, older people, even without drug contributions, are more prone to fainting, feelings of light-headedness, or falls when standing up abruptly. The orthostatic hypotension frequently caused by neuroleptics would obviously accentuate this difficulty. Moreover, elderly individuals are likely to suffer more from falls that might occur upon fainting, possibly suffering fractures that will be slower to mend or head trauma. Clients who tend to experience episodes of orthostatic hypotension need to be educated to avoid prolonged standing, especially in sunlight or hot showers, and to change positions more gradually.

Cardiotoxicity of neuroleptics derives from a depression of the myocardium—what pharmacologists call a quinidine-like action. Conduction blocks may occur, particularly in the atrio-ventricular node. Ectopic foci could develop in the conductile system or the ventricular muscle with consequent ventricular tachydysrhythmias. Since older clients are more likely to be suffering from cardiac abnormalities or diminished cardiac reserve, such neuroleptic-induced changes in cardiac function are more likely to culminate in clinically significant problems. When long-term therapy with neuroleptics is required for elderly clients, cardiac monitoring should be conducted frequently.

Many, though not all, neuroleptics also produce a package of early adverse reactions collectively referred to as **anticholinergic side effects** (see Table 9.3). Many of these potential problems exacerbate changes already in evidence as a result of aging. The drying of respiratory and nasal secretions and the inhibition of sweating, for example, may aggravate dryness of the skin and mucosal membranes brought on by reduced activity of secretory cells with aging. The constipation and urinary retention that occur as anticholinergic side effects likewise add to changes already evident with

Table 9.3 The Anticholinergic Syndrome

Organ system	Symptoms
CNS	Anxiety, agitation, restlessness, twitching, myoclonic contraction, hyperreflexia, amnesia, hallucinations, clouding of the sensorium, delirium, mania, impaired speech, impaired gait, seizures, coma, respiratory failure, circulatory collapse
Eyes	Mydriasis, photophobia, cycloplegia
Cardiovascular System	Tachycardia, vasodilation, weak pulse
Visceral Smooth Muscle	Urinary retention, decreased gastrointestinal motility
Exocrine Glands	Decreased salivation, decreased nasopharangeal secretions, difficulty talking or swallowing, decreased sweating, hyperpyrexia, decreased bronchial secretions
Skin	Flushing, rash, desquamation

Memory Aid for Learning Anticholinergic Effects:

Dry as a bone:	Inhibition of secretions
Red as a beet:	Flushing related to absence of sweating
Hot as a hare:	Temperature elevation from absence of sweating
Blind as a bat:	Cycloplegia and mydriasis
Mad as a hatter:	Mental confusion, delirium

aging. Older clients who are started on neuroleptic therapy should receive intake/output monitoring for evidence of constipation or urinary retention.

The two kinds of continuing side effects of antipsychotic drugs are a **lowering of the seizure threshold** and **suppression of hypothalamic homeostatic mechanisms.** Neuroleptics are specifically contraindicated for those undergoing sedative-hypnotic withdrawal, including delirium tremens associated with alcoholism, because of the increased seizure liability. In the latter category are impairments of sexual function, alterations in appetite and weight, and impairments of temperature regulation. Impairments in sexual functioning can be either more or less important for older clients than for younger counterparts. Some older clients will be less sexually active or have fewer opportunities for sexual interaction, but those male clients who are sexually active are likely to be more fully impacted by the ejaculatory impotence often caused by neuroleptics.

Extrapyramidal side effects of neuroleptics include four types:

1. acute dystonic reactions;
2. akathisia;
3. pseudoparkinsonism; and
4. tardive dyskinesias.

The first two types usually occur very early in therapy and are less common in geriatric clients than younger ones. Pseudoparkinsonism (drug-induced Parkinsonism) can develop at any stage of neuroleptic therapy and is characterized by the same triad of symptoms that occur in organic Parkinson's disease: tremor, rigidity, and weakness (with loss of mobility). Since elderly clients often suffer from diminished neuromuscular capacity, the motor deficits of drug-induced Parkinsonism will have proportionately more impact on an older person. Atypical neuroleptics, which have less or completely lack potential for extrapyramidal side effects, may be considered to have a special advantage for use in the older individuals. Anticholinergic drugs that are used in organic Parkinsonism are also effective in suppressing Pseudoparkinsonism, but other antiparkinsonian drugs, such as levodopa, are inappropriate because they will aggravate schizophrenia.

Tardive dyskinesias represent the worst of the extrapyramidal problems and, indeed, the worst of all of the side-effects of neuroleptics. Tardive dyskinesias consist of late-occurring abnormal, stereotypical movements, most often involving the tongue, mouth, jaw, eyes, trunk, and upper extremities. Since the likelihood and severity of tardive dyskinesias increase with duration of treatment, the incidence of such reactions is highest among elderly persons. Once these movements develop, they are likely to be irreversible (or, at the least, of prolonged persistence) even if neuroleptic therapy is discontinued, and they grow gradually more severe if neuroleptic therapy continues. Moreover, there are no certain methods for managing this disorder. Antiparkinsonian drugs do not alleviate tardive dyskinesias though dopamine-depleting drugs (alpha-methyl-para-tyrosine or tetrabenazine) have been helpful.

Interactions in the Elderly.   Interactions involving antipsychotic drugs are more likely to occur in the elderly because older individuals take, on average, more different medications (see Chapter 3). The most common interaction of neuroleptics is **additive CNS depression,** which can occur with any other CNS depressant. The interacting drug could be an anxiolytic or one of the sedative tricyclic antidepressants, perhaps being employed together with the neuroleptic for the client's psychiatric disorder. The interacting drug could be an hypnotic being administered for insomnia—a common complaint for older persons. The interacting drug might even be one not normally associated with effects on the CNS, such as an antiadrenergic compound being used to manage essential hypertension or a cardiac glycoside (e.g., digoxin) being used for a cardiovascular problem. Even though such drugs are classified as cardiovascular agents, they have significant effects on nervous tissue as well and contribute to CNS depression.

Another common interaction involving neuroleptics is **additive anticholinergic actions.** Many neuroleptics have substantial anticholinergic activity (see Table 9.2) and so too do many antidepressants, antiparkinsonian drugs, narcotics, and, of course, autonomic drugs expressly classified as anticholinergic. Once again, elderly individuals are substantially more likely than younger persons to be taking two or more drugs that contribute to anticholinergic toxicity.

Neuroleptics can also affect medications being taken by older persons for cardiovascular problems. Neuroleptics decrease the antihypertensive effectiveness of guanethidine (Ismelin) but, on the other hand, increase plasma concentrations of beta-blockers. Haloperidol combined with the antihypertensive drug methyldopa (Aldomet) has been noted sometimes to cause psychiatric reactions involving assaultiveness, irritability, or disorientation. Neuroleptics that have alpha-blocking properties can dangerously alter the action of sympathomimetics by allowing the beta-receptor effects to occur without the normally balancing effect of alpha-adrenergic activity.

Older people are more likely to require antacid therapy for problems of peptic ulcers and antacids that contain aluminum salts will inhibit absorption of the phenothiazine type of neuroleptic. Clients requiring both types of drugs should take the neuroleptic at least 1 hour, or preferably 2 hours, after taking the antacid.

Neuroleptics may increase requirements for antiepileptic medication because they lower the seizure threshold. The antiemetic action of neuroleptics may mask or even dangerously worsen the toxic effects of poisons or drugs that might otherwise be quickly removed from the stomach by emesis.

Administration in the Elderly.   Neuroleptic doses are quite variable and always require titration. This is all the more a necessity for the elderly client where the susceptibility to adverse effects is greater. Elderly clients receiving neuroleptics need to be monitored closely. Many of the side effects can be observed early on, but judgments regarding therapeutic response cannot be made too hastily, because therapeutic benefit with neuroleptics occurs only after 2–3 weeks of use. It is important that target symptoms be established and that they correspond to those that are known to respond to neuroleptic intervention. Florid symptoms such as agitation, hostility, and delusions can be expected to abate in 1–3 weeks, but cognitive and perceptual changes occur much more slowly.

Adherence to neuroleptic regimens by outpatients is often very poor for a variety of reasons. Neuroleptics do not produce the subjectively pleasant "buzz" associated with sedative-hypnotics or anxiolytics; indeed, the subjective effect has been described as mildly unpleasant. Moreover, the side effects may occur sooner than the therapeutic benefit. Also, clients with a history of psychosis are probably not the most reliable client population. Sometimes clients reason that they no longer need the drug because the symptoms have dissipated, when in fact the reduction in symptoms is a specific consequence of drug therapy. Chronic treatments with medication may serve as a drain on the client's financial resources—all the more so for some elderly clients trying to subsist on a fixed income during a time of inflation. For all these reasons, every effort needs to be made to promote and evaluate adherence to the regimen if indeed the regimen is one in which the therapeutic team has confidence and to adjust the regimen, if necessary, to improve adherence. Once-a-day regimens for outpatients requiring these drugs has been found to be optimum with respect to compliance and is only slightly inferior to divided doses, if only pharmacokinetics are to be considered. Therefore, in balance, the once-a-day approach is usually best. For clients with a history of nonadherence, special long-acting dosage forms (enanthate and decanoate esters) are available for fluphenazine (Prolixin) and haloperidol (Haldol). These formulations are injected intramuscularly or subcutaneously to provide sustained drug availability for up to 3–4 weeks, depending on the product.

Psychotropic drugs, such as neuroleptics, have been among the drugs most likely to be administered in excessive doses to elderly clients either because of failure to take into account age-dependent pharmacokinetics or because of unrealistic therapeutic objectives. The Omnibus Budget Reconciliation Act (OBRA) of 1987 sought to diminish this problem by establishing new guidelines for appropriate use of various psychotropic drugs, side effect monitoring, clinical contraindications, and, most importantly, maximum daily doses. The maximum daily doses, as specified for each drug covered by OBRA are included for each drug under Preparations and Administration. As regards neuroleptics in particular, the following conditions were specifically listed as *inappropriate* uses for these drugs: wandering, poor self-care, restlessness, impaired memory, anxiety, depression (without psychotic features), insomnia, indifference to surroundings, fidgeting, nervousness, uncooperativeness, or agitated behaviors which do not represent danger to the individual or others. Another provision of OBRA was that PRN doses of neuroleptics are no longer to be used more than twice in a seven-day period without further assessment and only in order to titrate dosage to optimize response or to manage unexpected behaviors that could not otherwise be managed.

Aminoalkyl Phenothiazines

CHLORPROMAZINE   (Thorazine, Promapar, Thor-Prom, and generic)

Recommended initial oral dose in the elderly: No specific recommendation, but substantially lower. Maximum 75 mg/day according to OBRA.

Young adult initial dosage for comparison: 10 mg 3–4 times daily or 25 mg 2–3 times daily.

PROMAZINE   (Sparine and generic)

Recommended initial oral dose in the elderly   No specific recommendation, but substantially lower. Maximum 150 mg/day according to OBRA.

Young adult initial dosage for comparison: 10–200 mg at 4–6 hr intervals.

TRIFLUPROMAZINE   (Vesprin)

Recommended initial oral dose in the elderly: No specific recommendation, but substantially lower. Maximum 20 mg/day according to OBRA.

Young adult initial dosage for cmoparison: 100 mg/day.

Piperazine Phenothiazines

ACETOPHENAZINE (Tindal)

Recommended initial oral dose in the elderly: No specific recommendation, but substantially lower. Maximum 20 mg/day according to OBRA.

Young adult initial dosage for comparison: 40–120 mg/day.

FLUPHENAZINE (Prolixin, Permitil)

Recommended initial oral dose in the elderly: 1–2.5 mg/day. Maximum 4 mg/day according to OBRA.

Young adult initial dosage for comparison: 0.5–10 mg/day in divided doses.

PERPHENAZINE (Trilafon)

Recommended initial oral dose in the elderly: One-third to one-half the adult dose. Maximum 8 mg/day according to OBRA.

Young adult initial dosage for comparison: 4–8 mg 3 times daily.

PROCHLORPERAZINE (Compazine, Chlorazine, and generic)

Recommended initial oral dose in the elderly: No specific recommendation, but substantially lower. Maximum 10 mg/day according to OBRA.

Young adult initial dosage for comparison: 5–10 mg 3–4 times daily.

TRIFLUPERAZINE (Stelazine, Suprazine, and generic)

Recommended initial oral dose in the elderly: No specific recommendation, but substantially lower. Maximum 8 mg/day according to OBRA.

Young adult initial dosage for comparison: 1–2 mg twice daily.

Piperadine Phenothiazines

THIORIDAZINE   (Mellaril, Millazine, and generic)

Recommended initial oral dose in the elderly: No specific recommendation, but substantially lower. Maximum 75 mg/day according to OBRA.

Young adult initial dosage for comparison: 50–100 mg 3 times daily.

MESORIDAZINE   (Serentil)

Recommended initial oral dose in the elderly: No specific recommendation, but substantially lower. Maximum 25 mg/day according to OBRA.

Young adult initial dosage for comparison: 50 mg 3 times daily.

Butyrophenones

HALOPERIDOL   (Haldol)

Recommended initial oral dose in the elderly: Lower initial doses and more gradual adjustment. Maximum 4 mg/day according to OBRA.

Young adult initial dosage for comparison: 0.5–5 mg 2–3 times daily.

Thioxanthenes

CHLORPROTHIXENE   (Taractan)

Recommended initial oral dose in the elderly: No specific recommendation, but substantially lower. Maximum 75 mg/day according to OBRA.

Young adult initial dosage for comparison: 25–50 mg 3–4 times daily.

THIOTHIXENE   (Navane)

Recommended initial oral dose in the elderly: No specific recommendation, but substantially lower. Maximum 7 mg/day according to OBRA.

Young adult initial dosage for comparison: 2 mg 3 times daily.

Dihydroindolones

MOLINDONE   (Moban)

Recommended initial oral dose in the elderly: No specific recommendation, but substantially lower. Maximum 10 mg/day according to OBRA.

Young adult initial dosage for comparison: 50–75 mg/day.

Dibenzoxazepines

LOXAPINE   (Loxitane)

Recommended initial oral dose in the elderly: No specific recommendation, but substantially lower. Maximum 10 mg/day according to OBRA.

Young adult initial dosage for comparison: 10 mg twice daily.

Atypical Neuroleptics

CLOZAPINE   (Clozaril)

Recommended initial oral dose in the elderly: No specific recommendation. Maximum 50 mg/day according to OBRA.

Young adult initial dosage for comparison: 25 mg once or twice daily.

REMOXIPRIDE   (Roxiam)

Investigational

RISPERIDONE   (Risperdal)

Recommended initial oral dose in the elderly: 0.5 mg twice daily in elderly or debilitated individuals, those with renal or hepatic impairment, or those predisposed to hypotension.

Young adult dosage for comparison: 1 mg twice daily on first day, increased by 1 mg per administration on second and third day to a target dose of 3 mg twice daily by the third day. Further dosage adjustments may be undertaken at 1 week intervals in increments of 1 mg twice daily. Maximum benefits occur in the range of 4 to 16 mg/day with 4 to 6 mg/day usual.

AFFECTIVE DISORDERS AMONG THE ELDERLY

The functional affective disorders include unipolar affective disorder—depression—and bipolar or manic-depressive disorder. Depression is common among the elderly, so much so that it could almost be considered the hallmark disturbance for older people. This is perhaps not surprising, because later life is rife with significant losses: death of close friends or the spouse; loss of mobility, bodily functions, or self-esteem; and financial difficulties represent but a few of the potential contributors. Depression often goes unrecognized and undiagnosed when it occurs in the elderly because too many people, both medical personnel and others, erroneously believe that depression is a normal aspect of aging. Somatic components of the disorder may be attributed to chronic illness already present. Onset of depression tends to be more gradual in elderly clients and therefore less likely to trigger notice.

Grief reactions occasioned by loss of loved ones are most certainly an event made more frequent by aging, but these reactions should not be confused with depressive syndromes. True depressive syndromes may be endogenous in the elderly, arising in neurochemical imbalances in the brain, but more often, as in younger people, are reactive conditions brought about by losses.

Certainly the hallmark psychological symptom of depression is dysphoric mood, which might be described by clients variably as sadness, depression, "feeling blue," or "down in the dumps." Other psychic symptoms include irritability, anhedonia (loss of pleasure responses to praise or previously enjoyed activities), pessimism or brooding, feelings of guilt, feelings of hopelessness, diminished libido, and suicidal ideation. The psychic symptoms may be expressed in such behaviors as withdrawal, crying, agitation, or conversely, psychomotor retardation, or suicide attempts. Suicide rates are higher in elderly people than among their younger counterparts. At age 80, yearly rates for men are approximately 50 per hundred thousand; for women approximately one-third that rate.

Somatic symptoms are usually evident as well, including changes in appetite and weight (more often anorexia than hyperphagia), sleep disturbances (insomnia more often than hypersomnia), and fatigue. In extreme cases, major depression can progress to a psychotic state with such features as delusions, hallucinations, impaired contact with reality, or ever depressive stupor.

Depression can also occur in elderly persons secondary to organic brain syndrome. When this happens it is sometimes difficult to make the correct diagnosis. Theoretically, concommitant cognitive impairments suggest that depression might be secondary to organic brain syndrome, but sometimes the relationship is the other way around. Some depressed individuals, especially among the elderly, exhibit cognitive deficits that are in fact secondary to severe depression—a phenomenon that has become known as **pseudodementia or pseudodementing depression.** The dysphoric mood of depression in these individuals results in negativistic behavior, so that the individual does not really cooperate with the effort to evaluate cognitive capabilities. Cognitive impairments of pseudodementia improve when antidepressant drug therapy is initiated to approximately the same extent that the depression improves. It is particularly tragic when functional depressions are erroneously assumed to be secondary to organic brain syndrome because evidence suggests that late-onset functional depressions are every bit as amenable to drug therapy as depressive conditions in younger people. In fact, when depression arises newly in an older person, it is highly likely that at least one of the positive prognostic indicators will be present—good premorbid functioning evidenced by a history of sound social, emotional, and psychosexual adjustment.

Manic episodes are probably less common among the elderly than in younger age groups, but occasionally manic episodes manifest for the first time in old age. When mania occurs, it typically indicates presence of bipolar disorder. Manic episodes consist of distinct periods of elevated, expansive, or irritable mood accompanied by at least three of the following: increased activity, pressure to keep talking, flight of ideas, grandiosity, decreased need for sleep, distractibility, or increased high-risk behaviors (reckless driving, buying sprees, sexual indiscretions, etc.). Lithium is the drug of choice for stabilization of mood swings. Unfortunately, the elderly are more prone to adverse reactions to lithium.

Antidepressant Drug Use in the Elderly

Antidepressants currently include three classes: (1) the tricyclic antidepressants; (2) the atypical (or second generation) drugs; and (3) the monoamine oxidase inhibitors. The last category rarely finds use today. The atypical drugs have overtaken the tricyclic antidepressants in recent years in terms of frequency of prescription.

Clinical Indications in the Elderly. Antidepressants are indicated for major depression, whether reactive or endogenous, though benefit is, on average, greater with the endogenous examples. The therapeutic benefit of tricyclic and second-generation antidepressants is, however, delayed, requiring approximately 2–3 weeks to be fully evident after treatment is initiated. Antidepressants can also provide symptomatic relief when used in clients with depression secondary to organic brain syndrome. Antidepressants are not consistently effective for dysthymic disorder, which is long-lasting, intermittent, mild depression.

There is generally a lack of evidence of significant differences in relative efficacy among the tricyclic antidepressants for depression. Therefore, selection of a particular drug for a specific client is usually based on other factors, such as the frequency of side effects in the various categories, cost, and availability. There is also little difference in relative efficacy when the newer atypical antidepressants are compared with the tricyclic group. The principal advantage of the newer drugs is a reduction in the variety and frequency of side effects rather than any increase in efficacy or in latency to development of that efficacy (see Table 9.4). A second-generation antidepressant is usually a better choice than a tricyclic, because of the smaller variety and severity of side effects, and perhaps all the more so in the elderly who are more likely to suffer from side effects.

Some of the antidepressants have distinctive profiles of effectiveness in some other psychiatric disorders. Some, but only some, of the antidepressants are uniquely effective for obsessive-compulsive disorder. Clomipramine is apparently most notably effective in this condition with some benefit also evident with fluoxetine (Prozac), but imipramine, amitriptyline,

Table 9.4 Pharmacological Properties and Adverse Effects of Antidepressants

| | Reuptake Block Release | | | | Major Adverse Effects | | |
Drug	NE	5HT	NE	DA	Anticho-linergic	Sedation	Orthostatic hypotension
Tertiary Amines							
Amitriptyline	+*	++++	0	0	++++	+++	++
Imipramine	+++*	+++	0	0	++	++	+++
Trimipramine	+	++	0	0	++	+++	++
Doxepin	+	+++	0	0	++	+++	++
Secondary Amines							
Nortriptyline	++	+++	0	0	++	++	+
Protriptyline	+++	+	0	0	+++	+/–	+
Desipramine	++++	0	0	0	+	+/–	+
Amoxapine	+++	++	0	0	+	++	+
Second-Generation Antidepressants							
Maprotiline	++	+	0	0	+	++	+
Trazodone	0	+++	0	0	+	+	++
Nomifensine	++	+	0	++	0	0	0
Bupropion	+/–	0	0	+	0	+	0
Stimulants							
Amphetamine	0	0	+++	+++	0	0	0

*Includes effect of secondary amine metabolites.
++++ greatest degree; +++ high degree; ++ moderate degree; + slight degree; +/– slight or not at all; 0 not at all.

and trazadone have little if any value. Both separation anxiety in children and panic disorder have been treated effectively with antidepressants. Imipramine is the antidepressant most often used in these conditions, though its efficacy in these disorders is not unique among the antidepressants.

Tricyclic antidepressants have been used over the years to augment the analgesic effect provided by narcotics for treatment of chronic pain. Tricyclic antidepressants, in effect, potentiate the action of the narcotic, allowing management of the pain with smaller doses. This is important because tolerance, and sometimes dependence, develops when narcotics need to be used for long periods of time for chronic pain. Concurrent use of tricyclic antidepressants will delay and reduce the development of these problems.

Monoamine oxidase inhibitors cannot be recommended as a first treatment approach for depression in any age group, but the elderly may actually be less responsive to these drugs than younger individuals, because some studies have indicated that activity of the enzyme monoamine oxidase increases with aging. Monoamine oxidase inhibitors have sometimes been recommended for a specific variety of depression—an **atypical depression** characterized by lethargy, fatigue, hypersomnia, overeating, and anxiety, often triggered by rejection.

Altered Pharmacokinetics or Pharmacodynamics in the Elderly.
Absorption, first-pass extraction, and metabolism of tricyclic antidepressants are all variable, from client to client, regardless of age. Therefore, doses need to be titrated to the requirements of the individual in every case. Tricyclic antidepressants exhibit what is called a "therapeutic window"—a range of plasma concentrations associated with effectiveness, below or above which benefit is unlikely to occur. Studies have confirmed that the therapeutic window for tricyclics does apply as well to elderly clients. However, starting doses need to be considerably lower for most elderly clients, because of altered pharmacokinetics, to achieve ultimate plasma concentrations that lie within the window. A minority of elderly clients may, however, require full doses for therapeutic plasma concentrations and will, in effect, be undertreated if doses are reduced. Thus, the only certain basis for determination of the optimal dose is periodic monitoring of plasma concentrations after administration.

Lethal doses of tricyclic antidepressants are also lower in the elderly than for younger adults. Lethal doses for young adults are in the range of 20 times the therapeutic dose. Some clients have hoarded tricyclic antidepressants for ultimate use in suicide attempts and fatal overdoses with these drugs do occur on a regular basis.

Pharmacokinetics are less problematic for the second-generation antidepressants than for the tricyclics, because the therapeutic window is not so narrow. Fluoxetine does, however, have a long elimination half-life as does its active metabolite (norfluoxetine). The main problem that derives from this characteristic is that the so-called **washout period** is rather long should the drug need to be discontinued either because of adverse reaction or a decision to change to another treatment approach. Paroxetine, which is very similar to fluoxetine in most respects, has a shorter half-life and, thus, a shorter washout period. The rate of inactivation of fluoxetine does not appear to be significantly different in elderly clients than for younger adults, but both sertraline and paroxetine, on the other hand, are metabolized slower (40% slower for sertraline) in the elderly.

Adverse Effects and Contraindications in the Elderly.   Side-effects of tricyclic antidepressants generally resemble those of neuroleptics. This is perhaps not surprising in that the two groups of drugs resemble one another in structure as well. Like the neuroleptics, tricyclic antidepressants cause allergies, dyscrasias, cardiovascular problems including orthostatic hypotension, and the cluster of anticholinergic side effects. Tricyclic antidepressants also share the propensity of neuroleptics for lowering the seizure threshold and suppression of certain homeostatic activities of the hypothalamic/pituitary axis (appetite and weight control, temperature regulation, sexual function). However, a major advantage of tricyclic antidepressants relative to the neuroleptics is that extrapyramidal side effects are rarer and considerably milder. Extrapyramidal reactions to tricyclic antidepressants are usually limited to mild pseudoparkinsonian reactions. Tardive dyskinesias occur only very rarely in response to antidepressants. The most usual manifestation of psuedoparkinsonism caused by antidepressants is a fine resting tremor. It will often resolve with continuation of drug therapy, but may be aggravated by caffeine or anxiety. Beta-blockers, such as propranolol, will suppress the tremor if necessary.

Tricyclic antidepressants of the tertiary amine subgroup produce considerable sedation, but those in the secondary amine subgroup produce little or none. Elderly persons, especially those with any degree of organic brain syndrome, will be more affected by depressant effects of drugs and need to be warned to avoid driving or other activities requiring mental alertness during peak drug action.

Anticholinergic side effects of tricyclics are perhaps even more severe than for neuroleptics. Elderly individuals are more susceptible to many of the anticholinergic problems, including visual impairments (mydriasis, blurred vision, aggravation of glaucoma), urinary retention and constipation, and dryness of skin and mucosal membranes from inhibition of normal secretions.

Cardiotoxicity (atrial dysrhythmias, decreased myocardial contractility, or, even cardiac arrest) is more likely with tricyclic antidepressants than with neuroleptics, and these drugs should therefore be used cautiously, if at all, in clients with a history of cardiac problems. Obviously elderly clients are much more likely to have such problems. A baseline electrocardiogram should always be obtained before initiating tricyclic antidepressant therapy in an older person, followed by subsequent frequent monitoring.

Sometimes antidepressants cause psychiatric side effects, which can include confusion, inability to concentrate, disorientation, hallucinations, or delusions. Other times clients may become agitated, even to the point of panic or mania. When an antidepressant causes a client's mood to change all the way from depression to mania, the effect is referred to as **mood switch.** The various antidepressants do vary somewhat in their likelihood of causing mood switch. Mania and, therefore, mood switch is less likely to be a problem in an elderly client. Most antidepressants suppress REM sleep initially; trimipramine is an exception and may therefore have special advantage for clients with sleep problems and depression. There have been reports with clomipramine of rebound worsening of preexisting psychiatric symptoms upon abrupt withdrawal of the drug.

An important issue for the antidepressants is their influence on suicide liability. Suicide attempts are, in any case, more common among depressed individuals than for any other client category. Although it is to be expected that antidepressant therapy will decrease likelihood of suicides to the extent that the medication succeeds in elevating mood, suicide liability reportedly increases when antidepressant therapy is first initiated. Most recently, this problem has been given a lot of attention and publicity as it relates to the widely used antidepressant fluoxetine, but the problem has been recognized for decades as one that applies to antidepressants in general. The significant inference to be drawn from the observation of increased suicide attempts with initiation of antidepressant therapy is that monitoring and nondrug components of treatment need to be intensified, not relaxed, when drug therapy with antidepressants is first undertaken. Prescriptions should not be written in such a manner as to provide an overly large supply of pills that might be used in suicide attempts. Suicide rates are higher among the elderly than among younger individuals, so the influence of medication on suicidal tendencies needs special attention when antidepressant therapy is begun in an elderly client.

Second-generation antidepressants are far less likely to cause side effects than tricyclic antidepressants and therefore must be considered the drugs of choice for initial therapy of elderly clients. Side effects are less with these drugs mainly because of their greater pharmacological specificity. Fluoxetine, sertraline, and paroxetine are virtually devoid of anticholinergic properties, for example, and trazodone has only weak actions at the cholinergic receptor. Cardiotoxicity and orthostatic hypotension are also far less likely to occur with the second-generation drugs. Second-generation drugs do, however, share some of the categories of adverse reactions with the tricyclics—they lower the seizure threshold, have potential for allergic reactions, can cause mood switch, and may increase suicidal attempts. Agitation and mood switch are more likely to be problems with many of the second-generation drugs than the tricyclic antidepressants.

Interactions in the Elderly. Anticholinergic side effects of tricyclic antidepressants are additive with those of other drugs. Elderly clients take, on average, more drugs, prescription and otherwise, so the likelihood of a given client inadvertently taking two or more anticholinergic drugs is much higher. Elderly persons receiving an antidepressant with anticholinergic properties should be alerted to avoid the nonprescription products that contain potent anticholinergic compounds such as diphenhydramine, atropine, or scopolamine.

A particularly difficult interaction to prevent in practice occurs between antidepressants and sympathomimetic amines, which, in combination, often cause agitation. One of the many uses of sympathomimetic amines is in remedies designed for colds or allergies where this component provides nasal decongestion. These products are available without prescription and are very widely used, both of which facts increase the likelihood and decrease control over the likely interaction. Clients should be advised to ask their pharmacist for help in choosing a product for relief of cold symptoms that will not interact adversely with their antidepressant regimen.

Those antidepressants that have sedative properties will have additive depressant influence with any other central nervous system depressant. Those antidepressants with high specificity for blocking serotonin reuptake (e.g., fluoxetine, paroxetine) should not be used with tryptophan, an amino acid that is the precursor of serotonin and which some depressed people purchase from health food stores. The combination of tryptophan with a selective serotonin reuptake inhibitor is especially likely to trigger reactions of agitation or mood switch.

Antidepressants may alter the efficacy of antihypertensive drug regimens required by elderly clients. Those antidepressants that block reuptake of norepinephrine will tend to elevate blood pressure and may necessitate an intensification of therapy for high blood pressure. On the other hand, antihypertensive drugs with antisympathetic activity tend to promote depression and should be avoided in a depressed person or may necessitate more vigorous treatment for depression.

Administration in the Elderly.   It is usually best to initiate therapy with antidepressants in an elderly client with small doses, to minimize early side effects. Doses can then be gradually titrated upward based on monitored serum concentrations and clinical response. Many elderly clients will ultimately respond best at doses approximately one-fourth to one-half those given to younger adults. The usual expectation with tricyclic or second-generation antidepressants is that benefit can be expected approximately 3 weeks after treatment is begun, but if therapy is begun cautiously in the elderly client, as we recommend, a slightly longer delay needs to be anticipated—perhaps even as long as 6 weeks.

If minor adverse responses occur, dosage reduction can be attempted. Other times, side effects can be addressed by change in the dosage schedule. If sedation poses a problem, for example, the largest part of the daily dose could be taken at bedtime. If discontinuation is undertaken, it should usually be conducted gradually to avoid withdrawal symptoms that can include nausea, vomiting, headache, chills, muscle aches, malaise, anxiety, and akathisias. Antidepressant therapy initiated as a result of an acute depressive episode should be viewed as a temporary measure and withdrawal should be planned after an appropriate recovery period.

Tertiary Tricyclics

AMITRIPTYLINE   (Elavil, Amitril, Emitrip, Endep, and generic)

Recommended initial oral dose in the elderly: 10 mg 3 times daily and 20 mg at bedtime.

Young adult initial dosage for comparison: 75–100 mg/day in divided doses.

CLOMIPRAMINE (Anafranil)

Recommended initial oral dose in the elderly: No specific recommendation.

Young adult initial dosage for comparison: 25 mg/day.

DOXEPIN (Adapin, Sinequan)

Recommended initial oral dose in the elderly: No specific recommendation.

Young adult initial dosage for comparison: 75 mg/day.

IMIPRAMINE (Tofranil, Janimine, SK-Pramine, Tipramine, and generic)

Recommended initial oral dose in the elderly: 30–40 mg/day.

Young adult initial dosage for comparison: 75–150 mg/day in divided doses.

TRIMIPRAMINE (Surmontil)

Recommended initial oral dose in the elderly: 50 mg/day.

Young adult initial dosage for comparison: 75–100 mg/day in divided doses.

Secondary Tricyclics

AMOXAPINE (Asendin, generic)

Recommended initial oral dose in the elderly: 25 mg 2–3 times daily.

Young adult initial dosage for comparison: 50 mg 2–3 times daily.

DESIPRAMINE (Norpramin, Pertofrane, generic)

Recommended initial oral dose in the elderly: 25–100 mg/day.

Young adult initial dosage for comparison: 100–200 mg/day.

NORTRIPTYLINE   (Aventyl, Pamelor)

Recommended initial oral dose in the elderly: 30–50 mg daily in divided doses.

Young adult initial dosage for comparison: 25 mg 3–4 times daily.

PROTRIPTYLINE   (Vivactil)

Recommended initial oral dose in the elderly: 5 mg 3 times daily.

Young adult initial dosage for comparison: 15–40 mg/day in 3 or 4 divided doses.

Second-Generation (Atypical) Antidepressants

BUPROPION   (Wellbutrin)

Recommended initial oral dose in the elderly: No specific recommendation.

Young adult initial dosage for comparison: 300 mg/day in 3 divided doses.

FLUOXETINE   (Prozac)

Recommended initial oral dose in the elderly: No specific recommendation.

Young adult initial dosage for comparison: 20 mg/day in the morning.

FLUVOXAMINE   (Floxyfral)

Investigational

MAPROTILINE   (Ludiomil, generic)

Recommended initial oral dose in the elderly: 50–75 mg/day.

Young adult initial dosage for comparison: 75–150 mg/day.

PAROXETINE   (Paxil)

Recommended initial oral dose in the elderly: 10 mg/day in the morning.

Young adult initial dosage for comparison: 20 mg/day in the morning.

SERTRALINE   (Zoloft)

Recommended initial oral dose in the elderly: No specific recommendation, but probably needs to be lower (see Pharmacokinetics).

Young adult initial dosage for comparison: 50 mg once daily.

TRAZODONE   (Desyrel, generic)

Recommended initial oral dose in the elderly: No specific recommendation.

Young adult initial dosage for comparison: 150 mg/day.

Monoamine Oxidase Inhibitors

ISOCARBOXAZID   (Marplan)

Recommended initial oral dose in the elderly: No specific recommendation.

Young adult initial dosage for comparison: 30 mg/day.

PHENELZINE   (Nardil)

Recommended initial oral dose in the elderly: No specific recommendation.

Young adult initial dosage for comparison: 15 mg 3 times daily.

TRANYLCYPROMINE   (Parnate)

Recommended initial oral dose in the elderly: No specific recommendation.

Young adult initial dosage for comparison: 30 mg/day.

ANXIETY DISORDERS AMONG THE ELDERLY

Anxiety can occur in the elderly either as a primary disorder or as a symptom complex secondary to physical illness, other categories of psychiatric disorders, or inappropriate drug use. Anxiety is most often recognized as such by the client and by medical personnel, but the cause is often misidentified. In particular, anxiety that is secondary to physical illness or drug use is often misidentified as a primary anxiety disorder. When an elderly client complains of or exhibits anxiety that is discomforting or that impairs ability to function, medical intervention should begin with a complete medical examination and inventory of drugs in use. Anxiety may be secondary, for example, to hyperthyroidism, parathyroid disease, pheochromocytoma, or hypertension. Brief episodes of anxiety may occur during attacks of angina pectoris, bronchial asthma, or paroxysmal atrial tachycardia. Psychiatric conditions that often include anxiety as a symptom include depression, hysteria, schizophrenia, paraphrenia, sleep disturbances, and drug dependencies.

The most frequent drug contributor to anxiety symptoms is caffeine and any evaluation relating to anxiety should include a careful inventory of caffeine consumption. Although the major source of caffeine consumption for most clients will be from coffee ingestion, other significant contributions can derive from tea, cola and certain other soft drinks, stay-awake pills, chocolate, migraine medications, or certain combination cold remedies. Consumption in excess of 250 mg per day should be considered a potential contributing factor when anxiety is present.

Anxiety that occurs independent of other psychiatric problems, drug use, or physical illness is classified as **primary anxiety.** Primary anxiety disorders that affect the elderly include phobias, posttraumatic stress disorder, obsessive-compulsive disorder, panic disorder, and generalized anxiety disorder. The characteristics of these disorders as they occur in the elderly are not substantially different than when they occur in younger adults.

Generalized anxiety is by far the most prevalent type of primary anxiety disorder among the elderly. Generalized anxiety disorder includes manifestations in four categories: subjective, behavioral, motor, and autonomic. The subjective feelings, which the client might characterize as stress, worry, apprehensiveness, edginess, or tension, are the hallmarks of the disorder. The intensity of subjective symptoms can be ascertained only by the client's verbal or written report, but evaluating personnel need to keep in mind that the client may have one or more reasons to either downplay or exaggerate the intensity of his subjective distress.

Behavioral symptoms, which can include distractibility, insomnia, irritability, impatience, inability to relax, exaggerated need for reassurance, or hypervigilance, provide a more objective basis for evaluation by medical personnel.

Motor symptoms can include tremor, trembling, shakiness, jumpiness, fidgeting, or elevated muscle tone—the last of which can result in tension headaches or muscle aches.

Autonomic symptoms derive from both elevated sympathetic tone (increased heart rate, increased blood pressure, sweating, cold and moist palms, pallor) and elevated parasympathetic tone (upset stomach, "butterflies in the stomach," diarrhea, and frequent urination). Chronically elevated autonomic tone can, in time, result in or aggravate various medical problems.

Generalized anxiety can be reactive, situational, or chronic. The elderly are especially prone to reactive anxiety in relation to losses or anticipation of loss because of the increased variety of sources of stress that are encountered with aging (see Table 9.1). Situational anxiety is anxiety that occurs periodically in response to one or a few specific stressful circumstances. Chronic anxiety is anxiety that has become part of the fabric of that individual's personality. It will usually be evident from a review of the client's history, but may be worsened by the additional stresses of aging.

Anxiolytic Drug Use in the Elderly

Antianxiety drugs (or anxiolytics) are the second most widely prescribed category of drugs for the elderly. This massive level of application for this class of drugs has resulted in heated controversy about their appropriate place in medicine. Many critics argue that the use of anxiolytics is excessive, while a smaller number argue that irrational fear of addiction is depriving many clients of needed relief. In the best instances, anxiolytics can provide much needed relief from anxiety, not only alleviating subjective distress, but also improving ability to function. In the worst of applications, anxiolytics given for inappropriately long periods of time result in psychological and physical dependence, while providing little if any continuing benefit. As in virtually all areas of medicine involving drug therapies, what is needed here is the knowledge and judgment to correctly distinguish the appropriate from the inappropriate applications for these drugs.

The dominant class of antianxiety drugs in current medial practice is the benzodiazepines. Benzodiazepines have many uses in medicine— sleeping pills, antiseizure drugs, adjuncts for anesthesia, and muscle relaxation are some of the other important uses. A half-dozen or so of the drugs from this family are marketed primarily for anxiety, including diazepam, chlordiazepoxide, and alprazolam (see Table 9.5). These drugs are most familiar by their tradenames Valium, Librium, and Xanax, respectively. The major alternatives today to benzodiazepines for anxiety are diphenylmethane antihistamines (hydroxyzine and diphenhydramine) and azaspirodecanediones (busprione and gepirone).

Table 9.5 Comparisons of Benzodiazepines

Drug	Equivalent dose	Plasma half-life* (HR)
Alprazolam	0.5	12
Chlordiazepoxide	10	8–28
Clorazepate	7	30–100
Diazepam	5	20–42
Halazepam	20	14
Lorazepam	1	12–15
Oxazepam	15	10–14
Prazepam	10	30–100

*For drug or active metabolite.

Clinical Indications in the Elderly.   Antianxiety drugs are indicated for management of primary anxiety disorders or for short-term relief of symptoms of anxiety secondary to physical or other psychiatric ailments. Those most likely to benefit from anxiolytic mediation are those with anxiety that is severe, has been evident for only a short-time, and is reactive, and those who have had few previous drugs or good previous drug response.

The main controversial aspect of anxiolytic use in current medical practice is their role in management of long-term anxiety—chronic, or trait, anxiety. Most carefully controlled clinical trials have failed to demonstrate that anxiolytics provide benefit beyond approximately 3 months of use when employed on a regular daily basis. Although physical dependence can develop in response to normal therapeutic doses after as little as 4–6 weeks of regular daily use of benzodiazepines, it is most likely to occur when use has extended beyond 3 months. The risk of dependence is even greater when doses exceed therapeutic recommendations; for example, high doses of alprazolam have resulted in physical dependence in as little as a week. The balance between benefits and risks shifts sharply with chronic use both because benefits are less evident and because risks increase. Although some will disagree, we believe that continuous daily use of benzodiazepines for more than approximately 3 months is ill-advised. At the very least, the usefulness of the benzodiazepine as part of the treatment regimen should be periodically reassessed for each individual client. Nondrug measures for anxiety such as relaxation techniques or psychotherapy to improve coping mechanisms should be utilized whenever possible in lieu of drug therapy or as a means of facilitating dosage reduction.

In contrast to the benzodiazepines, neither the diphenylmethane antihistamines nor the azaspirodecanediones cause physical or psychological dependence. The antihistamines used as anxiolytics are, however, far less selective for anxiety and provide less maximum antianxiety potential. These drugs will usually not provide an adequate treatment for severe anxiety. Buspirone, the only currently available azaspirodecanedione, on the other hand, provides an anxiolytic action comparable to that of the benzodiazepines without abuse liability. Moreover, its benefit is demonstrable after at least 6 months of daily use and there is no evidence, at present, that the benefit is other than indefinite.

Some clients given buspirone improve in as little as 7–10 days, but most show maximum response only after 3–4 weeks of regular daily use. Therefore, buspirone cannot be considered a useful alternative to benzodiazepines for as-needed use in situational anxiety.

Altered Pharmacokinetics or Pharmacodynamics in the Elderly.
Benzodiazepines are inactivated mainly by liver metabolism although, for many of the compounds, not before production of intermediate active metabolites. Those that produce active metabolites (by hepatic oxidative metabolism), including diazepam and chlordiazepoxide, are metabolized more slowly in the elderly with a consequent increase in the half-life of these drugs and a greater likelihood of clinically significant sedation, lethargy, ataxia, or confusion. Alprazolam likewise has a longer and more variable half-life in older individuals. Doses of these drugs should be lower when

used in the elderly. Those benzodiazepines inactivated directly (by liver conjugation), including oxazepam and lorazepam, do not exhibit age-dependent changes in rate of metabolism (in the absence of specific liver disease) and therefore can be considered safer for use in the elderly.

Although buspirone has not been systematically tested in the elderly, several hundred elderly individuals were included in the clinical studies that preceded approval and no age-related change in rate of inactivation or dosage requirements were reported.

Adverse Effects and Contraindications in the Elderly.   The most common adverse responses to benzodiazepine anxiolytics are indications of **excess depression:** sedation, drowsiness, fatigue, lethargy, muscle weakness, ataxia, confusion, or disorientation. The elderly are more susceptible to such effects, especially if there is any degree of psychoneurological impairment or other depressant drugs must be used concurrently. Since excess depression is a dose-dependent side effect, dosage reduction should be undertaken when this problem is evident. Elderly clients receiving benzodiazepines need to be warned to avoid driving or other potentially dangerous activities during times when symptoms of excess depression are occurring. Excess depression can also occur with diphenylmethane antihistamines, but is not a problem with buspirone.

Benzodiazepines can cause **paradoxical reactions** of restlessness, agitation, confusion, aggressiveness, and even rage. Outbursts of anger in elderly clients receiving benzodiazepines may suggest the need to consider an alternative medication.

Benzodiazepines can cause **urinary retention** in the elderly. When this occurs, the urine may have a peculiar musty odor. Elderly clients should be taught to report any obvious alteration in urinary frequency, color, or odor. Some clients taking benzodiazepines will experience minor gastrointestinal disturbances such as **nausea.** If so, they can be advised to take the drug with or shortly after a meal or snack to reduce gastrointestinal discomfiture.

When benzodiazepines have been used for longer than approximately 3 months or at doses higher than the recommended ranges, **physical dependence** will develop and **withdrawal symptoms** will occur if the drug is discontinued abruptly. Typical symptoms include anxiety, photophobia, paresthesias, flu-like body aches, fatigue or restlessness, irritability and difficulty concentrating, insomnia or hypersomnia, and muscle twitches. Seizures may even occur. Whenever possible after prolonged use of a benzodiazepine, doses should be decreased gradually over 4–8 weeks to minimize withdrawal symptoms. Success rates for benzodiazepine discontinuation can be improved if carbamazepine, imipramine, or buspirone is given before, during, and after withdrawal of the benzodiazepine.

Buspirone does not cause physical or psychological dependence and does not exhibit cross-tolerance with benzodiazepines. Therefore, abruptly switching a client from a benzodiazepine to buspirone will not prevent benzodiazepine withdrawal. Before initiating buspirone therapy, clients need to be carefully withdrawn from the benzodiazepine as outlined above.

Adverse responses to buspirone are infrequent. The only problems occurring in significantly more than 1% of clients are CNS problems in about 3.4% (dizziness, insomnia, nervousness, drowsiness, or light-headedness), and gastrointestinal problems in about 1.2% (mainly nausea). The main category of adverse reactions to the diphenylmethane antihistamines, such as hydroxyzine, are anticholinergic side effects (e.g., dry mouth) and excess depression (e.g., drowsiness).

Interactions in the Elderly.   The most important interaction of benzodiazepine and antihistamine anxiolytics is certainly the potential for **additive CNS depression** with all other kinds of CNS depressants. The interacting drug might be a narcotic, a sedative-hypnotic, an antipsychotic drug, an antihistamine being used for cold symptoms or allergy, an antihypertensive drug, or an antidepressant with sedative properties, but it is most likely to be alcohol because of its unusually widespread use.

Diphenhydramine and hydroxyzine have substantial anticholinergic properties and should not be used in elderly clients if any other anticholinergic compounds are already required. Tobacco smoking or use of anxiogenic drugs such as cocaine, caffeine, sympathomimetics, or levodopa will naturally decrease the effectiveness of anxiolytic medications.

Administration in the Elderly.   Reactive anxiety is best treated for a brief period of time—a few weeks at most—with a fixed regimen. For example, diazepam taken 3 times per day on a regular schedule for 2 weeks could be appropriate to help an elderly person recover from an additional stress of recent development. Situational anxiety, for example, anxiety associated with some needed but stressful medical procedure, is best treated with individual doses or a short series of administrations during or shortly before the stressful event. Since the benefit provided by benzodiazepines in anxiety disorder is evident from the first administration, the benzodiazepines provide the treatment of choice for reactive or situational anxiety symptoms. For management of chronic generalized anxiety, use of benzodiazepines should normally be limited to 3–4 months with daily doses titrated to the lowest effective level.

Benzodiazepines

ALPRAZOLAM   (Xanax)

Recommended initial oral dose in the elderly: 0.25 mg 2–3 times daily. Maximum 0.75 mg/day for anxiety or 0.25 mg/day for sleep according to OBRA.

Young adult initial dosage for comparison: 0.25–0.5 mg 3 times daily.

CHLORDIAZEPOXIDE   (Librium, A-poxide, SK-Lygen, Sereen, Murcil, Lipoxide, etc.)

Recommended initial oral dose in the elderly: 5 mg 2–4 times daily. Maximum 20 mg/day for anxiety according to OBRA.

Young adult initial dosage for comparison: 5–10 mg 3 or 4 times daily.

CLORAZEPATE   (Tranxene, Gen-xene, generic)

Recommended initial oral dose in the elderly: 7.5–15 mg/day. Maximum 15 mg/day for anxiety according to OBRA.

Young adult initial dosage for comparison: 30 mg/day.

DIAZEPAM   (Valium)

Recommended initial oral dose in the elderly: 2–2.5 mg 1 or 2 times daily. Maximum 5 mg/day for anxiety according to OBRA.

Young adult initial dosage for comparison: 2–10 mg 2–4 times daily.

HALAZEPAM   (Paxipam)

Recommended initial oral dose in the elderly: 20 mg once or twice daily. Maximum 40 mg/day for anxiety or 20 mg at bedtime for sleep according to OBRA.

Young adult initial dosage for comparison: 20–40 mg 3–4 times daily.

LORAZEPAM   (Ativan, generic)

Recommended initial oral dose in the elderly: 1–2 mg/day in divided doses. Maximum 2 mg/day for anxiety or 1 mg/day for sleep according to OBRA.

Young adult initial dosage for comparison: 2–3 mg/day in 2 or 3 doses.

OXAZEPAM   (Serax, generic)

Recommended initial oral dose in the elderly: 10 mg 3 times daily. Maximum 30 mg/day for anxiety or 15 mg/day for sleep according to OBRA.

Young adult initial dosage for comparison: 10–15 mg 3–4 times daily.

PRAZEPAM   (Centrax)

Recommended initial oral dose in the elderly: 10–15 mg/day in divided doses. Maximum 15 mg/day for anxiety according to OBRA.

Young adult initial dosage for comparison: 30 mg/day in divided doses.

Diphenylmethane Antihistamines

HYDROXYZINE   (Atarax, Vistaril, generic)

Recommended initial oral dose in the elderly: No specific recommendation. Maximum 50 mg/day for anxiety or sleep according to OBRA.

Young adult initial dosage for comparison: 50–100 mg 4 times daily.

Azaspirodecanediones

BUSPIRONE   (Buspar)

Recommended initial oral dose in the elderly: No specific recommendation. Maximum 30 mg/day for anxiety according to OBRA.

Young adult initial dosage for comparison: 15 mg/day (5 mg tid).

GEPIRONE

Investigational

REFERENCES AND RECOMMENDED READINGS

Anderson G: Benzodiazepines. *Nurse Practitioner,* 1980; 47(1):50–51.

Baldessarini RJ: *Chemotherapy in Psychiatry, ed 2.* Cambridge, Mass., Harvard University Press, 1985.

Bellantuono C, et al.: Benzodiazepines:clinical pharmacology and therapeutic uses. *Drugs,* 1980; 19:195–219.

Cattabeni F, et al. (eds): *Long-term Effects of Neuroleptics, Advances in Biochemical Psychopharmacology, Vol. 24.* New York, Raven, 1980.

Coleman JH, & Dorevitch AP: Rational use of psychoactive drugs in the geriatric patient. *Drug Intell. Clin. Pharm.* 1981; 15(12):940–944.

Costa E, & Racagni G (eds): *Typical and Atypical Antidepressants. (Adv. Biochem. Psychopharm. Vol. 31 & 32).* New York, Raven, 1982.

Coyle JT, & Enna SJ (eds): *Neuroleptics: Neurochemical, Behavioral, and Clinical Perspectives.* New York, Raven, 1983.

DeGennaro MD, et al.: Antidepressant drug therapy. *Am. J. Nurs.,* 1981; 81:1304–1310.

DeVane CL, & Tingle D: Psychiatric disorders, in Delafuente, Stewart: *Therapeutics in the Elderly.* Baltimore, Williams & Wilkins, 1988, pp. 189–195.

Diamond JM, & Santos AB: Unusual complications of antipsychotic drugs. *Am. Fam. Physician,* 1982; 26(4):153–157.

Feighner JP: The new generation of antidepressants. *J. Clin. Psychiat.,* 1983; 44(11):49–55.

Greenblatt DJ, Shader RI, & Abernethy DR: Current status of benzodiazepines. *N. Engl. J. Med.,* 1983; 309:354–358, 410–416.

Harris B: Drugs and depression. *Am. J. Nurs.,* 1986; 86(3):292–293.

Harris E: Antidepressants: old drugs, new uses. *Am. J. Nurs.,* 1981; 81:1308–1310.

Harris E: Lithium. *Am. J. Nurs.,* 1981; 81(7):1310–1315.

Hollister LE: Current antidepressant drugs: Clinical use. *Drugs,* 1981; 22:129–152.

Hollister LE: Depression: The delicate art of lifting it with drug Rx. *Mod. Med.,* 1982; 50(1):110.

Hollister LE, et al.: Long-term use of diazepam. *JAMA,* 1981; 246(14):1568–1570.

Itil TM, Soldatos C: Epileptogenic side effects of psychotropic drugs. *J. Amer. Med. Assoc.,* 1980; 244:1460–1463.

Jann MW, et al.: Alternative drug therapies for mania: A literature review. *Drug Intell. Clin. Pharm.,* 1984; 18:577–589.

Jefferson JW: Lithium carbonate-induced hypothyroidism: Its many faces. *JAMA,* 1979; 242:271–272.

Johnson FN: *Handbook of Lithium Therapy.* Baltimore, University Park Press, 1980.

Lassler LB, Gauiria JM: Depression in old age. *J. Am. Geriatr. Soc.,* 1978; 26:471–475.

Lippman S: Antidepressant pharmacotherapy. *Am. Fam. Physician,* 1983; 25(6):145–153.

Mackinnon GL, Parker WA: Benzodiazepine withdrawal syndrome: A literature review and evaluation. *Am. J. Drug Alcohol Abuse,* 1982; 9:19–33.

Malick JB, Enna SJ, Yamamura HI: *Anxiolytics: Neurochemical, Behavioral, and Clinical Perspectives.* New York, Raven, 1983.

Marks J: *The Benzodiazepines: Use, Overuse, Misuse, Abuse.* Baltimore, University Park Press, 1978.

Maletta GJ: Neuropsychiatric problems in the elderly, in Gambert (ed): *Contemp. Geriatric. Med.,* Plenum, 1983, pp. 331–374.

Pfeiffer RF, Murrin LC: Pathogenesis and treatment of neuroleptic malignant syndrome. *Gen. Pharmacol.* 1990; 21:267–286.

Prien RP: Lithium in the treatment of affective disorders. *Clin. Neuropharm.,* 1978; 3:113–132.

Rickels K: Benzodiazepines in the treatment of anxiety. *Am. J. Psychother.,* 1982; 36(3):358–370.

Rosenberg JM, Kirschenbaum HL: Lithium. *RN,* 1981; 44:44–46.

Tosteson DC: Lithium and mania. *Sci. Am.,* 1981; 244(4):164–174.

Usdin E, et al. (eds): *Pharmacology of Benzodiazepines.* London, Macmillan Press Ltd., 1982.

White S, Williamson K: What to watch for with minor tranquilizers. *RN,* 1979; 11:57–59.

Williamson J: Depression in the elderly. *Age, Aging,* 1978; 7(suppl):35–40.

CHAPTER 10

Sleep Problems in the Elderly and Related Drug Therapies

The incidence of sleep problems among the elderly is so high as to suggest that a full night of sound sleep may indeed be a blessing that is largely a unique privilege of the young. Most studies indicate that the elderly require less sleep than the young, but these measures are confounded by the fact that elderly individuals are more likely to take naps during the day, and some studies have even suggested that, in fact, total sleep time may be greater for elderly persons. What is certain is that periods of sleep tend to be shorter but more frequent and less sound and refreshing. Some elderly complain about poor sleep incessantly, while others will not discuss it. Relatives who attend the individual may notice that sleep appears to be fitful and restless. Elderly people wake up many more times during the night than younger people, a phenomenon known as **fragmentation**. Although the changing pattern of sleep is sufficiently universal as to suggest that it is an inherent aspect of aging of the nervous system, the fragmentation of sleep for the elderly may be aggravated in a given person by individual factors, including added sources of stress, more frequent nocturia, more frequent daytime naps, or too much coffee consumed too late in the day. The full measure of impact that sleep deficits impose on the elderly can only be appreciated from a perspective of the role that sleep plays in physical and psychological rejuvenation.

SLEEP AND DREAMING

Sleep is a time during which consciousness is temporarily suspended so as to allow the body to undertake activities that provide for mental and physical restoration. To support this period of inactivity, muscle tone decreases along with heart rate, respiration, blood pressure, and body temperature. Basal metabolic rate decreases, allowing for a diminished rate of urine production. Oxygen consumption by the brain slows, allowing for a reduction in blood flow to the brain.

One of the most persistent but erroneous societal myths is that the normal sleep requirement for all people is 8 hours. This comes closest to being the case for young and middle-aged adults, but even then sleep requirements depend in large measure on the level of both physical and mental activity, personality, and life circumstances. Children and adolescents require more than 8 hours for adequate rest, while older adults generally require less. Those providing clinical services for the elderly need to abandon stereotypes regarding sleep expectations and to focus instead on the individual client's sleep pattern and requirements and whether or not the current pattern is adequate to the client's health needs.

Sleep is part of a daily rhythm, the sleep-wake cycle. Since this cycle repeats in a 24-hour period, it is a **diurnal rhythm,** or 24-hour rhythm. Daily rhythms impact each of us a bit differently; some of us are most alert in the morning; others are most alert in midafternoon or evening. The sleep-wake cycle is also, however, a **circadian rhythm,** meaning that it is linked to and driven by the day-night light cycle. One factor that can weaken the sleep-wake cycle for the elderly who are confined to bed is diminished contact with the outside world and increased exposure to artificial lighting. Lack of occupational demands after retirement and fewer social contacts may also cause an elderly person to develop a more free-running rhythm, such as occurs in laboratory studies when environmental cues are eliminated. When this occurs, regularity of rhythm needs to be restored by consistent synchronizing of activities such as scheduling bedtime, waking time, and exercise periods.

Within the sleep phase, two distinct sleep states occur, called **dreaming** (paradoxical or rapid-eye-movement (REM)) **sleep** and **nondreaming** (slow-wave) **sleep.** Nondreaming sleep is further divided into four stages labeled 1 through 4. Stages 1 and 3 are brief transitional stages that need not concern us overly much here. Stage 1, in fact, may not be true sleep and corresponds to the common language phrase "falling asleep." During Stage 1, a person can still be alerted by someone calling his or her name.

Stage 2 of nondreaming sleep is how the largest part of the night is spent and serves as a launching pad, so to speak, for periodic excursions into either Stage 4 or dreaming. Episodes of either Stage 4 or dreaming always begin and end in Stage 2 unless the person awakes abruptly directly out of a Stage 4 or dream episode. Stage 4 and dream episodes provide for the basic work of sleep: physical and psychological rejuvenation.

Stage 4 of Nondreaming Sleep and the Elderly

Stage 4 of nondreaming sleep is characterized by continuous high-amplitude sawed-toothed slow-waves called **delta waves.** Stage 4 episodes are pronounced in children and young adults, occurring predominately during the first half of the night. Stage 4 provides for physical rejuvenation and answers the need that is manifest as physical tiredness. Athletes engaged in an intensive regimen of physical training experience more Stage

4 sleep than do others. Intensive exercise close to bedtime increases the time spent in Stage 4. During Stage 4, replenishment of macromolecules (anabolism) proceeds at maximum rates. A sharp peak in the rate of secretion of growth hormone (which in adults provides mainly for tissue repair) occurs during Stage 4. Renewal of the skin proceeds at its maximum rate during this stage, as well, as evidenced by increased proliferation and keratinization of epidermal cells.

The elderly, however, exhibit little and sometimes a complete absence of Stage 4 sleep. Whether this change in the sleep pattern is a **consequence** of diminished physical activity or whether it is a **cause** of lessened ability to rejuvenate the physiology are open questions. The fact remains that the near absence of Stage 4 sleep in the elderly is one of the two major changes in their sleep pattern; the other is fragmentation described earlier.

Dream Sleep and the Elderly

Dream sleep is accompanied by several distinctive events: more frequent brain waves (increasing into the beta range), rapid eye movements, increased pulse and respiratory rates, penile erections in males, but further decrease in the tone of postural muscles. Mental activity increases along with physiological adjustments to support increased mental activity, yet the muscles are more fully depressed to ensure that the mental activity has no opportunity to manifest as behavior.

That dreaming provides some kind of crucial service to health is evident from the fact that the brain carefully preserves its total dream time. When an individual is deprived of dreaming for one or more nights, by whatever circumstance, a compensatory increase in the percentage of sleep time spent dreaming will occur on the first night that the person's sleep is undisturbed—a phenomenon known as **REM rebound.** If REM deprivation occurs excessively without the opportunity for compensation, severe psychiatric disturbances will develop, starting with irritability and diminished ability to process information, progressing to aggressiveness, persecutory delusions, and hallucinations.

Dreaming provides for the mind what Stage 4 sleep provides for the body. It provides psychological rejuvenation. During the course of each waking period, experiences are stored in our neural circuits in the form of electrophysiological potentials in what neuroscientists call **short-term memory.** Like the random access memory of a computer, however, short-term memory has limited capacity and would soon be exhausted without transfer of neural representations into a more permanent format. Dreaming appears to be the major opportunity for that transfer (or consolidation) of experience into long-term memory. In contrast to short-term memory, long-term memory is neuroanatomic (or structural) in form with relatively unlimited capacity.

The activity of dreaming can be likened to the process that a secretary goes through to file papers no longer in active use. The secretary's effort actually promotes two different advantages: (1) the papers are stored away in a systematic manner that ensures their retrievability should that be necessary in the future; and (2) the active work area—the desktop—is cleared of noncurrent material so that new activities can be undertaken without interference. Thus, in the case of the neural system, the process of consolidation of memory during dreaming not only ensures a long-term record of experience but, perhaps even more crucial, clears and refreshes the limited-capacity neural circuits for the encounters of a new day.

The time that a person requires for dreaming has been shown to depend on life circumstances that reflect the magnitude of challenges confronting him. For example, dream time increases when people change jobs, start or quit school, marry or divorce, or increase intellectual activity. People who have a fixed, stable lifestyle exhibit less dream time, while those with fluid, flexible, changing life circumstances dream more. When long-sleepers are compared with short-sleepers of the same age, the difference in total sleep time can be accounted for entirely by the difference in dream time—the time spent in nondreaming sleep is the same.

Elderly people show less change in dream time than they do in Stage 4 of nondreaming sleep. In fact, elderly people spend as much time dreaming as younger people, if taken as a percentage of total sleep time—about 20%. Were it not for the fact that total nighttime sleep is less for older people than their younger counterparts, dream time would be the same.

On the other hand, given the increased use of medications with aging, elderly people are more likely to be taking one or another drug that interferes with dreaming. Such drugs are called **REM suppressants.** Ironically, some of the very drugs that are used for sleep disorders have this detrimental effect, but so too do many other classes of psychotropic agents. Given the importance of dreaming to psychological functioning and mental health, REM suppressant medications should be avoided whenever possible and preference given to drugs of comparable benefit that lack this effect.

Those providing clinical services for the elderly need to reflect on the importance of adequate sleep and adequate opportunity for each stage of sleep to the health of clients. Complaints regarding sleep need to be fully assessed and changing sleep patterns monitored. Attention needs to be paid to controllable factors that influence opportunity for sleep—ensuring quiet, darkness, and a comfortable temperature for appropriately long time periods and providing opportunity for performance of presleep rituals (bathing, brushing teeth, reading, prayer). Every effort should be made to ensure that institutional activity schedules and schedules for medical procedures not interfere with the opportunity for needed sleep.

CLASSIFICATION OF SLEEP DISORDERS AND EPIDEMIOLOGY IN THE ELDERLY

Primary sleep disorders include insomnias, excess daytime sleepiness, disorders of the sleep-wake cycle, and parasomnias (Table 10.1). Many of these are more common for elderly persons. Although it is not known if jet lag affects the elderly more than younger people, there is evidence that aging

Table 10.1 Major Sleep Disorders

Diagnostic category	Incidence	Sex ratio	Drug treatments
Insomnias	More in elderly	F > M	Hypnotics, sleep-aids, or L-tryptophan
Psychophysiological	Common all age groups	?	As above
Due to sleep apneas	Very common; less in elderly	M > F	Imipramine
Due to nocturnal myoclonus or akathisias	?	M = F	Diazepam
Drug-induced	Usually caffeine	?	Cut back late day coffee.
Secondary to depression	More common among elderly	F > M	Treat depression.
Excess daytime sleepiness	More common among elderly	?	
Associated with insomnia	Common	F > M	Determined by type of insomnia
Associated with insufficient sleep	Common	?	None
Narcolepsy	Rare	M > F	Stimulants
Disorders of the sleep-wake cycle			
Transient (e.g., jet lag, work schedule shifts)	Common; less in elderly	M = F	None
Persistent	Rare	None	
Parasomnias			
State 4-related (e.g., sleepwalking, night terrors)	Less in elderly	M > F	Diazapam
REM-related (nightmares)	Common	M = F	None

weakens the circadian rhythm. For example, elderly people adjust less well to shifts in work schedules. There is also an increase in many kinds of parasomnias, including nocturnal dyspnea and orthopnea brought on by congestive heart failure, nocturnal angina, and even dysrhythmias.

Insomnia

For the elderly, insomnia and associated daytime sleepiness are the main issue. All people experience isolated episodes of insomnia when anticipating or recovering from an emotionally difficult event. Bereavement, which occurs with greater frequency for elderly people, may cause periods of insomnia that last as much as a year. Elderly people are more likely to have chronic medical problems which, because of pain, discomfort, fever, cough, dyspnea, itchiness, or anxiety, interfere with sleep. Sleeplessness itself may become a cause of worry. So stress clearly contributes to insomnia, but how much of a role stress plays in the insomnia of elderly people is a difficult question to answer. Certainly there can be no doubt that stress exacerbates the changing sleep pattern that is inherent in aging and no doubt aging is associated with added categories and added frequency of stressful circumstances. However, the exceedingly high incidence of sleep problems among the elderly suggests that part of the problem is a direct expression of the neurophysiological consequences of aging.

The incidence of insomnia is neglible during childhood and adolescence, though many children experience isolated and unpredictable instances of poor sleep. Approximately 15% of young adult women and men experience insomnia, and that incidence remains nearly constant until the mid-forties. In the late forties, a sharp gender differential develops in the incidence of insomnia, with about 40% of women but only 20% of men experiencing difficulties with sleep. After age 65, the incidence of insomnia in men climbs, but only to approximately 25%, while the incidence in women continues at the higher level of approximately 40%.

The term *insomnia* actually subsumes two rather distinct kinds of problems. It can occur at the beginning of the night as **difficulty getting to sleep** or it can occur later during the night in the form of **early morning awakenings.** Although most people think of insomnia in terms of the first problem, it is actually the early morning awakenings that are more common and troublesome, especially for the elderly. Estimates in the United States are a 15% incidence of frequent difficulties getting to sleep, but a full 37% of adults have problems of early morning awakenings. One important difference between the two problems is the kind of drug that might be employed (if any is required at all). Difficulties in initiating sleep are best treated with short- and quick-acting hypnotics, while early morning awakenings are best managed with intermediate-acting drugs that persist well into the night.

Sleep Apnea

For some elderly clients, sleep apnea is frequently a factor contributing to fragmentation of sleep. **Sleep apnea** is characterized by marked reduction or cessation of respiration during sleep. It occurs in approximately 28% of elderly people. It may be due to depression of the central respiratory center or obstruction of air flow. In the latter case, periods of loud snoring typically alternate with periods of silence and apnea, typically lasting 20 to 40 seconds. The lack of air exchange during apnea interferes with deep sleep, because partial arousal is necessary to terminate each episode. Sometimes hundreds of such episodes occur nightly, resulting in sleeplessness, which can then be a cause of nocturnal confusion and wanderings or excess daytime sleepiness the following day. Sleep apneas are sometimes position-dependent and therefore come and go throughout the night as the person shifts position. Frequency also increases as the night goes on. Elderly clients suffering from this kind of insomnia should not be treated with standard hypnotic drugs, because all of these depress the respiratory center and can potentially aggravate sleep apnea. Antidepressants with sedative properties, such as imipramine, are a useful alternative.

Restless Leg Syndrome and Nocturnal Myoclonus

Restless leg syndrome and nocturnal myoclonus are two other kinds of events that are more common among the elderly and contribute to sleep fragmentation. **Restless leg syndrome** is also known as **nocturnal akathisias.** Individuals with this condition describe creeping, crawling sensations in their legs (or less often the arms) along with an irresistable urge to move. In severe cases the person may feel compelled to stand up, walk about, pace rapidly, or stomp their feet. Massage provides only brief respite. Others may have severe **nocturnal myoclonus**—an exaggeration of the jerky movements that occur asymptomatically in many people as they fall asleep, but which cause arousal and sleep fragmentation when overly severe.

SEDATIVE-HYPNOTIC USE IN THE ELDERLY

Before initiating treatment for insomnia with a sedative-hypnotic, a full clinical examination should be undertaken with the aim of determining the likely cause of the insomnia, its severity, and the presence of disease that might alter the response to a sedative-hypnotic compound. Studies conducted in sleep labs indicate that elderly persons may overestimate the severity of their sleep problems. Many elderly spend more time in bed than is necessary for their sleep requirements without realizing it. They may cling to the expectation that 8 hours sleep is the right amount or they may feel that they have nothing to get up for. Inevitably, people are more aware of the time they spend awake than that which they spend sleeping. Elderly people studied in sleep labs often report having been awake when awakened out of sleep. Nondrug alternatives should be considered rather than reflexive prescription of a sleeping pill, especially for the elderly who are more likely to experience adverse effects of hypnotics than are younger adults.

Drugs available for management of insomnia are classified as hypnotics or sleeping pills; sometimes they are more fully characterized as sedative-hypnotics, because at lower doses the same drugs can be used to provide daytime sedation of an agitated individual. The term *hypnotic* in pharmacology does not imply anything resembling the concept of hypnosis as it is encountered in psychiatry, but rather a drug-induced state more or less resembling natural sleep. How much the drug-induced state resembles natural sleep depends, in large part, on the specific drug selected for use, for most of the hypnotics suppress one or another of the states of sleep with a corresponding increase in other components of sleep. Most non-benzodiazepine hypnotics suppress dreaming, while many of the benzodiazepines reduce the quantity of Stage 4 of nondreaming sleep. While the detrimental effects of dream suppression have been well-documented, less is known about the health consequences of suppressing Stage 4 of nondreaming sleep.

The sedative-hypnotics taken as a whole are a rather homogenous class of drugs, sharing more elements in common than differences. The drugs currently available are loosely grouped into three categories:

1. benzodiazepines, which are currently most widely used;
2. barbiturates, which were the major hypnotics during the 1940s through the mid-sixties;
3. miscellaneous other drugs.

For the elderly, the benzodiazepines are the clear drugs of choice, at least as an initial treatment approach. However, certain individual clients will be unable to tolerate a benzodiazepine, for one reason or another, giving the alternative drugs a continuing, limited role in treatment of insomnia.

Clinical Indications in the Elderly.   Hypnotics are indicated for short-term management of insomnia. The emphasis in that statements needs to be placed on **short-term,** because no hypnotic currently available provides continuing benefit if used on a regular nightly basis for more than an appropriate period of time. How long a period of time is appropriate depends on which drug is selected, but for the most part nonbenzodiazepines are limited to approximately 14 consecutive nights of use, while the benzodiazepines range from 3–5 weeks of effectiveness on that basis. These limitations of period of usefulness do not apply to situations where the drugs is taken as-needed if the client limits use to 2–3 times per week or less. With that kind of irregular use, benefit can be maintained indefinitely.

Clients who have difficulty only with getting to sleep initially need a drug that will act as a sleep inducer. A short-acting drug will usually be most appropriate, because these drugs are also quick-acting and will result in no measurable residual action the next day. On the other hand, clients who suffer from frequent early-morning awakenings with inability to get back to sleep need a drug whose action persists well into the night—an intermediate-acting drug which can act as a sleep sustainer. Clients who experience both kinds of problems may benefit from products with the specific ability to both act quickly and sustain their action for many hours. The drugs available, today, in the benzodiazepine category provide a full range of options with respect to duration of action, allowing physicians to carefully select a drug with respect to both potential benefits and certain side effects that are related to duration.

Altered Pharmacokinetics or Pharmacodynamics in the Elderly. All of the sedative-hypnotics, regardless of group, are inactivated mainly by metabolism prior to excretion. Except for aprobarbital and phenobarbital, which may be eliminated up to 25–50% by renal excretion, all but neglible amounts of administered barbiturates are metabolised in the liver before elimination. The same can be said for the benzodiazepines except that flurazepam and quazepam produce an active metabolite, *N*-desalkylflurazepam, which is excreted largely unchanged by the kidneys. Thus, renal impairment will have little impact on plasma levels of most hypnotics, but changing capacity for liver metabolism in the elderly must be taken into account. The barbiturates and the longer-acting benzodiazepines are metabolized by oxidation utilizing the liver microsomal enzyme system, which clearly undergoes a diminishment in capacity with aging. The shorter-acting benzodiazepines, such as temazepam and triazolam, are inactivated in the liver by conjugation, which is not much altered as a result of aging. Therefore, the pharmacokinetics of these drugs will be little different in elderly than in younger individuals. Zolpidem, a new, miscellaneous hypnotic drug that pharmacologically resembles the benzodiazepines, was specifically tested for age-dependent pharmacokinetics during clinical trials, revealing a 32%-longer half-life in clients over age 70.

Barbiturates and benzodiazepines both exhibit age-dependent changes in pharmacodynamics as well. Put simply, the effects of a given plasma concentration of either type of drug will be greater in an elderly person than a younger person. Apparently, the central nervous system of the elderly person is more sensitive, in some respect, to the depressant action of hypnotic drugs.

Adverse Effects and Contraindications in the Elderly.   Adverse effects of hypnotics fall in mainly in six categories, though the specific drug selected will determine the liability for certain categories of problems (Table 10.2):

1. excess depression;
2. paradoxical excitation;
3. increased early morning awakenings and next day anxiety;
4. REM suppression;
5. hypersensitivity reactions;
6. tolerance and dependence.

Excess depression is a categorical term that encompasses a wide range of possible reactions, including somnolence, lethargy, weakness, ataxia, loss of equilibrium, confusion, lack of concentration, depressed respiration, and psychiatric depression. One potential manifestation of excess depression requiring specific mention in relation to hypnotics is **residual depression.** This refers to the potential for continuing drug effects of the depressive variety during the waking hours the day following the use of a sleeping pill the previous night. The extent to which this will occur is a predictable consequence of drug selection; it will be a major problem if a long-acting drug was used; a potentially significant one if an intermediate-acting drug was selected; and no problem at all if the drug was a short-acting one. If the elderly client is one who may benefit from rather than be impaired by a modest sedative effect continuing into the next day, then residual depression can be viewed as an added therapeutic benefit rather than an adverse effect. Elderly people who experience excess depression from use of a hypnotic drug need to be advised to avoid driving or other tasks requiring mental alertness during the period of depression. Concurrent use of alcoholic beverages should be avoided. Clients should be observed for indications of drug-induced psychiatric depression, suicidal tendencies, or hoarding of medications for suicide attempts.

Paradoxical excitation caused by hypnotics can be manifested as anxiety, excitement, nervousness, or agitation. The term *paradoxical* al-

Table 10.2 Comparison of Attributes of Sedative-Hypnotics

Attribute	Benzodiazepines			Barbiturates		Piperidine-diones	Ethchlorvynol	Chloral Derivatives
	Short-acting	Intermediate-acting	Long-Acting	Short-Acting	Intermediate-Acting			
Sleep effects								
Acute effectiveness as sleep inducer	++	++	++	++	0	++	++	++
Acute effectiveness as sleep sustainer	0	+	++	0	++	0	0	++
Effectiveness after 2 weeks	+	++	++	0	0	0	0	0
Acute REM suppression	0	0	0	++	++	++	++	0
Elevated REM during withdrawal	0	0	0	++	++	++	++	0
Suppression of slow-wave sleep	++	++	++	+/-	+/-	+/-	+	+
Abuse potential								
Psychological dependence	+	+/-	+/-	++	++	++	++	++
Physical dependence	+	+/-	+/-	++	++	++	++	++
Induction of liver enzymes	0	0	0	++	++	++	++	++
Suicide potential	0	0	0	++	++	++	++	++
Adverse effects								
Residual depression	0	+	++	+	++	+	+	++
Increased early morning awakenings	++	+	0	+	0	+	+	0
Paradoxical excitation	++	++	++	++	++	++	+	++
Acute intoxication	0	0	0	+	+	++	+	+

0, does not produce indicated effect; +/-, equivocal tendency toward effect; +, moderate tendency to produce effect; ++, strong likelihood or severity of effect.

ludes to the fact that these symptoms are opposite to those that one normally associates with this class of drugs. Paradoxical reactions are more frequent among the elderly and more frequent when depressant drugs are used repeatedly. Inpatients should be protected from self-injury during paradoxical reactions to the extent possible.

Short-acting hypnotics frequently produce such a rapid depressant effect and subsequent rebound that the rebound occurs in the form of anxiety during the next day or even as an increased likelihood of early morning awakenings. These phenomena have been noted in particular with the short-acting benzodiazepine, triazolam. These problems are practically nonexistent with intermediate-acting hypnotics.

REM suppression occurs with all barbiturate sedative-hypnotics and most of the miscellaneous ones as well (chloral hydrate and zolpidem are two exceptions). Benzodiazepine hypnotics produce little or no REM suppression. Tolerance develops to the REM-suppressant effects of those hypnotics that cause this problem, however, only after the same time span associated with loss of therapeutic benefit. If a REM-suppressing hypnotic is used long enough for tolerance to develop, REM elevation will inevitably occur later when the drug is discontinued (i.e., as a withdrawal symptom).

Allergic reactions occur in a small percentage of individuals with nearly all drugs, and hypnotics are no exception. Allergic reactions are generally not dose-dependent; that is, they can occur to a major extent even when doses are small. Allergic reactions are among the least predictable side effects with only the client's personal history of drug reactions providing significant predictive value. Allergic reactions to hypnotics can include angioderma, skin rashes, and even life-threatening skin problems. Any occurrence of allergic reaction needs to be carefully recorded in the client's medication history, and the client needs to be informed regarding the problem so that personnel involved in future medical care can be informed.

Tolerance and **dependence** are unquestionably the limiting features for this class of drugs. Were it not for these problems, hypnotics would find much greater favor in clinical practice. The development of tolerance creates a built-in limit on the usefulness of these drugs, in particular, the period of time over which they can be used successfully on a nightly basis. All hypnotics have the ability to cause intoxication resembling that produced by alcohol, with consequent risk of injury from poorly controlled behavior. Long-term use promotes both psychological and physical dependence. A withdrawal syndrome, possibly even life-threatening when extreme, follows when the drug is discontinued. The severity of the withdrawal syndrome is directly proportional to the degree of tolerance and physical dependence that has been allowed to develop. Withdrawal symptoms include anxiety, muscle twitches, tremor, weakness, dizziness, nausea and vomiting, insomnia, weight loss, orthostatic hypotension, and psychiatric symptoms ranging from delusions and hallucinations to paranoia and delirium. The life-threatening component of withdrawal is the possibility of seizures. Although short-term use of normal therapeutic doses of hypnotics should not result in a full-blown withdrawal syndrome, a lesser form called **rebound hyperexcitability** may occur, resulting in one or more nights of diminished sleep. Among the benzodiazepines, triazolam, the short-acting agent, is more likely to cause rebound insomnia than the intermediate or long-acting drugs. Clients need to be forwarned and reassured that this effect is expected and will go away with continued abstinence.

Benzodiazepines provide a number of distinct advantages in comparison with barbiturates and most of the miscellaneous agents. One major advantage is that therapeutic doses are much lower than the doses that cause either intoxication or death. Thus, episodes of inadvertant intoxication and the likelihood that a prescribed benzodiazepine will be used successfully in a suicide attempt are much less common. Benzodiazepines have rarely if ever been implicated as the sole drug involved in a suicide, although they have frequently been used in combination with other CNS depressants. Should overdose occur, a benzodiazepine antagonist called flumazenil (Romazicon) is available for use in emergency room treatment. No comparable antidote exists for barbiturates.

Benzodiazepines also have the advantage of altering REM sleep to a much smaller extent than most other hypnotics. Benzodiazepines do not alter activity of liver enzymes in the manner of barbiturates, and thus have one less set of drug interactions. Finally, their abuse liability, though well-documented and all too frequently encountered, is less than that of barbiturates and most miscellaneous hypnotics. The down side for benzodiazepines is the occurrence of two kinds of side effects not evident with most other hypnotics: vivid, sometimes annoying, dreams or nightmares and, occasionally, suppression of ovulation in female clients (a drawback that is irrelevant for most elderly women).

Most miscellaneous hypnotics, including paraldehyde, glutethimide, methyprylon, and ethchlorvynol, resemble the barbiturates in their general characteristics and cannot be recommended for use in elderly clients. One exceptional drug among the miscellaneous agents is zolpidem, a hypnotic newly approved in 1993. Although not a benzodiazepine, it resembles that subgroup in its pharmacology. The benzodiazepine receptor in the brain exists in at least three subtypes. While benzodiazepines act on all three types, zolpidem is relatively selective for one type. Possibly as a result, it lacks the muscle relaxant and antiseizure activity of benzodiazepines, but shares the hypnotic action and, unfortunately, the same abuse liability.

Interactions in the Elderly.   Interactions of sedative-hypnotics fall into three main categories:

1. additive CNS depression,
2. induction of liver enzymes,
3. inhibition of metabolism of the sedative-hypnotic by drugs that inhibit liver enzyme activity.

The first of these occurs with virtually any sedative-hypnotic when the drug is used with alcohol, antihistamines, narcotics, anxiolytics, neuroleptics, antidepressants with sedative properties, or antihypertensive drugs with depressive influences. Elderly clients use more different drugs, on average, than do younger individuals, so the likelihood of additive CNS depression is higher. Oversedation, dizziness, ataxia, confusion, and cognitive impairments are examples of excess depression that occur more often in elderly persons than younger adults.

Induction of liver enzymes occurs with all of the hypnotics except the benzodiazepines. Dosage schedules for other medications may have to be altered as a result if regular, nightly use of a nonbenzodiazepine hypnotic is undertaken. Certain drugs inhibit the metabolism of particular hypnotics; for example, sodium valproate and monoamine oxidase inhibitors slow metabolism of barbiturates.

Administration in the Elderly.   Every effort should be made to seek alternatives to hypnotic therapy for long-term management of insomnia. Hypnotics should not be prescribed for regular, nightly use for periods in excess of the accepted limits: 2 weeks for barbiturates and miscellaneous hypnotics, 3–5 weeks for benzodiazepines, depending on the specific drug selection.

Most elderly clients will respond to lower doses of hypnotics and they require lower doses because of greater sensitivity to adverse effects. However, elderly clients suffering from confusion may be more resistant to the sedative action afforded by these compounds.

Benzodiazepine Hypnotics

CLOBAZAM   (Frisium)

Duration: Long-acting

Investigational.

ESTAZOLAM   (ProSom)

Duration: Intermediate-acting.

Recommended initial oral dose in the elderly: 1 mg at bedtime; 0.5 mg if small or debilitated.

Young adult initial dosage for comparison: 1 mg at bedtime.

Recommended maximum duration of nightly use: Not determined.

FLURAZEPAM   (Dalmane)

Duration: Long-acting.

Recommended initial oral dose in the elderly: 15 mg at bedtime. Maximum 15 mg/day according to OBRA.

Young adult initial dosage for comparison: 15–30 mg at bedtime.

Recommended maximum duration of nightly use: 4 weeks.

NITRAZEPAM   (Mogadon)

Duration: Long-acting.

Investigational.

QUAZEPAM   (Doral)

Duration: Long-acting.

Recommended initial oral dose in the elderly: 15 mg at bedtime; attempt to reduce dose to 7.5 mg after first 1 or 2 nights. Maximum 7.5 mg/day according to OBRA.

Young adult initial dosage for comparison: 15 mg at bedtime; possibly reduce to 7.5 after individual response is determined.

Recommended maximum duration of nightly use: not determined.

TEMAZEPAM   (Restoril, generic)

Duration: Intermediate-acting.

Recommended initial oral dose in the elderly: 15 mg at bedtime. Maximum 15 mg/day according to OBRA.

Young adult initial dosage for comparison: 15–30 mg at bedtime.

Recommended maximum duration of nightly use: 5 weeks.

TRIAZOLAM   (Halcion)

Duration: Short-acting.

Recommended initial oral dose in the elderly: 0.125–0.25 mg at bedtime. Maximum 0.125 mg/day according to OBRA.

Young adult initial dosage for comparison: 0.125–0.5 mg at bedtime.

Recommended maximum duration of nightly use: 3 weeks.

Barbiturate Hypnotics

AMOBARBITAL   (Amytal, generic)

Duration: Intermediate-acting.

Recommended initial oral dose in the elderly: No specific recommendation, but substantially lower.

Young adult initial dosage for comparison: 65–200 mg at bedtime.

Recommended maximum duration of nightly use: 2 weeks.

APROBARBITAL   (Alurate)

Duration: Intermediate-acting.

Recommended initial oral dose in the elderly: No specific recommendation, but substantially lower.

Young adult initial dosage for comparison: 40–160 mg at bedtime.

Recommended maximum duration of nightly use: 2 weeks.

BUTALBITAL   (Butazem, Butisol, Butal, Butalan, Sarisol, Soduben, generic)

Duration: Intermediate-acting.

Recommended initial oral dose in the elderly: No specific recommendation, but substantially lower.

Young adult initial dosage for comparison: 50–100 mg at bedtime.

Recommended maximum duration of nightly use: 2 weeks.

PENTOBARBITAL   (Nembutal, generic)

Duration: Short-acting.

Recommended initial oral dose in the elderly: No specific recommendation, but substantially lower.

Young adult initial dosage for comparison: 100 mg at bedtime.

Recommended maximum duration of nightly use: 2 weeks.

PHENOBARBITAL   (Luminal, generic)

Duration: Long-acting.

Recommended initial oral dose in the elderly: No specific recommendation, but substantially lower.

Young adult initial dosage for comparison: 100–320 mg at bedtime.

Recommended maximum duration of nightly use: 2 weeks.

SECOBARBITAL   (Seconal)

Duration: Short-acting.

Recommended initial oral dose in the elderly: No specific recommendation, but substantially lower.

Young adult initial dosage for comparison: 100 mg.

Recommended maximum duration of nightly use: 2 weeks.

TALBUTAL   (Lotusate)

Duration: Intermediate-acting.

Recommended initial oral dose in the elderly: No specific recommendation, but substantially lower.

Young adult initial dosage for comparison: 120 mg at bedtime.

Recommended maximum duration of nightly use: 2 weeks.

Miscellaneous Hypnotics

CHLORAL HYDRATE (Noctec, generic)

Duration: Short-acting.

Recommended initial oral dose in the elderly: Maximum 750 mg/day for anxiety or 500 mg at bedtime for sleep according to OBRA.

Young adult initial dosage for comparison: 500–1000 mg at bedtime.

Recommended maximum duration of nightly use: 2 weeks.

ETHCHLORVYNOL (Placidyl)

Duration: Short-acting.

Recommended initial oral dose in the elderly: Smallest effective dose.

Young adult initial dosage for comparison: 500 mg at bedtime.

Recommended maximum duration of nightly use: 1 week.

ETHINAMATE (Valmid)

Duration: Short-acting.

Recommended initial oral dose in the elderly: 500 mg at bedtime.

Young adult initial dosage for comparison: 500–1000 mg at bedtime.

Recommended maximum duration of nightly use: 7 nights.

GLUTETHIMIDE (Doriden)

Duration: Short-acting.

Recommended initial oral dose in the elderly: Not greater than 500 mg at bedtime.

Young adult initial dosage for comparison: 250–500 mg at bedtime.

Recommended maximum duration of nightly use: 3–7 nights.

METHYPRYLON   (Noludar)

Duration: Short-acting.

Recommended initial oral dose in the elderly: No specific recommendation.

Young adult initial dosage for comparison: 200–400 mg at bedtime.

Recommended maximum duration of nightly use: 7 nights.

PARALDEHYDE   (Paral, generic)

Duration: Intermediate-acting.

Recommended initial oral dose in the elderly: No specific recommendation.

Young adult initial dosage for comparison: 5–10 mg at bedtime.

Recommended maximum duration of nightly use: 2 weeks.

ZOLPIDEM   (Ambien)

Duration: Short-acting.

Recommended initial oral dose in the elderly: 5 mg at bedtime.

Young adult initial dosage for comparison: 10 mg at bedtime.

Recommended maximum duration of nightly use: 7–10 days.

REFERENCES AND RECOMMENDED READINGS

Bevier WC, Bliwise DL, Bliwise NG, Bunnell DE, Horvath SM: Sleep patterns of older adults and the effects of exercise. *J. Clin. Exp. Gerontol.* 1992; 14(1): 1–15.

Borkovec TD: Insomnia. *J. Consult. Clin. Psychol.* 1982; 50:880–895.

Castleden M: Management of insomnia in the elderly, in K. O'Malley and JL Waddington (eds): *Therapeutics in the Elderly,* New York, Elsevier Sci. Publ, 1985, pp. 163–167.

Erman MK: Insomnia: treatment approaches. *Drug Ther.* 1984; 14(8):103.

Gillin JC, Mendelson WB, Sitaram N, Wyatt RJ: The neuropharmacology of sleep and wakefulness. *Annu. Rev. Pharmacol. Toxicol.* 1978; 18:563–579.

Harris E: Sedative-hypnotic drugs. *Am. J. Nurs.* 1981; 81(7):1329–1334.

Hartmann EL: *The Functions of Sleep.* New Haven, Yale University Press, 1977.

Hauri P: *The Sleep Disorders.* Kalamazoo, Mich., The Upjohn Company, 1977.

Kales A, et al.: Rebound insomnia and rebound anxiety: a review. *Pharmacology* 1983; 26:121–137.

Lader M, Lugaresi E, Richardson RG (eds): The benzodiazepines and insomnia. *Clin. Neuropharm.* 1985; 8(Suppl. 1).

Lader MH, Petursson H: Long-term effects of benzodiazepines. *Neuropharmacology* 1983; 22:527–533.

Lerner R: Sleep loss in the aged: Implications for nursing practice. *J. Gerontol. Nurs.* 1982; 8:323–326.

Mendelson WB: *The Use and Misuse of Sleeping Pills: A Clinical Guide.* New York, Plenum, 1980.

Millman RP, Weaver TE: Broken sleep. *Am. J. Nurs.* 1986; 86(2):146–150.

Pollak CP: Sleep disorders and sleep dysfunctions in the elderly, in Rossman: *Clin. Geriatr.,* Lippincott, 1986, pp. 693–700.

Prinz P, Raskind M: Aging and sleep disorders, in Williams, R, Karacan I (eds): *Sleep Disorders: Diagnosis and Treatment,* 1978, John Wiley & Sons, New York, pp. 303–321.

Quan SF, Bamforn CR, Beutler LE: Sleep disturbances in the elderly. *Geriatrics* 1984; 39(9):42–47.

Roehrs T, Zorick F, Roth T: Sleep disorders in the elderly. *Geriatr. Med. Today,* 1984; 3(6):78–86.

Simon C: Benzodiazepine hypnotics for insomnia. *American Journal of Nursing* 1983; 83(9):1330–1332.

Walsleben J: Sleep disorders. *Am. J. Nurs.* 1982; 82(6):936–940.

Weitzman ED: Sleep and its disorders. *Annu. Rev. Neurosci.* 1981; 4:381–417.

Zarcone VP Jr: Diagnosis and treatment of excessive daytime sleepiness. *Clin. Neuropharmacol.* 1977; 2:87–97.

CHAPTER 11

Drug Abuse and Drug Misuse among the Elderly

Drug abuse and drug misuse among the elderly share many features in common with the drug problems of younger persons, but also they present some very distinctive characteristics. For the most part, the principles are the same, but the patterns of occurrence differ. It is best in any discussion of drug abuse and misuse to start with a definition of terms and an elaboration of concepts, because terminology continues to be used inconsistently and misconceptions persist regarding the nature of the drug abuse problem.

THE NATURE OF DRUG ABUSE AND DRUG MISUSE

It is popular these days to extend the concept of drug abuse to include the many misapplications of medicines that result either from poor medical practices or limited wisdom of lay persons regarding appropriate use of medications. There are indeed some similarities in the health consequences and even the motivational factors that lead to overly frequent use of, for example, laxatives or antacids and more conventional examples of drug abuse, such as chronic excessive consumption of alcohol. Yet, several of the most basic mechanisms that operate to maintain compulsive patterns of drug abuse are not applicable to the more general instances of misuse. For purposes of clarity, it is probably best to limit the term *drug abuse* to the classic examples characterized by the **self-administration of a chemical substance for the purpose of producing an altered mental state to an extent that significantly impairs the user's physical or mental health or ability to function in a social context.** The broader term, *drug misuse,* can then be used to allude to **the full range of drug misapplications where the intention, however misguided, is health care benefits.**

155

Drug misuse includes the many examples of misguided self-administration, as well as errors in medical judgment pertaining to drug selection, dosage, duration of use, or mode of use. This distinction between drug abuse and drug misuse is a valuable one for discussing drug problems among the elderly, in particular, because by any realistic assessment the incidence of drug abuse among the elderly, while troublesome, is less than among younger people. But, the incidence of drug misuse clearly outstrips anything seen among younger individuals.

The concept of drug abuse, as we have defined it, applies to certain classes of drugs with abuse potential: sedative-hypnotics, narcotics, stimulants, and psychedelics. Mainly the first two of these classes of drugs have major relevance for older individuals. The potential sources for drugs of abuse are grocery and liquor stores (for alcohol, tobacco, and caffeine), illicit drug sources ("pushers"), and prescription medications. The concept of drug misuse, on the other hand, relates to a much broader variety of drug categories and the drugs are obtained from the same three sources plus over-the-counter medications purchased without prescription from the pharmacy.

DRUG ABUSE AMONG THE ELDERLY

Drug abuse is a problem that invariably has antecedents in the biopsychosocial hardships that the individual has needed to endure. For the elderly, one need not search too deeply to suggest that some of the factors leading to drug abuse might include chronic illness, loss of a spouse or child, feelings of uselessness, rejection or isolation, family problems, depression, loss of social status after retirement, poverty, disappointments upon reflecting on one's life, and loss of independence. Some studies have suggested that the loss of structured activity, following from retirement and the emptying of the nest, may be a major factor. Yet, it is a mistake to view drug abuse merely as a symptom of unresolved psychosocial stresses. Whatever the circumstances that led originally to the cycle of abuse, once activated, the abuse pattern introduces additional problems for the abuser. Put simply, drug abuse is both a symptom of underlying problems and a problem in its own right. Most drug abuse treatment specialists believe that it is not possible to skip past the abuse problem to treat the antecedents directly in the hopes that removal of the antecedents will eliminate the abuse problem. The conventional wisdom is that the drug abuse must be dealt with up front either before or simultaneously with efforts to address underlying psychosocial antecedents. The abuser is chemically impaired by the abuse itself and is poorly prepared to deal with deeper-lying issues until the abuse problem is under control.

Psychological Dependence

The problems that the abuse itself can bring to the table include psychological dependence, physical dependence, damage to bodily tissues, alterations in mental function, legal confrontations, and risks of injury or even death. A persistent misconception regarding drug abuse concerns the relationship between so-called psychological dependence and physical dependence. The idea that psychological dependence means *weak* dependence and that physical dependence means *severe* dependence is, quite simply, wrong. The two phenomena are qualitatively different matters and are largely independent. There are examples of drugs that cause physical dependence without psychological dependence, ones that cause psychological dependence without physical dependence, ones that cause neither, and ones that cause both.

The term *psychological dependence* is an unfortunate one, in some respects, because it suggests that the phenomenon does not have a physiological basis. In fact, its basis is just as firmly rooted in neuroanatomic mechanisms as is physical dependence. Psychological dependence occurs with drugs that act on one or the other of two systems in the brain, called the reward and punishment systems. Drugs that either activate the reward system or suppress the punishment system are perceived as pleasant and, in the terminology of behavioral psychology, reinforce the drug-taking behavior. Whatever behaviors were instrumental in procuring and taking the drug are given added emphasis as the brain gradually prioritizes and reorganizes its synaptic relationships. With enough repetitions of the drug-taking experience, the person becomes preoccupied with the procuring and taking of the drug to an extent that interferes with and ultimately displaces other activities requisite to psychological health and social functioning. Psychological dependence is the mechanism that is most basic to the phenomenon of drug abuse. The **abuse liability** of a drug reflects its ability to promote psychological dependence.

Physical Dependence

Physical dependence, when it occurs, can add a second motivation for continuation of drug abuse. It is not a prerequisite for abuse, but can add to the difficulties of confronting abuse. Physical dependence is best understood as part of a triad of problems that begins with tolerance, advances to physical dependence, and culminates in withdrawal symptoms if the drug is later discontinued. **Tolerance** has become a familiar enough concept in modern society, but many people are unaware that it encompasses two components. One part of tolerance is called **drug-disposition tolerance,** involving an increase in the rate at which the liver metabolizes a drug that it is confronted with on a daily basis. This pharmacokinetic alteration is an important matter for clinicians who must anticipate drug interactions and dosage adjustments, but it plays no role in the development of physical dependence. It is the second component of tolerance, **pharmacodynamic tolerance,** that leads directly to physical dependence. Pharmacodynamic tolerance is an adaptive adjustment on the part of the brain to the chronic challenge posed by a drug taken daily. The activities of the brain are delicately balanced in the absence of drug influence and maintained by vigorous homeostatic mechanisms. When a drug influence emerges and then recurs day after day, the homeostatic processes of the brain seek to cancel the primary effect of the drug, as best they can, by adjustments in the contrary direction. Thus, the pharmacodynamic adjustment of the brain to the chronic presence of a depressant drug, like alcohol, is hyperexcitability, or hyperirritability. Now the abuse problem has completed its vicious circle—the victim feels compelled to continue use of the drug just to feel "normal" or to escalate the dose to retrieve the "high" once obtained at the original low dose.

Withdrawal

Withdrawal is the withholding of a drug that a person has been taking on a regular basis (chronically). If the drug is one that causes physical dependence, the result will be one or more withdrawal symptoms, which together comprise the **withdrawal syndrome.** The withdrawal syndrome is basically the behavioral and physiological consequences of unmasking the neurochemical adaptations that have occurred in the brain with the development of physical dependence. Only certain categories of drugs produce symptoms upon withdrawal (see Table 11.1). Withdrawal syndromes are different for each class of drugs, but the same for any two drugs in the same class except for matters of timing.

Long-acting drugs produce withdrawal syndromes that are more protracted, but less severe at any one point. Short-acting drugs produce abrupt, severe withdrawal syndromes. For the most part, measurable physical symptoms of withdrawal and many of the most dramatic behavioral and subjective consequences dissipate within a period of approximately 2 weeks, for most drug classes. This period of intense symptoms is called the **acute withdrawal phase.** A longer period of more subtle symptoms follows, lasting up to six months for the major categories of abused substances. This so-called **postacute withdrawal** period is often characterized by cognitive deficits, poor concentration, memory problems, exaggerated sensitivity to stress, and increased emotionality. These are some of the same kinds of mental stress that often contribute to drug abuse problems in the first place and can play a major role in recidivism after initially successful responses to drug abuse treatment programs.

Other Hazards of Drug Abuse

In addition to the risks of psychological or physical dependence, drug abuse is associated with other hazards. Damage can occur to bodily tissues from chronic use of any drug, but most evidently with some of the drugs of abuse. The elderly person is more liable to many of these risks, such as cirrhosis or fatty liver from alcohol use; gastritis or ulceration from alcohol, tobacco, or caffeine; or cardiovascular problems from any of the same drugs. Tobacco is responsible for an estimated 340,000 premature deaths in the United States, and alcohol for another 125,000 (from medical problems alone).

Drugs of abuse alter mental functioning in the healthiest of individuals. The elderly are more likely to suffer cognitive impairments from alcohol such as delirium, depression, or memory loss. The elderly are more likely also to suffer excess depression from narcotics or sleeping pills. The elderly are more prone, as well, to drug effects that can culminate in fatality, such as seizures, respiratory arrest, cardiac dysrhythmias, or cardiac arrest.

The Elderly Drug Abuser

Two distinct patterns of drug abuse are reported among the elderly, both with respect to alcohol and narcotics. One is the **early onset type,** in which the history of abuse of alcohol or another drug dates from the early or middle years of the person's life. The early onset elderly abuser is most often male and destitute. Elderly people with this pattern exhibit significant personality changes related to their near lifelong history of abuse. They are usually alone and abandoned, having long since worn down any family support that might have been offered in the early days. They are detached from their pasts, generally have few or no momentos of their life, have lost track of family members, and often depend on charitable handouts for survival. They typically have multiple medical complications caused or exacerbated by their drug abuse, such as cognitive impairment, liver disease, peptic ulcer, and chronic obstructive pulmonary disease. They are, however, in one sense, survivors because they have already outlived their life-expectancy based on their chronic pattern of drug abuse. Some studies have reported that early onset elderly drug abusers often exhibit remnants of a previous social charm that contributes to their continuing survival. Given a history of abuse spanning several decades, the person with the early onset pattern of abuse is unlikely to respond significantly to any kind of intervention in our current arsenal.

The other pattern of drug abuse among the elderly is the **late onset type.** These one-time social drinkers or casual drug users, male and female alike, have recently developed a new level of problem with use of alcohol or other drugs. They are less likely to have physical impairment caused by the drug problem, but they may suffer chronic illnesses which, together with psychosocial stresses, provide new inducement for overuse of drugs. Such a person may live alone or with a spouse, but remains in contact with family. He or she may be recently depressed, hostile, or withdrawn because of deteriorating circumstances; but he or she once enjoyed a normal range of social, occupational, and family affiliations. If there were periods of drug abuse earlier in life, they were during periods of unusual hardship and were not identified as problems. Drug abuse may have begun in response to a sharp increase in unstructured time brought on by retirement and children leaving home.

The late onset elderly drug abuser often responds well to treatment. Afterall, he or she has a long life of functioning in society and successful adaptations to changing life circumstances. If the current stresses seem, for the time being, to have strained those skills to the breaking point, there is still strong possibility that a reorientation of existing support systems, educational efforts about the hazards of drug abuse, introduction to new social support systems and drug counseling programs such as Alcoholics Anonymous, or added attention to structuring free time, can help such

Table 11.1 Characteristics of Drug Withdrawal Syndromes

Drug class	Onset	Duration	Symptoms	Clinical management
Sedative-Hypnotics				
Barbiturates and similar drugs	8–12 hr	5–10 days	Anxiety, irritability, insomnia, REM elevation, weakness, tremor, nausea, vomiting, hypotension, hallucinations, delirium, convulsions, cardiovascular collapse, possible death	Gradual withdrawal and symptomatic treatment; supportive and psychiatric treatment
Benzodiazepines	2–12 days	9–14 days		
Alcohol	12–72 hours	5–7 days		For alcohol, in addition to the above, substitution of chlordiazepoxide; vitamins (especially thiamine), fluid, and electrolytes, as needed; diazepam for convulsions
Narcotics	2–24 hr	7–10 days	Lacrimation, rhinorrhea, perspiration, mydriasis, yawning, anxiety, irritability, insomnia, REM elevation, anorexia, nausea, vomiting, diarrhea, piloerection, slight hypertension, muscle spasms	Methadone substitution and gradual withdrawal, or clonidine substitution; symptomatic treatment; supportive and psychiatric treatment
Stimulants				
Amphetamine-like drugs	12–24 hr	3–7 days	Fatigue, depression, suicidal ideation, decreased appetite, disturbed sleep, REM sleep elevation	Supportive therapy and tricyclic antidepressants for depression, if necessary
Caffeine	8–12 hr	1–2 days	Headache, drowsiness, poor concentration, irritability, lethargy	Gradual withdrawal
Nicotine	3–24 hr	1–20 wk	Anxiety, irritability, restlessness, poor concentration, headache, drowsiness, nausea, anorexia	Supportive therapy; nicotine gum

Table 11.1 Continued

Drug class	Onset	Duration	Symptoms	Clinical management
Psychiatric Drugs				
Antipsychotics	2–3 days	12–14 days	Withdrawal dyskinesias, nausea, vomiting, diarrhea, sweating, rhinorrhea, increased appetite, insomnia, agitation, delirium, headache, schizoid symptoms	Gradual withdrawal
Tricyclic antidepressants	1–2 days	A few days	Malaise, chills, headache, dizziness, nausea, vomiting, muscle aches, akathisias, anxiety	Resume medication and withdraw gradually
Neurologic Drugs				
Antiepileptics	1–2 days	A few days	Seizures, status epilepticus	Resume medication and withdraw gradually
Methysergide	1–2 days	A few days	Headaches	Resume drug and withdraw over 2–3 weeks
Endocrine Drugs				
Glucocorticoids	A few days	Indefinite	Depression, fatigue, hypotension, anorexia, nausea, vomiting	Resume drug and withdraw gradually over several months
Cardiovascular Drugs				
Antihypertensives	2–3 hr	1–2 days	Agitation, insomnia, headache, nausea, hypertension	Resume drug and withdraw gradually; treat hypertension
Antianginal drugs	10 min–2 wk	Variable	Angina attacks, anxiety, trepidation, increased blood pressure	Resume drug and withdraw slowly

persons reestablish their previous sense of self-worth, dignity, and purpose. The late onset elderly abuser has good prognosis.

Incidence of Drug Abuse among the Elderly

The extent of drug abuse among the elderly is hard to ascertain for a number of reasons. Awareness that abuse occurs in this age group as in younger individuals has increased in recent years; yet, it remains far more likely to be overlooked. The elderly abuser is less likely than younger counterparts to come to legal attention for drug-related crimes of violence. They are less likely to be employed, where drug abuse problems are often identified because of their impact on job performance. The problem may be hidden from the family or hidden by the family. Confusion, memory impairment, or cognitive impairments caused by alcohol or other depressants may be misattributed to changes in mental function in relation to normal aging or onset of Alzheimer's disease. Depression, irritability, and sleep disorders caused by drugs could be reasonably misattributed to aging, because all are more frequent among the elderly even without drug abuse. Adverse effects on organ system functions, such as gastritis, hepatitis, renal failure, hypertension, angina, or impairments of sexual function caused by drugs, could be misidentified as health problems associated with aging.

The available estimates may therefore considerably understate the incidence of drug abuse among the elderly, but for what they are worth, the typical projections are 2–10% of the entire elderly population in the United States. Presumably such estimates exclude tobacco or caffeine abuse. Among those elderly in hospitals or clinics estimates are higher, ranging from 20–40%. These two sets of estimates are not necessarily at variance given that drug abuse contributes so heavily to health problems that might necessitate hospitalization. If the first range is accurate, then drug abuse is certainly less prevalent among the elderly than younger individuals, because alcohol alone affects an estimated 9% of adult males in the United States.

There is also a difference between abuse among the elderly and younger individuals as pertains to the categories of drugs most often abused. For example, psychedelic abuse is almost a nonissue for the elderly, although that could change when we reach the point when the elderly consist of people who were young adults or adolescents after the advent of psychedelics in about 1960. Stimulants, such as cocaine and amphetamine, are also much less likely to be available to the elderly person for purposes of abuse. So, of the four major classes of drugs that are abused by young adults and adolescents, two continue as major problems among the elderly: the sedative-hypnotics, which include alcohol, and the narcotics. Even then, as regards the last category, there is a major change in the nature of the abuse problem. Narcotics abused by the elderly are obtained mostly by prescription, while those abused by young people are purchased mainly from the black market. Abuse of narcotics by the elderly is mainly by the oral route, while the common mode of abusing street narcotics is intravenous. Thus, only the abuse of the sedative-hypnotics retains substantially the same characteristics for both the elderly and younger persons.

Alcohol Abuse

Alcohol is by far the most serious drug problem among the elderly. Even in younger age groups, only tobacco abuse can compare in terms of medical costs and cannot compete with alcohol with respect to social, family, and economic costs. Moreover, tobacco takes such a heavy toll on life-expectancy that the incidence of its use is lower among the elderly because their contemporaries who smoked have died in disproportionate numbers.

Adverse effects of alcohol take a greater and faster toll on the elderly abuser. Since lean body weight and body fluid volume decline with aging, the volume of distribution for alcohol, which is mainly soluble in the aqueous compartment, decreases. Hence, a given amount of alcohol consumption will produce a higher plasma concentration than it did when the same person was younger. Liver metabolism of alcohol changes little with aging except to the extent that the elderly person has liver dysfunction or is taking a concurrent medication that inhibits alcohol metabolism, both distinct possibilities for elderly persons. So, alcohol blood levels will be at least somewhat higher in an elderly person for a given quantity consumed and perhaps a whole lot higher. What was once "social drinking" for the young person is now problem drinking for the same individual as a senior citizen.

Nearly all of the major adverse effects of alcohol are ones that interrelate with adverse physiological changes associated with aging. Alcohol promotes gastritis, pancreatitis, and peptic ulcers that add to gastrointestinal problems of the elderly. Alcohol irritates the myocardium, exacerbating cardiac problems. Alcohol depresses the brain, adding to cognitive impairment of organic brain syndrome and the psychiatric depression so common among the elderly. Alcohol is toxic to the liver, inducing hepatitis, fatty liver, or cirrhosis and adding to whatever hepatic dysfunction has developed with aging. Alcohol speeds development of atherosclerosis, increasing hypertension and liability of strokes, angina, or myocardial infarction. Alcohol suppresses the bone marrow production of white blood cells, increasing the elderly person's already elevated susceptibility to infection. Alcohol depresses libido in both sexes and promotes impotence and testicular atrophy in males, adding to already declining sexual function in the elderly. Alcohol-induced myopathy adds to developing weakness and impairments of motor control for the elderly. The elderly are more prone to injury from falls caused by intoxication.

Even one of the seemingly most favorable attributes of alcohol can be a two-edged sword for the elderly person. Like other sedative-hypnotics, alcohol promotes sleep. If consumed within a couple of hours of bedtime, latency to onset of sleep is decreased. Insomnia is common among the elderly and this action of alcohol might seem to hold an appeal. Rated against hypnotics available for medical use, however, alcohol does not rate very well. It suppresses REM sleep as well as Stages 3 and 4 of nondreaming sleep. These latter stages are already diminished among the elderly, who can little tolerate further reductions. As discussed in Chapter 10, the phases of sleep depressed by alcohol are the very ones that provide for psychological and physiological rejuvenation. Therefore, sleep after consumption of alcohol to the point of inebriation is virtually devoid of restful or restorative quality.

Moreover, any period of nonuse of alcohol long enough to precipitate the beginnings of a withdrawal syndrome will be associated with restlessness, anxiety, and insomnia. Withdrawal symptoms emerge after a rather brief period of abstinence from alcohol, because it is a short-acting drug.

Abuse of Prescription Drugs

The two most prevalent examples of abuse of prescription drugs among the elderly involve sedative-hypnotics and narcotic analgesics. The reason, of course, is that sleep problems and pain are pervasive problems in this age group. Well-intentioned efforts to control these problems too easily culminate in overuse of and then dependence on the respective drug.

The point is made in Chapter 10 that no hypnotic drug currently available provides the benefits of sleep induction and/or sleep prolongation indefinitely if used on a regular nightly basis. The available drugs range from a low of 10 consecutive nights of established benefit to a high of 5 weeks for flurazepam, but no hypnotic works indefinitely if used night after night. In spite of this limitation and its specification in drug literature, physicians still persist in prescribing hypnotics for nightly use for months or years on end, especially for institutionalized elderly. Other times, the client is complicit, using prescriptions from several different physicians to circumvent reasonable efforts on the part of the healthcare providers to prevent dependence. When the drug is continued in this way for an unrealistic and excessive period, the only continuing "benefit" of the drug is prevention of withdrawal that would now follow upon discontinuation. Physical dependence has inadvertently developed. The client who does now discontinue the hypnotic, at the urging of a family member or the physician, invariably experiences restless nights of fitful sleep and quickly concludes that the drug was doing something useful afterall.

As with alcohol, elderly clients have greater than typical susceptibility to the health consequences of excessive use of these other sedative-hypnotics. Confusion, cognitive impairment, psychiatric depression, and daytime anxiety can occur and add to existing mental alterations that occur with aging. If withdrawal is ultimately undertaken, the syndrome for this class of drugs is a potentially life-threatening one, especially for elderly or debilitated clients, because of the possibility of seizures.

Narcotic analgesics used for pain are extraordinary drugs and nearly all that medicine could require when pain is acute. The limitations inherent in this class of drugs become apparent mainly when pain is chronic, necessitating long-term management. In this circumstance, the limitations of narcotics become all too apparent. Elderly who are dependent on narcotics most usually arrive at that state as a result of treatment for pain associated with various medical conditions. Approximately 10% of drug dependence among the elderly is to narcotics prescribed for medical purposes. Like other central nervous system depressants, narcotics add to mental confusion and motor incoordination. Clients receiving narcotics are more prone to falls and motor vehicle accidents as a result.

Careful use of narcotics can delay the rate at which dependence develops and extend the period of effective clinical use (see Chapter 15). Concurrent use of nonnarcotic analgesics, stimulants, or antidepressants allows a reduction in the dosage of the narcotic. Doses can be titrated to the minimum level at which the chronic pain can be endured. Clients can be involved in their own pain management by use of patient-controlled analgesia. Yet, even with the most diligent effort on the part of the medical team, some instances of dependence will need to be condoned in the interest of pain relief. If a time arrives when the necessity for the drug diminishes, management of withdrawal will need to be considered. Clients and the family may need to be educated about the advantage of tapering doses to minimize the discomfort of withdrawal. Although narcotic withdrawal is seldom life-threatening, the psychological distress of abrupt withdrawal together with any renewal of pain can be unbearable.

Recognition and Intervention

An elderly person with an alcohol or drug problem may choose to hide it, as best he can, if he feels ashamed, weak, or guilty and unable to reach out for help. Those who work with the elderly often find that the family provides the first indication of the problem by their complaints. Other episodes that should alert the clinician to likely drug abuse include falls, motor vehicle accidents, an increase in argumentative behavior, distruction of property, fires, forgetfulness, or run-ins with authority.

The elderly abuser is likely to respond to an intervention as straight forward as frank discussion of the potential problems that the abuse poses to his or her health only if the problem is addressed early on, before the abuser becomes enmeshed in guilt and denial. After that, treatment is best conducted by referral to programs expressly designed to cope with abuse problems.

Financial considerations are likely to come into play in selecting between residential programs, individual counseling, or self-help groups such as Alcoholics Anonymous or Narcotics Anonymous. Getting the abuser into a program is more important than is frequently recognized and how they are gotten in is less important than often contended. Evidence does not support the claim that abusers will benefit from treatment programs only if they themselves provide the impetus for undertaking the treatment. There can even be a kind of benefit in the family's message that the well-being of the abuser is important enough to them to insist on a recovery effort.

Relapses are frequent among drug abusers, partly because the initial period without the drug is associated with a whole new set of psychophysiological stressors that are superimposed on the preexisting ones. Treatment, in effect, must cope with both the problems of withdrawal and the biopsychosocial antecedents that brought on abuse—a tall order. If, however, progress has been made during treatment, relapse should not be viewed by family or treatment personnel as a complete failure or reversion. Clients and family need to be taught to recognize and respond to relapses promptly. When this is done, the recovery process can frequently be put back on track.

DRUG MISUSE AMONG THE ELDERLY

While drug abuse, in the conventional meaning of the term, may be less prevalent among the elderly than younger persons, there can be no doubt that the broader problem, drug misuse, is far more evident. This should come as no surprise to those who have surveyed the data presented in Chapter 3, regarding the extent of drug use among the elderly. To recapitulate briefly, the elderly use prescription drugs at twice the level of younger people, averaging 3.7 prescriptions per person. That number has continued to rise in recent years. In 1987, approximately 25% of the elderly received more than 21 drug prescriptions for the year, and only slightly more than that received less than 5. Elderly women average slightly more active prescriptions than elderly men. The exact rank of the various categories of prescriptions drugs varies a bit from study to study and from year to year, but the twelve most widely prescribed categories for the elderly seem clear:

    beta-blockers
    antiarthritics
    cardiac glycosides
    thiazide, and related diuretics
    high-ceiling diuretics
    potassium-sparing diuretics
    other antihypertensive agents
    nitrite/nitrate vasodilators
    benzodiazepine hypnotics and anxiolytics
    oral antidiabetic drugs
    narcotic analgesics (mainly codeine)
    xanthine bronchodilators

Retail pharmacies fill more than one prescription per year for every two elderly people in the country for each of the top seven of these drug classes! Elderly people also use many more nonprescription drugs than younger people; the nonprescription drugs account for 40% of all medicines that they take. If nonprescription drugs are added to the mix of most widely used drug categories by the elderly, three categories join the elite group of most widely used drugs:

    vitamins
    laxatives
    antacids

All of this drug use adds up to a lot of potential for drug misuse, adverse effects, and drug interactions. The population of individuals most at risk for drug-related problems is also the population that uses the largest number of drugs.

Analysis of the hazards relating to drug misuse reveals that about two-thirds of drug overdoses reaching emergency rooms involve drugs obtained by prescription. Adverse drug reactions (ADRs) severe enough to culminate in hospitalization are almost all in response to prescription drugs. Digoxin ranks first or second in nearly every study of drugs that most commonly cause ADRs. Aspirin, warfarin, and prednisone also appear consistently in the top five in most studies. Other leading causes of ADRs include diuretics, other antihypertensives, insulin, oral hypoglycemics, quinidine, and antibiotics—all prescription drugs. ADRs account for approximately 5% of hospital admissions. Patients in hospitals have somewhere between an 18% and a 30% chance of a severe ADR during that hospitalization. It has been estimated than 70–80% of these ADRs are avoidable consequences of poor medical practice. The elderly confront a higher incidence of ADRs because they are more vulnerable and because physicians seldom account for age-dependent changes in drug kinetics.

In spite of efforts to educate physicians regarding the most prevalent errors relating to drug use in medical practice, certain errors persist year after year (see Table 11.2). In spite of similar efforts to educate drug consumers, certain errors in use of nonprescription medications likewise persist year after year (see Table 11.3). Most consumers of nonprescription drugs fail to recognize their potential for harm, while overrating the potential for health benefits. Personnel providing clinical or support services to the elderly need to intensify education for elderly clients regarding appropriate use and judicious nonuse of over-the-counter products. The following paragraphs offer some guidelines that might be incorporated into educational efforts.

Laxatives may be the most abused class of nonprescription drugs. The point is often made, for example, that laxatives cause more hospitalizations due to adverse reactions than the total number of persons with conditions for which laxative use is appropriate by conservative medical standards. In one large study, 15% of subjects between 65 and 74 and 26% of those over 75 had used a laxative in the last 2-week period. Another large survey found that 58% of residents in nursing homes had an order written for a laxative. Approximately 16.4% of elderly women and 12.2% of elderly men use laxatives on a regular basis. Laxatives are the most widely used class of drugs by residents of nursing homes. What is probably even more alarming than the overuse of laxatives is the choice of which one to use. There are four subgroups of laxatives:

1. bulk-forming drugs
2. osmotic/saline agents
3. contact agents
4. emollient agents.

Some classify stool softeners as a separate, fifth group, but they really differ very little from contact agents and should be included in that group. Regardless, it is well-established that the only type of laxative safe and appropriate for regular long-term use is the bulk-forming type. Other laxatives present serious risks and are appropriate only for promoting intestinal evacuation in preparation for surgical or diagnostic procedures. Nevertheless, the ten laxatives or laxative combinations most often used in one large study

Table 11.2 Prescription Drugs Commonly Misused in the Elderly

Drug category	Nature of misuse
Antibiotics	Use for nonresponsive organisms; identity of infecting pathogen not determined; premature discontinuation; allergic reaction not anticipated
Anticoagulants	Unrecognized drug interactions
Antidepressants	Unnecessary use of multiple drug regimens; dosage titration not systematically conducted; dose not reduced for elderly; inadequate monitoring for suicide potential during initiation
Antihypertensives	Less than optimal drug selection; inadequate monitoring; unanticipated drug interactions
Antipsychotics	Use for nonresponsive conditions; overuse for agitation; unnecessary use of multiple drug regimens; dosage titration not systematically conducted; reassessment for discontinuation not planned; dose not reduced for elderly
Anxiolytics	Unnecessary use; use for nonresponsive conditions; duration of treatment too long
Digitalis	Inappropriate dosage; unanticipated interactions; age-dependent pharmacokinetics not anticipated
Diuretics	Unnecessary use before nondrug measures exhausted; K^+ depletion not anticipated
Hypnotics	Unnecessary use; duration of treatment too long; dose not reduced for elderly; excessive use leading to dependence
Narcotics	Unnecessary use when nonnarcotic analgesic, antitussive, or antidiarrheal would suffice; overuse leading to dependence
Steroids	Unnecessary use; duration of treatment too long

Table 11.3 Over-the-Counter Drugs Commonly Misused

Drug Category	Nature of Misuse
Vitamins	Unnecessary expense when not required or beneficial; occasional hypervitaminosis
Laxatives/Cathartics	Widely overused; electrolyte or nutritional problems as a result; use of unnecessarily harsh agents instead of a bulk-forming laxative (e.g., fiber)
Antacids	Overuse for nonspecific symptoms of indigestion; undercompliance in severe peptic ulcers; use of sodium bicarbonate for nonsystemic applications
Antihistamines	Excessive use for cold symptoms and as sleep aids; use for asthma (contraindicated because of increased viscosity of bronchial secretions)
Aspirin/acetaminophen	Overdoses; overuse for minor aches and pains resulting in significant adverse effects
Cough suppressants	Inappropriate use for productive cough
Anorexics	Dubious value in achieving long-term weight loss; addiction liability

include only one bulk-forming agent—psillium hydrophilic mucilloid. It was the single most widely used choice, yet accounted for less than half of orders.

Approximately 9% of elderly people in nursing homes are therefore taking laxatives on a regular basis that are not safe for long-term use. Whenever possible, elderly persons with problems of constipation should try to remedy such problems, first, by treatment for underlying causes when possible; second, by increased attention to dietary and defecatory habits; third, by added dietary fiber; and fourth, by use of a laxative of the bulk-forming type. Use of other laxatives on a regular basis should be discouraged.

Next most widely abused of the nonprescription drugs is probably the antihistamines. Although these drugs provide significant, even dramatic, benefits when used for conditions such as urticaria or hay fever, the bulk of their use is for unreasonable applications. Clients should be discouraged from regular use of antihistamines for cold symptoms, sleeplessness, or asthma.

Antacids are both underused and overused by elderly persons. They are often underused due to nonadherence in the sometimes intensive and tasking regimens required for active peptic ulcers. At the same time, they are much overused by self-administration for nonspecific gastric symptoms, loosely described as heartburn or indigestion. Inappropriate use of antacids risks significant adverse effects as well as interference with prescribed regimens due to drug-drug interactions.

Vitamins are another widely overused but sometimes underused class of drugs. Sometimes physicians fail to recognize marginal deficiency states brought about by poor nutritional habits or debilitating disease. Consumers are justified in seeking the safeguard of vitamin supplementation when there is reason to believe that their vitamin levels might be marginal or inadequate. The actual prevalence of use of supplements, however, far exceeds what can be justified based on any reasonable appraisal of medical necessity. In one large study of elderly persons, 45.5% of women and 34% of men used a vitamin supplement. Mineral products were used by 22.4% of women and 15% of men. Except for the occasional occurrences of hypervitaminosis, the main price paid for this fanciful, excessive indulgence in vitamins is financial. The same expense might be better applied to improving diet. As a general guideline, vitamin supplementation should be recommended only for treatment of frank vitamin deficiencies or the following circumstances that contribute risk:

1. poor vitamin intake due to poverty, cultural, or religious dietary restrictions; alcoholism; fasting; anorexia; poor eating habits; or over reliance on foods processed in such a manner as to eliminate or destroy vitamins;
2. poor vitamin absorption due to maldigestion, malabsorption syndrome, prolonged diarrhea, use of drugs with antivitamin effects, or inflammatory diseases of the gastrointestinal system;
3. diminished ability to activate or utilize vitamins due to liver or renal disease or genetic abnormalities;
4. increased nutrient losses due to renal failure, hemodialysis, or hypermetabolic states (such as fever or hyperthyroidism);

5. increased nutrient requirements, such as in childhood, pregnancy, chronic disease, or periods of intense exertion.

Iron and calcium deficiencies are probably the two most frequently justifiable reasons for supplementation.

Three additional problem applications of nonprescription drugs are less prevalent among the elderly:

overuse of anorexics as diet aids

routine use of aspirin or aspirin-like analgesics for minor aches and pains

use of cough suppressants when cough is productive.

CONCLUSION

Although *drug abuse* involving the full gamut of tolerance, physical dependence, and psychological dependence is undoubtedly less common among the elderly than younger people, it does occur. Two distinct patterns have been identified—early and late onset. Drug abuse among the elderly almost always involves either sedative-hypnotics (especially alcohol) or narcotics. Sleeping pills or pain-killers obtained by prescription often play a role. *Drug misuse,* a far broader phenomenon than classic drug abuse, is much more prevalent among the elderly than younger persons and, indeed, constitutes the essential subject matter of this book.

REFERENCES AND RECOMMENDED READINGS

Bakdah D: Essentials the nurse should know about chemical dependency. *J. Psychiatr. Nurs.* 1978; 16(10):33–37.

Blum K: *Handbook of Abused Drugs.* New York, Gardner Press, Inc., 1984.

Casselman G: Breaking the cycle of abuse. *Can. Nurse* 1980; 76(10):30–33.

Dupont RI, Goldstein A, O'Donnell J (eds): *Handbook on Drug Abuse.* Washington, D.C., National Institute on Drug Abuse, 1979.

Ellor JR, Kurz DJ: Misuse and abuse of prescription and nonprescription drugs by the elderly. *Nurs. Clin. North Am.* 1982; 17:319–330.

Fitzpatrick E: Primary nursing: Treatment that works for the hospitalized drug dependent client. *Can. Nurse* 1980; 76(10):29–30.

Flynn WE, Batzer GB: Alcoholism and Drug Abuse, in Reichel: *Clinical Aspects of Aging,* 3rd ed., Baltimore: Williams & Wilkins, 1989, pp. 132–136.

Holden KL et al.: Accelerated mental aging in alcoholic patients. *J. Clin. Psychol.* 1988; 44(2):286–292.

Jaffe JH: Drug addiction and drug abuse, in Gilman AG, Goodman LS, Gilman A (eds): *The Pharmacological Basis of Therapeutics, ed 6.* New York, Macmillan, 1980, pp. 535–584.

Khantzion E, McKenna J: Acute toxic and withdrawal reactions associated with drug use and abuse. *Ann. Intern. Med.* 1979; 90:361–372.

Krasnegor NA (ed): *Behavioral Analysis and Treatment of Substance Abuse. NIDA Research Monograph.* 1979; 25 (GPO No. 017-024-00939-3).

Leporati NC, Chychula LH: How you can really help the drug-abusing patient. *Nursing (Horsham)* 1982; 12(6):46–49.

Milkman H, Sunderwith S: Addictive processes. *J. Psychoactive Drugs* 1982; 14(3):177–192.

Pradhan SN, Dutta SN (eds): *Drug Abuse: Clinical and Basic Aspects.* St. Louis, C.V. Mosby Co., 1977.

Ray OS: *Drugs, Society, and Human Behavior, ed 6.* St. Louis, C. V. Mosby, 199?.

Shomaker DM: Use and abuse of OTC medications by the elderly. *J. Gerontol. Nurs.* 1980; 6(1):21–24.

Yowell S, et al.: Working with drug abuse patients in the ER. *Am. J. Nurs.* 1977; 77:82–85.

CHAPTER 12

Antiparkinsonian Drug Use for the Elderly

Parkinsonism, or Parkinson's disease, is a clinical syndrome that derives from dysfunction of the corpus striatum. The healthy corpus striatum acts to maintain stability of movement, to provide certain simple movements, and to balance the tone elevating influence of the cerebellum. The absence of adequate output from the corpus striatum causes the classic triad of symptoms that characterize parkinsonism: tremor, weakness (or akinesia), and rigidity. The combination of weakness and rigidity results in various symptoms, including a thrusting forward of the trunk and head; compensatory flexion of the knees, hips, neck, and elbows; diminished facial expressiveness (the *masked facies* or *Diplomat's expression*); difficulty with chewing and swallowing; jerky movement of the arm (*cogwheel motion*); shuffling gait; and absence of reflex arm swinging. Trembling, tremor, and pill-rolling motion of the hands are additional features.

Parkinsonism is sometimes a purely motor syndrome, particularly in early stages, but later dementia, memory loss, and depression may be added features. The autonomic nervous system may be involved as well, producing such symptoms as salivation, lacrimation, excess sweating, constipation, incontinence, and decreased sexual function. Clients with predominantly motor symptoms respond better to treatment, on average, than those with a wider array of adverse features.

Autopsy studies of brains of victims of this disorder reveal a deficiency of dopamine associated with a dopaminergic pathway, the nigrostriatal pathway, that originates in the brainstem and terminates in the corpus striatum. It is believed that this dopamine deficiency is the common pathogenesis in all cases of parkinsonism. Deficiency of function of this input pathway for the corpus striatum ultimately translates into deficient output as well. Cholinergic activity in the corpus striatum, on the other hand, is excessive because cholinergic neurons in this region are normally under inhibitory restraint exerted by dopamine. Thus, parkinsonism entails too little dopaminergic action and too much cholinergic action in this brain region.

Though the pathogenesis may be common in all cases of parkinsonism, the etiologies can be quite varied. One type of parkinsonism, found almost exclusively in people born prior to 1930, was triggered by exposure to a particular strain of encephalitis virus that circulated through the United States during the 1920s. This post-encephalitic type did not always appear immediately upon exposure, but sometimes developed after a delay of several decades. More recently, a time-linked cause of parkinsonism occurred in mid-1982 and again in late 1983 when a novel illicit drug appeared on the black market, touted as a variety of heroin called "China White." In reality, the drug was a so-called designer drug—an original chemical entity produced in some unknown, clandestine laboratory. This drug, MPTP, turned out to be a potent neurotoxin with special toxic potential for dopaminergic neurons. MPTP was capable of producing such rapid damage that some users were discovered in a state of parkinsonian rigidity with a needle still inserted into a vein.

A small percentage of instances of parkinsonism are hereditary, but parkinsonism as a whole is not a mainly hereditary disorder in the manner of, say, Huntington's disease. The majority of cases are caused by various traumatic circumstances that damage the corpus striatum: cerebrovascular disorders (cerebral arteriosclerosis, thrombosis, embolism, or hemorrhage), brain tumors, neurosyphilis, or near lethal poisonings with carbon monoxide or heavy metals. Neuroleptics and, less often, antidepressants can produce a syndrome, called **pseudoparkinsonism** or **drug-induced parkinsonism,** that shares the same triad of symptoms as organic parkinsonism.

Parkinsonism is usually, but not always, progressive. The typical progression can be described as four stages.

- In Stage 1, the disorder is not disabling and seldom requires drug intervention. Speech therapy, physical therapy, or occupational therapy may be helpful.
- In Stage 2, drug intervention is initiated, usually with good results. Responsiveness is dose-related and treatment protocols are individualized to the needs of the individual case.
- In Stage 3, dose-related responsiveness continues, but clients begin to exhibit a wearing off of drug benefit shortly before the next scheduled drug administration. This phenomenon is often called **end-of-dose failure.**
- Stage 4 is end-stage parkinsonism and introduces a raft of new treatment difficulties.

The balance between beneficial effects of medications and their adverse effects becomes tenuous at best in Stage 4. Drug-induced dyskinesias may occur with doses of levodopa barely adequate to sustain mobility at other times of the day. Clients may exhibit "on-off" phenomena, alternating between periods of peak-dose dyskinesias and trough-period immobility. Psychiatric side effects may occur at treatment levels minimally sufficient to sustain mobility and independent function. Additional drugs may be required in Stage 4 to improve the balance between benefits and drug-related problems. Drugs such as antinausea medications or antipsychotics may need to be added specifically to alleviate side effects of antiparkinsonian medications if dosage levels are at the minimum required to sustain mobility.

On-off phenomena may be caused by peaks and troughs in plasma concentration of antiparkinsonian medications, or may be due in part to the client's natural diurnal rhythm. The client or a family member should be encouraged to keep a log of on-off events, including date, time of day, duration of the event, and any usual concurrent circumstances, to aid in identifying the contributing factors.

Some 1–2% of individuals over 60 years of age suffer from parkinsonism, and the incidence increases with age. Although parkinsonism in elderly people generally resembles the appearance of the condition in younger persons, a larger fraction of older clients with the disease will have reached end-stage with its consequent treatment difficulties. Elderly clients who have reached this stage will need to be monitored more closely to observe for treatment-related dyskinesias or mental symptoms. On the other hand, if an elderly client first develops parkinsonism at an advanced age, there need be less reservation about starting levodopa therapy relating to the long-term risk of producing dyskinesias.

Parkinsonism among the elderly is more likely to be associated with defects of the cerebral vasculature. These individuals may be treated with more complicated regimens that add an antithrombotic drug (e.g., aspirin) or a cerebral vasodilator to slow the progressive decline in blood flow to the brain.

Given the neurochemical pathogenesis of parkinsonism, it is no surprise that the two kinds of drugs that have provided effectiveness in its management are anticholinergic and dopaminergic compounds. Dopaminergic transmission in the vicinity of the corpus striatum can be enhanced by any of three different strategies:

1. administration of the precursor, levodopa;
2. administration of a dopamine agonist; or
3. inhibition of the breakdown of dopamine by the enzyme monoamine oxidase.

ANTICHOLINERGIC DRUGS FOR ELDERLY CLIENTS WITH PARKINSONISM

Anticholinergic drugs were the first drugs found useful for parkinsonism and were the sole method of treatment from 1867 to 1961. These drugs work by blocking cholinergic receptors, reducing excess cholinergic transmission in the corpus striatum. Their major benefit is reduction of resting tremor and rigidity, but they provide little improvement with respect to akinesia or action tremor. Since akinesia is the symptom that most threatens the independence and quality of life for clients with parkinsonism, anticholinergic drugs are seldom satisfactory as the sole medication beyond the early stages of parkinsonism.

Anticholinergic drugs currently used for parkinsonism are

benztropine (Cogentin)
biperiden (Akineton)

diphenhydramine (Benadryl)
ethopropazine (Parsidol)
orphenadrine (Disipal)
procyclidine (Kemadrin)
trihexyphenidyl (Artane, Tremin).

Some readers may wonder at the listing of diphenhydramine as an anticholinergic drug, because it is better known as an antihistamine. Diphenhydramine is a potent antihistamine, but also possesses anticholinergic properties equal to those of conventional anticholinergics, such as atropine. Only those antihistamines that have strong anticholinergic activity provide benefit in parkinsonism, so it is evident that it is diphenhydramine's anticholinergic action that is operative in this application.

Clinical Indications in the Elderly.   Anticholinergic drugs provide only modest benefit in parkinsonism, but provide that benefit in both organic and drug-induced parkinsonism. Anticholinergic drugs can provide a means of postponing the introduction of levodopa therapy for younger clients in the early stages of parkinsonism, to delay risks that accrue from long-term levodopa therapy. In this context, the qualifier *younger* needs to be understood to include those in the first geriatric decade, from 65 to 75. After parkinsonism has progressed to Stage 3 or 4, anticholinergic drugs may be useful in combination with dopaminergic drugs, because the two classes afford somewhat different benefits with respect to which symptoms of the disorder are most alleviated.

Altered Pharmacokinetics or Pharmacodynamics in the Elderly.
There are many anticholinergic drugs available for use in medicine, but only those with a high ratio of central to peripheral activity are employed for parkinsonism. Trihexyphenidyl is completely absorbed after oral administration, but biperiden, diphenhydramine, and procyclidine have less than complete bioavailability. Trihexyphenidyl has a half-life of 5.6–10.2 hours; procyclidine's is 11.5–12.6 hours, diphenhydramine's is 4–15 hours; and biperiden's is somewhat longer at 18.4–24.3 hours. There is no documentation thus far for these drugs regarding age dependent pharmacokinetics, but clients over age 60 are demonstrably more susceptible to the adverse effects of anticholinergic compounds (refer to *Adverse Effects and Contraindications*).

Adverse Effects and Contraindications in the Elderly.   Anticholinergic drugs produce a family of side effects known collectively as the **anticholinergic syndrome.** This set of side effects includes ones related to both the central and peripheral nervous systems, since acetylcholine is an important neurotransmitter in both of these locales. Cardiovascular manifestations of anticholinergic activity include tachycardia, palpitations, flushing, and orthostatic hypotension. Elderly persons will be more susceptible to all of these problems because of weaker homeostatic mechanism and especially if other cardiovascular problems preexist. For example, elderly individuals are much more prone to dangerous falls caused by dizziness or syncope that occurs due to orthostatic hypotension when the client stands abruptly from a prone or seated position. Elderly clients prone to orthostatic hypotension should be taught to avoid rapid changes in position, prolonged standing, and exposure to extremes of heat such as hot showers or hot sunlight. Elderly clients receiving anticholinergic drugs will be more susceptible to heat exhaustion due to inhibition of sweating caused by these drugs.

Ocular side effects in the anticholinergic set include mydriasis, diplopia, blurred vision, and increased intraocular pressure. The last of these actions as well as the mydriasis are potential aggravating factors for glaucoma. Elderly clients with preexisting glaucoma should usually not receive an anticholinergic drug. Elderly clients who require anticholinergic drugs should be advised to have yearly ophthalmic evaluation.

Elderly persons are often more susceptible to the gastrointestinal problems that derive from anticholinergic activity. Dry mouth, constipation, and urinary retention are more likely to develop in response to these drugs for elderly clients. Urinary retention may be added to existing problems of bladder control for elderly clients. Many elderly clients experience constipation more often even in the absence of drug treatments. Elderly clients who require anticholinergic medication need to be encouraged to maintain high fiber content in their diet to provide the natural laxative effect of added bulk. It may be helpful to provide clients with a list of foods that can help prevent constipation. Fluid intake of at least eight glasses of water per day will help overcome any drug-induced tendency toward urinary retention or urinary hesitancy. Another tactic for avoiding potential urinary hesitancy or dysuria is for the client to void immediately prior to each drug administration. Elderly clients should be taught to observe for signs of paralytic ileus, such as abdominal distention or persistent constipation, that might occur in response to anticholinergic drugs.

Psychiatric side effects due to anticholinergic drug actions are far more common for elderly clients. Confusion, disorientation, agitation, memory impairment, and toxic psychosis are frequent events when anticholinergic drug action is superimposed on a degree of cerebrovascular insufficiency, chronic organic brain syndrome, or other mental impairments that occur commonly with aging. Depression caused by anticholinergics may add to preexisting depression that is common among elderly people. **Because the elderly are especially prone to anticholinergic side effects, doses must be titrated carefully.**

Ethopropazine (Parsidol) has some unique adverse effects not shared by other anticholinergic drugs used for parkinsonism. It is a phenothiazine derivative and shares some of the potential problems of that class (see Chapter 9), including risk of seizure, endocrine disturbances, allergic jaundice, and hematological reactions. It can also cause abnormal pigmentation of the cornea, lens, retina, or skin. There would seem to be little justification for its selection.

Interactions in the Elderly. Additive anticholinergic side effects are among the most common of drug interactions to impact seriously on elderly clients. Elderly clients are at considerably elevated risk for this interaction, because they take many more drugs, on average, than younger persons and because so many different drug classes contribute anticholinergic influences. Other drugs with anticholinergic activity include many of the narcotic analgesics, most neuroleptics, tricyclic antidepressants, many antihistamines, some antidysrhythmic drugs, and, of course, the belladonna alkaloids and other drugs specifically classified as anticholinergic drugs. Many nonprescription products contain drugs with anticholinergic activity, so elderly clients need to be encouraged to ask their pharmacist about products they are planning to purchase.

The depressant effect of anticholinergic drugs on the central nervous system adds to depressant influences of any other CNS depressant. Additive depression could occur with any sedative-hypnotic, sleep aid, narcotic, neuroleptic, anxiolytics, antiepileptic, most antihistamines, and antidepressants with sedative properties. Clients receiving anticholinergic drugs need to be reminded to abstain from alcoholic beverages and to avoid other CNS depressants. They will also need to be reminded to avoid driving or other hazardous activities during times of peak depressant action.

Anticholinergic drugs delay gastric emptying, which delays absorption of many drugs, if administered concurrently. Ultimate extent of absorption is not usually affected unless the drug is one that is degraded by stomach acid. Anticholinergic drugs also decrease intestinal motility, which increases absorption of drugs like digoxin or beta-blockers that benefit from prolonged intestinal transit time. Absorption of drugs subject to intestinal metabolism, such as haloperidol, is decreased by anticholinergic drugs due to decreased intestinal motility.

Administration in the Elderly.   Anticholinergic drugs are best taken with meals to minimize potential gastrointestinal upset, nausea, or vomiting. Dryness of mouth caused by these drugs is also often less troublesome if the drug is taken at mealtime.

BENZTROPINE   (Cogentin, generic)

Recommended initial oral dose in the elderly: Patients over 60 years of age are often more sensitive to anticholinergic side effects. Mental confusion, disorientation, agitation, hallucinations, or psychotic-like symptoms may develop. Strict dosage regulation is required. Start with a low dose and titrate upward slowly.

Unspecified adult initial dose for comparison: 1 or 2 mg/day PO for organic parkinsonism; 1–4 mg once or twice daily for drug-induced parkinsonism.

BIPERIDEN   (Akineton)

Recommended initial oral dose in the elderly:
See comments for benztropine.

Unspecified adult initial dose for comparison: 2 mg PO 3 or 4 times daily for organic parkinsonism; 2 mg PO 1–3 times daily for drug-induced parkinsonism.

DIPHENHYDRAMINE   (Benadryl)

Recommended initial oral dose in the elderly:
See comments for benztropine.

Unspecified adult initial dose for comparison: 25–50 mg
orally, 3 or 4 times daily.

ETHOPROPAZINE   (Parsidol)

Recommended initial oral dose in the elderly:
See comments for benztropine.

Unspecified adult initial dose for comparison: 50 mg PO, once
or twice daily.

ORPHENADRINE   (Disipal)

Recommended initial oral dose in the elderly:
See comments for benztropine.

Unspecified adult initial dose for comparison: 50 mg PO, three
times daily after meals.

PROCYCLIDINE   (Kemadrin)

Recommended initial oral dose in the elderly:
See comments for benztropine.

Unspecified adult initial dose for comparison: 2.5 mg PO 3
times daily with meals.

TRIHEXYPHENIDYL   (Artane, Tremin, Aphen, Trihexane)

Recommended initial oral dose in the elderly:
See comments for benztropine.

Unspecified adult initial dose for comparison: 1–2 mg PO
daily, increased by increments of 2 mg at intervals of 3–5 days to a
maximum of 6–10 mg for organic parkinsonism or 5–15 mg for drug-
induced parkinsonism.

LEVODOPA FOR ELDERLY CLIENTS WITH PARKINSONISM

Levodopa therapy for parkinsonism dates from 1961. Levodopa is the substance that dopaminergic cells convert to dopamine, what neurochemists call a **precursor.** Levodopa therapy is a kind of replacement therapy, not unlike insulin therapy for type I diabetes, because parkinsonism is a dopamine deficiency disorder. Levodopa will have benefit only so long as a significant number of dopaminergic neurons remain intact in the corpus striatum to provide the conversion of levodopa to dopamine. Dopamine itself cannot be used effectively, because it does not cross the blood-brain barrier to any appreciable extent. Even with levodopa, transit across the blood-brain barrier is problematical and is usually facilitated by coadministration of a peripheral decarboxylase inhibitor as described below in the section pertaining to pharmacokinetics.

Levodopa is most active in alleviating the muscle weakness (akinesia or immobility) and the action tremors of parkinsonism. Anticholinergic drugs work better for resting tremor and rigidity, so it is not at all uncommon to include both kinds of drugs in regimens for advanced parkinsonism.

Clinical Indications in the Elderly.   Levodopa is indicated for organic parkinsonism but is contraindicated for neuroleptic-induced parkinsonism, because it will aggravate the psychosis for which the neuroleptic is required. Response to levodopa in Stage 2 or 3 of parkinsonism is dose-dependent, though the severity of symptoms at presentation is not a good predictor of the dose that will ultimately be required. Response to levodopa is less satisfactory in end-stage (Stage 4) parkinsonism because adverse motor and psychiatric effects begin to occur at doses close to or even below those required for alleviation of immobility. The effectiveness of levodopa therapy dimishes gradually over a period of 2 to 5 years of use. Response time after initiation of levodopa therapy varies from as little as 2 to 3 weeks to as much as 3 to 4 months. Elderly clients are more susceptible to the adverse effects of levodopa, therefore, treatment should be initiated at a low dose with only very gradual upward titration.

Altered Pharmacokinetics or Pharmacodynamics in the Elderly.
Levodopa is absorbed quickly after oral administration, reaching peak concentration in the blood after 0.5 to 2 hours. Concurrent administration of anticholinergic drugs, which delay gastric emptying, not only delays absorption of levodopa, but even decreases extent of absorption because levodopa is degraded by gastric enzymes.

Levodopa is nearly 70% metabolized by enzymes in the gastrointestinal tract under normal circumstances and further metabolized by enzymes in the blood, liver, and sympathetic nerve terminals before passage into the brain can occur. The elimination half-life is about 1 to 3 hours. In the absence of special measures, 97–99% of an administered dose of levodopa will fail to reach the brain. This circumstance can be greatly improved by coadministration of a peripheral dopa-decarboxylase inhibitor, such as carbidopa. Coadministration of carbidopa reduces gastrointestinal metabolism to about 30% of the administered dose enabling about 10% of the dose to reach the brain. Although still a small fraction, it is a big improvement over the 1% to 3% that would otherwise occur. Peripheral side effects, mainly orthostatic hypotension, are greatly reduced. Levodopa and carbidopa are formulated together in the product Sinemet.

Levodopa is stored in body fat from which it is released sporadically when blood levels decline. Therefore, it will be harder to regulate dosage for elderly clients who are obese. Such clients will require especially close monitoring for blood pressure, pulse, respiratory rate, and gastrointestinal disturbances.

Adverse Effects and Contraindications in the Elderly. Levodopa therapy initially produces dramatic benefits, usually at doses that cause few side effects, particularly if carbidopa is coadministered. As parkinsonism progresses and particularly when it reaches the end-stage, the benefits decline while the adverse reactions increase. Among the most common problems are levodopa-induced dyskinesias (choreiform or dystonic movements). Examples that often occur first are muscle twitches and blepharospasm. Oculogyric crisis may occur if the problem advances. Doses will need to be titrated to optimal levels, but even then dyskinesias or other side effects may occur at doses below those required to provide adequate mobility.

There is no treatment strategy for Stage 4 that is uniformly successful, but several strategies have been found successful in individual cases. Gradual dosage reduction or scheduling of periodic drug holidays may help improve the balance between benefits and adverse effects. Lower but more frequent doses can help to alleviate adverse effects, if they occur predictably at peak plasma concentrations. Other clients may benefit from addition of a dopamine agonist or selegiline together with a reduction in the dose of levodopa.

Nausea and vomiting as well as dry mouth, impaired taste sensitivity, or impaired appetite occur frequently in response to levodopa. Such symptoms can be diminished in many cases if the drug is taken with food or an antacid. If constipation occurs, an increase in dietary fiber and water consumption will help. Levodopa can cause upper gastrointestinal hemorrhage in those with preexisting peptic ulcers.

Like the anticholinergic medications, levodopa can cause visual problems, including blurred vision, mydriasis, and aggravation of glaucoma. Clients should be taught to observe for incidents of eye or head pain that might indicate glaucoma and to arrange for annual visual examination.

Cardiovascular side effects are reduced by concurrent use of carbidopa with levodopa but may nevertheless occur. Orthostatic hypotension is the most likely problem and is especially troublesome for older persons. Elderly individuals, especially those with parkinsonism, have poorer motor control and balance and are more prone to falls from the dizziness provoked by orthostatic hypotension. Cardiac irregularities are also a possible problem with levodopa and can aggravate preexisting cardiac problems of elderly clients. Dopamine produced peripherally from levodopa is a potent cardiac stimulant and, in fact, dopamine is used clinically, from time to time, as a positive inotropic agent. Caution must be exercised when using this drug in clients with a history of myocardial infarction, because an increase in cardiac output triggered by dopamine might outstrip oxygen supply.

Psychiatric side effects of levodopa can be a limiting feature and are much more common for elderly clients. Some of the possible psychoneurological problems are confusion, anxiety, agitation, insomnia, nightmares, hallucinations, delusions, increased libido, fatigue, and depression. Depression is sometimes severe to the extent of suicide liability. Levodopa can also increase cognitive impairment of chronic organic brain syndrome.

Interactions in the Elderly.   The uptake of levodopa into the brain is inhibited by large amounts of vitamin B_6 (pyridoxine). Oral doses in excess of 5 mg for this vitamin can significantly impair therapeutic response to levodopa. Clients need not abnormally reduce pyridoxine intake, but should resist taking multivitamins with large amounts of pyridoxine or over-reliance on foods (lima beans, navy beans, kidney beans, and fortified cereals) especially rich in vitamin B_6. High protein meals can also interfere with uptake of levodopa into the brain, because such foods furnish large quantities of amino acids that compete for carriers that transport levodopa across the blood-brain barrier.

Drugs with dopamine depleting (reserpine) or blocking (all neuroleptics) properties will antagonize levodopa. Among the neuroleptics, thioridazine (Mellaril) produces less antagonism, because its action is greater on limbic system dopamine receptors than those in the corpus striatum. When a neuroleptic is required to control psychiatric side effects of levodopa, thioridazine is therefore the drug of choice.

Orthostatic hypotension caused by levodopa is additive with hypotensive effects of other drugs. This would include vasodilators, diuretics, and anticholinergic agents. The cardiac stimulating effect of dopamine produced peripherally from levodopa is dangerously additive with other sympathomimetic amines with beta-agonist properties or tyramine contained in food substances. Levodopa should not be used with conventional nonselective MAO-inhibitors because the combination can result in hypertensive crisis.

Administration in the Elderly.   When clients are switched from levodopa to levodopa plus carbidopa (Sinemet), the latter drug should not be initiated sooner than 8 hours after discontinuing the levodopa.

LEVODOPA   (Dopar, Larodopa, generic)

Recommended initial oral dose in the elderly: Initial dose should be small and the rate of increments slow.

Unspecified adult initial dose for comparison: 0.5–1 g/day PO initially in 2 or more divided doses. Titrate in increments of 0.75 g/day at intervals of 3–7 days.

LEVODOPA/CARBIDOPA (Sinemet)

Recommended initial oral dose in the elderly: Initial dose should be small and the rate of increments slow.

Unspecified adult initial dose for comparison: one 10/100 tablet (consisting of 10 mg levodopa and 100 mg carbidopa) or one 25/250 tablet PO, 3 times daily. Titrate in increments of 1 tablet each day or every other day up to 6 tablets per day.

DOPAMINE AGONISTS FOR ELDERLY CLIENTS WITH PARKINSONISM

Dopamine receptor agonists were added to the array of drugs available for management of parkinsonism in the 1980s. The three dopamine agonists currently available for clinical practice are amantadine (Symmetrel), bromocriptine (Parlodel), and pergolide (Permax). A half-dozen other drugs in this family are in development. Ciladopa and terguride are a bit different from the other members of this family in that they are partial agonists. It is thought that partial agonists might be less apt to exhibit long-term loss of benefit or drug-induced dyskinesias. In contrast to levodopa, dopamine agonists act directly on postsynaptic receptors and therefore continue to have activity even after most dopaminergic neurons of the nigrostriatal pathway have degenerated. Amantadine differs a bit from the other drugs for three reasons: (1) a large part of its mechanism is by release of dopamine from stores in dopaminergic nerve terminals; (2) it is more active on neurons of the corpus striatum than those of the limbic system and is therefore less likely to exacerbate psychosis; and (3) it has an additional unrelated application as an antiviral drug.

Clinical Indications in the Elderly. Dopamine agonists in small doses are usually employed as add-ons to a regimen that already utilized levodopa and/or an anticholinergic drug. They are quicker acting and can be used to reduce end-of-dose failure when levodopa effects do not sustain mobility throughout the day. Dopamine agonists can also be used in end-stage management as a means of reducing the dose of levodopa and the associated dyskinesias and psychiatric side effects. Although bromocriptine and pergolide in high doses (i.e., 60–300 mg/day for bromocriptine) can provide benefits comparable to those of levodopa, side effects at these dosage levels are greater than those occurring with comparably effective doses of levodopa. Amandatine alone among these drugs can also be used for drug-induced parkinsonism, as an alternative to anticholinergic drugs, because it has less of a dopaminergic influence on limbic system pathways than in the corpus striatum.

Altered Pharmacokinetics or Pharmacodynamics in the Elderly.
Age-dependent pharmacokinetics have yet to be determined for these drugs.

The half-life of amantadine increases sharply in relation to renal impairment and a specific schedule for dosage reduction in renal failure has been established based on creatinine clearance. For example, in the absence of diminished creatinine clearance (i.e., a value of 100 mg/min/1.73 m²), 200 mg/day of amantadine is appropriate but at 50 mg/min/1.73 m², the recommended dose is 100 mg/day. Consult the drug literature for this product for other values. Both bromocriptine and pergolide are metabolized in the liver to multiple metabolites, but it is not known which of these metabolites, if any, are active. Presumably dosage reduction would need to be affected in clients with hepatic dysfunction.

Adverse Effects and Contraindications in the Elderly.   Dopamine agonists cause central nervous system side effects not unlike those of levodopa. Fatigue and depression may occur or, alternatively, insomnia, hallucinations or confusion. Neurological problems can include ataxa, dizziness, seizures, slurred speech, or oculogyric crisis. Choreoform movements, blephorospasm, and other dyskinesias can occur as with levodopa.

Peripheral side effects of bromocriptine include urinary frequency, incontinence, or retention; edema; nasal stuffiness; paresthesias; headache; or skin rash. Amantadine can cause orthostatic hypotension, edema, congestive heart failure, visual problems, seizures, or hematological deficits.

Interactions in the Elderly.   The action of dopamine agonists is diminished by dopamine antagonists, including all neuroleptics and metoclopramide, an antiemetic.

Administration in the Elderly.   Administration with meals will help to minimize gastric irritation.

AMANTADINE   (Symmetrel)

Recommended initial oral dose in the elderly: 50 or 100 mg/day, increased every fourth day to a maximum of 100 mg/day. Reduce dose for renal impairment.

Unspecified adult initial dose for comparison: 100 mg PO twice daily, increased up to 400 mg daily for organic parkinsonism or up to 300 mg daily for drug-induced parkinsonism.

BROMOCRIPTINE   (Parlodel)

Recommended initial oral dose in the elderly: 0.625–1.25 mg/day initially, increased every 3–4 days by 0.625–1.25 mg/day to a maximum of 15 mg/day to supplement levodopa therapy for organic parkinsonism.

Unspecified adult initial dose for comparison: One-half of a 2.5-mg tablet initially, twice daily with meals, increased by 2.5 mg/day at intervals of 2–4 weeks. If withdrawal is required, withdraw at increments of 2.5 mg/day.

CILADOPA

Investigational.

LERGOTRILE

Investigational.

LISURIDE

Investigational.

MESULERGINE

Investigational.

PERGOLIDE   (Permax)

Recommended initial oral dose in the elderly: No specific recommendation.

Unspecified adult initial dose for comparison: 0.05 mg once daily for the first 2 days, increased by 0.1–0.15 mg/day at 3-day intervals for 12 days, then 0.25 mg/day at 3-day intervals until optimum response is achieved.

PIRIBEDIL   (Trivastal)

Investigational.

TERGURIDE

Investigational.

SELEGILINE FOR ELDERLY CLIENTS WITH PARKINSONISM

Selegiline is a new approach to treatment of parkinsonism introduced in 1989. Selegiline inhibits type B monoamine oxidase (MAO). Many nonselective MAO inhibitors (drugs that inhibit both type A and type B MAO) have been available for medical practice, mainly as antidepressants, since the 1950s, but nonselective MAO inhibitors suffer from excessive risk of drug-drug and drug-diet interactions. Nonselective drugs interact with a substance called tyramine found in a wide variety of foods, most notably cheeses, beer, and certain wines. The task of avoiding all the foods that contain tyramine as well as other drugs that interact with nonselective MAO inhibitors is too much for most clients. Selegiline largely avoids the drawbacks of nonselective MAO inhibitors by inhibiting only the B type. Since most MAO in the intestines is type A, ingested foods and drugs continue to be metabolized normally after selegiline is given. MAO in the brain is about evenly divided between the two forms, so selegiline substantially reduces brain MAO activity without completely eliminating it.

Clinical Indications in the Elderly.   The currently approved indication for selegiline is for addition to a regimen already including levodopa/carbidopa for parkinsonism. Addition of selegiline to the regimen allows for a dose reduction for the levodopa/carbidopa and helps to prolong responsiveness, while reducing levodopa-induced dyskinesias.

Some researchers believe that the progression of parkinsonism is caused by continuing degeration of dopaminergic neurons of the nigrostriatal pathway and that oxidative metabolites of dopamine contribute to the damage. The further argument is that levodopa therapy, by increasing production and subsequent breakdown of dopamine, may actually hasten the deterioration even while alleviating motor deficits in the short run. If this theory proves valid, selegiline could be expected to help prevent progression of parkinsonism, whether occurring as a natural process or in response to treatment with levodopa, by slowing degradation of dopamine and allowing the corpus striatum to get more use out of less dopamine. Accordingly, selegiline is currently undergoing clinical testing for prophylaxis against the progression of parkinsonism. Since progression has to be measured over many months or a few years, the trial period will necessarily be long and results are not yet available.

Altered Pharmacokinetics or Pharmacodynamics in the Elderly.
Selegiline is rapidly absorbed after oral administration, with an ultimate bioavailability of about 75%. Selegiline is metabolized into desmethyldeprenyl, amphetamine, and methamphetamine. Inhibition of MAO type B by selegiline is irreversible. It is not known how rapidly MAO type B is replaced when selegiline is discontinued. Age-dependent pharmacokinetics have yet to be evaluated for selegiline.

Adverse Effects and Contraindications in the Elderly.   Adverse effects of selegiline include gastrointestinal irritation (mainly nausea or abdominal pain), cardiovascular side effects (dysrhythmias, angina, edema, orthostatic hypotension or, conversely, hypertension), skin reactions, sexual dysfunction, visual problems (diplopia or blurred vision), and neurological symptoms (confusion, hallucinations, vivid dreams, or dyskinesias). Elderly individuals have elevated liability to cardiovascular and neurologic side effects of drugs.

Interactions in the Elderly.   There is no evidence at present that selegiline shares the large variety of interactions characteristic of nonselective MAO inhibitors. No instances of hypertensive crisis caused by dietary tyramine have been reported. Nevertheless, as a precaution, dietary precautions are advised when large doses of selegiline are required. Similarly, caution should be taken to avoid drugs, such as meperidine, known to interact dangerously with nonselective MAO inhibitors.

Some clients receiving selegiline will experience a worsening of levodopa side effects, presumably reflecting an increase in dopaminergic activity at peak-dose. Doses of levodopa/carbidopa may need to be reduced by 10–30% when selegiline is added to the regimen.

Administration in the Elderly.   Daily doses above 10 mg usually do not provide additional benefit.

SELEGILINE   (Endepryl)

Recommended initial oral dose in the elderly: 2.5 mg/day, increased every fourth day up to a maximum of 5 mg twice a day.

Unspecified adult initial dose for comparison: 10 mg/day in 2 divided doses with breakfast and lunch, as adjunct to levodopa/carbidopa therapy for parkinsonism. The dose of levodopa/carbidopa will usually need to be reduced an average of 10–30%, 2–3 days after addition of selegiline to the regimen.

REFERENCES AND RECOMMENDED READINGS

Calne D, et al.: Advances in the neuropharmacology of parkinsonism. *Ann. Intern. Med.* 1979; 90(2):219–229.

Carroll JD, Savundra PA: The management of parkinsonism in the elderly, in K. O'Malley and JL Waddington (eds): *Therapeutics in the elderly,* New York, Elsevier Sci. Publ, 1985, pp. 153–162.

Fischback F: Easing adjustment to Parkinson's disease. *Am. J. Nurs.* 1978; 78(1):66–69.

Hahn K: Management of Parkinson's disease. *Nurse Practitioner* 1982; VV:13–25.

Parkes JD: Adverse effects of antiparkinsonian drugs. *Drugs* 1981; 21(5):341–353.

Quinn NP: Antiparkinsonian drugs today. *Drugs* 1984; 28:236–262.

Yahr MD (ed): Parkinsonism: Current perspectives and new horizons. *Clin. Neuropharm.* 1986; 9(Suppl. 1).

CHAPTER 13

Drug Therapies for Cardiovascular Problems of the Elderly

Cardiovascular problems can arise with aging as a result of several factors. In many cases, first among these is the gradually developing renal failure that is evident to some extent even in healthy elderly people and more pronounced in those with cardiovascular problems. As clearance of salt and water diminishes, excess electrolytes and fluid are retained. At the same time, slowly developing arteriosclerosis begins to interfere with good flow through the arteries. Together, these factors raise blood pressure. Though high blood pressure itself is an asymptomatic condition, it sets the stage for the life-threatening cardiac events that follow. Elevated arterial pressure increases **afterload,** which is the resistance of the arteries to receiving the blood the heart pumps into them. The result is that the heart must work harder, but cardiac output nevertheless declines. Congestive heart failure occurs when the heart wears down under this added workload.

Even as the work of the heart increases, there is profound risk that its supply of energy will be impaired. The heart must compete with the needs of other tissues for the now diminished flow of blood and even though it is given first priority, along with the brain, perfusion may suffer. If the blood vessels supplying the heart have themselves been overlayed with sclerotic deposits, local or global deficiencies in oxygen delivery may gradually develop, producing the pain of angina. The narrowed vessels become increasingly prone to formation of clots or other occlusion, leading to myocardial infarctions. **Angina** and **myocardial infarction** comprise the two varieties of **ischemic heart disease.** The combination of myocardial infarction and hypertension is particularly lethal in the elderly.

If atherosclerosis is also at work in peripheral blood vessels, the elderly person will be at increased risk of thromboembolism, as well. Thromboembolism is occlusion of a peripheral vessel that curtails blood supply to the lungs, the brain, or perhaps a deep vein in the calf.

Then, too, the conductile system of the heart may begin to suffer from accumulated scar tissue, small infarcts, or blockages. These changes, as well as drugs that the elderly might require, establish the conditions that might lead to cardiac dysrhythmias, including tachycardia, AV block, flutter, fibrillation, or arrest. Thus, the elderly are more prone than younger people to all of the five major kinds of cardiovascular problems: hypertension, congestive heart failure, ischemic heart disease, dysrhythmias, and thromboembolisms. These are the subject matter of the four sections of this chapter.

HYPERTENSION IN THE ELDERLY

Hypertension is the most common disorder of the cardiovascular system, occurring in nearly 10% of Americans, and is a factor in each of the kinds of cardiac disturbances discussed in subsequent sections of this chapter. Hypertension is defined as an elevation in either systolic or diastolic pressure, or both. The criteria for hypertension change with age as does normal blood pressure. For young adults, 120/80 is normal, and 135/90 is considered hypertension. For middle-aged adults, normal is 135/85 and hypertension is 140/90. For the elderly (over 65), normal is 150/85, while hypertension is defined as 160/90. Many clinicians believe that diastolic pressure is the more telling of the two measures because it reflects afterload or peripheral resistance to blood flow. Other clinicians believe that systolic pressure may be an equally or more important parameter.

Hypertension can be secondary to a wide variety of endocrine, renal, or other health problems. If not, it is **essential hypertension,** meaning that it is a primary health problem in its own right. Hypertension is essential in approximately 85–90% of cases. The two main factors thought to contribute to essential hypertension are excess activity of the renin-angiotensin-aldosterone system and excess sympathetic tone. Renin and its cohorts promote sodium and fluid retention, increasing body fluid volume. Excess sympathetic tone, usually related to stress, promotes vasoconstriction and vascular resistance to flow. Epidemiological factors in hypertension include age, gender, race, weight, exercise, dietary sodium, dietary fat and cholesterol, and smoking tobacco. Incidence of essential hypertension increases dramatically with age. It is more common in blacks than whites, males than females, and in those with diabetes mellitus or, of course, atherosclerosis.

Hypertension is itself asymptomatic, which is one factor making it so difficult to control. Clients have minimal immediate incentive to adhere to therapeutic regimens. Yet hypertension is a major risk factor for various cardiovascular diseases, such as ischemic heart disease, congestive heart failure, and chronic renal failure, as well as overall mortality rates.

Treatments for hypertension, if well planned, adhered to, and objectively monitored, can not only lower blood pressure, but also can reduce the occurrence of many of the complications of high blood pressure. Major cardiac events, strokes, and mortality rates all decline with effective therapy. Yet countless studies have indicated that only a small minority of those with hypertension receive appropriate therapy and less than 50% of them have adequately controlled pressure. The deficiencies in treatment include inappropriate drug selection, failure to individualize doses, failure to adjust doses with changing client status, nonadherence by the client, and inadequate monitoring of drug response by the client and/or physician.

Treatment of hypertension needs to be matched to the severity of the problem. There is little evidence at present that drug treatment for **borderline hypertension** is warranted. Nondrug measures such as discontinuation of smoking tobacco, drinking alcohol, using oral contraceptives, restrictions on dietary sodium, and weight control are appropriate interventions at this stage. Drug therapy is clearly indicated when hypertension is moderate or severe, with drug combinations often necessitated in the later category. The decision whether or not to resort to drug therapy is difficult, then, only for clients in the middle—those with mild hypertension. For these clients, nondrug approaches might be explored first, but drug intervention needs to be considered if a positive response to nondrug measures is not soon evident. Risk factors should also be considered in the decision, namely, high cholesterol, diabetes mellitus, male, black, or early onset (prior to age 45). One guideline often used is that therapy should be initiated at a diastolic pressure above 100 if two risk factors are present, above 95 with three risk factors, and above 90 with four or five risk factors.

When drug combinations are required (for moderate or severe hypertension), the **step approach** is often used in the United States to guide therapy (see Table 13.1). Therapy is first initiated with a diuretic, usually a thiazide. A beta-blocker or a sympatholytic is added, if needed, in Step two. If response is still not adequate, a vasodilator is added in Step three. If a fourth drug is required, a sympatholytic drug compatible with other drugs in the regimen can be added in Step 4. The following sections discuss the six classes of drugs that find widespread use for treatment of hypertension:

1. diuretics
2. angiotension-converting enzyme inhibitors
3. beta-blockers
4. other sympatholytics
5. calcium channel blockers
6. other vasodilators

Table 13.1 The Step Approach to Treatment of Essential Hypertension

Step 1 Thiazide diuretic or High-ceiling diuretic if azotemia is present
Step 2 Add Beta-blocker[1] or other sympatholytic:
　　　　　Methyldopa
　　　　　Clonidine
　　　　　Reserpine
Step 3 Add Vasodilator:
　　　　　Prazosin[2]
　　　　　Hydralazine
　　　　　Minoxidil
Step 4 Add Sympatholytic:
　　　　　Guanethidine[3]
　　　　　Clonidine[4]
　　　　　Phenoxybenzamine[5]

1. Sometimes used as Step 1.
2. Sometimes used as Step 2.
3. Not if reserpine was used in Step 2.
4. Not if methyldopa was used in Step 2.
5. Only if a beta-blocker was selected in Step 2.

Diuretic Drug Use in the Elderly

Diuretics work by stimulating the ability of the kidneys to remove salt from filtered plasma and transfer it into the urine. Water follows the movement of salt passively as a result of osmotic pressure, so salt elimination automatically means water elimination. Four classes of diuretics have current clinical importance, but of these, one, the osmotic diuretic manitol finds use only for short-term purposes in clinical settings. It will not be discussed here. The three classes that find widespread, long-term use in elderly clients for the standard purpose of reducing body fluid volume are

1. thiazides and related diuretics
2. high-ceiling diuretics
3. potassium-sparing diuretics

Unfortunately, the action of diuretics is seldom limited to promoting salt and water elimination. Each of these drugs has the potential for altering potassium levels and hydrogen ion concentration (pH) of body fluids. Many times diuretics alter glucose tolerance, uric acid levels, and calcium levels, as well.

Clinical Indications in the Elderly.   Common uses of diuretics in the elderly are for volume depletion in hypertension and congestive heart failure. They are prescribed for clients unable to correct sodium and water retention through nondrug measures alone—mainly restrictions on dietary salt.

Altered Pharmacokinetics or Pharmacodynamics in the Elderly.
Thiazide, high-ceiling, and potassium-sparing diuretics are well-absorbed from the intestines after oral administration. Absorption is little affected by other drugs except for anion exchange resins, which should not be given within an hour of most any drug. Thiazides and high-ceiling diuretics are eliminated mainly by renal excretion. Among the potassium-sparing agents, spironolactone is a prodrug requiring hepatic metabolism to an active metabolite, which is then inactivated by renal excretion. Triamterene depends on both hepatic metabolism and renal excretion for inactivation. No solid information is available regarding age-dependent kinetics for diuretics. Diuretics need to be used cautiously, however, for clients with acute renal insufficiency because inactivation is mainly by renal excretion.

Adverse Effects and Contraindications in the Elderly.   Whenever diuretics are used, thought must be given to the likely effect that the treatment will have on potassium balance for the client. Elderly persons are especially likely to develop potassium depletion in response to thiazide or high-ceiling diuretics, because their dietary intake of potassium (see Table 13.2) is often

Table 13.2 Potassium-Rich Foods

Greater than 350 mg/portion	Greater than 150 mg/portion
Baked Potato	Cod
Avocado	Beef liver
Raisins	Apricots, fresh
Dates	Sirloin, trimmed
Sardines, drained	Steak, round
Flounder	Haddock
Orange juice	Pork
Banana	Lamb, leg
Apricots, dried	Turkey
Winter squash, cooked	Perch
Cantaloupe	Tomato, raw
Skim milk	Prunes
Sweet potato	Tuna, dried
Salmon, fillet	Artichoke
Buttermilk	Chicken
Whole milk	

Also high in potassium but not quantified: Honeydew melon, molasses, lima beans, apples, peaches, peanuts, chocolate, and cola.

decreased and because they are less likely to adhere to taking prescribed potassium supplements. Severe potassium depletion is life-threatening. When clients are unable to maintain adequate potassium levels through dietary adjustments or adherence to prescribed potassium supplementation, concurrent use of a potassium-sparing diuretic is indicated. Determination of serum electrolytes needs to be conducted periodically.

On the other hand, when a potassium-sparing diuretic is used as the sole diuretic, care must be taken that hyperkalemia does not develop. Hyperkalemia develops in 10% of clients receiving a potassium-sparing diuretic alone. Symptoms indicative of hyperkalemia are fatigue and weakness, flaccid paralysis, bradycardia, and paresthesias. Hyperkalemia occurs most often in elderly clients and those with diabetes mellitus, renal impairment, or acidosis.

Thiazide and high-ceiling diuretics can cause magnesium depletion and magnesium supplements may be indicated. Thiazide diuretics cause calcium retention, but high-ceiling diuretics cause calcium depletion. Calcium supplements may be necessary in the latter case.

The intended effect of diuretic therapy for hypertension is to reduce body fluid volume and thereby reduce blood pressure. Sometimes diuretics provide too much of a good thing, resulting in hypovolemia, dehydration, and orthostatic hypotension. This is especially likely for elderly clients, because total body water content decreases with age. Normal doses of thiazide or high-ceiling diuretics are likely to cause dehydration in an elderly individual. Orthostatic hypotension is accompanied by a tendency to faint or to experience dizziness upon standing abruptly from a prone or sitting position. The elderly are more liable to fall because of poorer balance and motor control, are more likely to experience severe injury from falls, and take longer to recover from fractures and bruises. Clients receiving diuretics who experience orthostatic hypotension need to be educated to avoid rapid changes in position, so as to avoid concommitant problems. Dehydration caused by diuretics can cause xerostomia (dry mouth), especially for the elderly. Clients on diuretics who experience dry mouth should be advised to maintain thorough oral hygiene to protect oral membranes from irritation and to protect the teeth from the demineralization that can accompany reductions in salivary secretions.

All three major categories of diuretics have the potential to cause gastro-intestinal irritation, resulting in such symptoms as upset stomach, heart-burn, nausea, constipation, cramps, or anorexia. Diuretics are best taken with meals to minimize gastrointestinal problems. The elderly are more likely to experience gastrointestinal difficulties from drug effects than younger individuals.

Diuretics that are taken once per day are best taken in the morning. If taken at bedtime, diuretics will often cause nocturia, interfering with a good night's sleep. Moreover, some elderly persons are at risk of falls and injury if nocturia necessitates frequent getting up during the night.

Thiazide diuretics can alter insulin or sulfonylurea requirements for individuals with diabetes mellitus by promoting hyperglycemia. Moreover, cardiovascular mortality rates may actually be higher in hypertensive diabetics treated for hypertension than those not treated. If treated at all for hypertension, clients with diabetes should be reassessed if thiazide administration is begun or discontinued. Thiazide diuretics and especially high-ceiling diuretics, can aggravate preexisting hyperuricemia (gout), because they inhibit uric acid secretion. Elderly clients are more likely to suffer from gout and are therefore more prone to this side effect of diuretics.

Interactions in the Elderly.   Elderly clients receiving a thiazide or high-ceiling diuretic together with a steroid (glucocorticoids with mineralocorticoid activity) or digoxin are most likely to experience significant hypokalemia. Hypokalemia intensifies the action of digoxin, with potentially serious consequences. Hypokalemia also prolongs and intensifies neuromuscular blockade produced by neuromuscular blockers that might be required during surgery.

Volume depletion produced by diuretic therapy contributes to a usually therapeutic reduction in blood pressure, but can sometimes result in hypovolemia, hypotension, and dehydration. The hypotensive effect of diuretics is additive with that produced by other hypotensive drugs, including sympatholytics and vasodilators. Many central nervous system depressants also cause orthostatic hypotension, if not as obviously so as drugs used expressly for that purpose, and such hypotensive actions are additive with those of diuretics.

Clients with diabetes may require increased doses of insulin due to the hypoglycemic action of thiazides. Lithium clearance is decreased by concurrent use of a thiazide, high-ceiling, or potassium-sparing diuretic with a corresponding increase in its potential for toxicity. Phenytoin interferes with absorption of high-ceiling diuretics.

High-ceiling diuretics are highly bound to plasma proteins and will compete for binding sites with other highly bound drugs, including warfarin and digoxin. The result is a greater free fraction for the interacting drug and a potentiation of its activity.

Administration in the Elderly.   Frequency of administration is determined by the duration of action of the various drugs. Drugs with durations longer than 18 hours are given once a day in the morning, those with durations from 6 to 18 hours are given twice a day, with the second dose no later than 3:00 PM to avoid nocturia. Peak effects of diuretics typically occur approximately 3 to 6 hours after drug administration, and some clients may want to schedule activities or time of drug administrations so that peak drug action does not interfere with work or leisure plans.

Thiazide Diuretics

BENDROFLUMETHIAZIDE   (Naturetin)

Recommended initial oral dose in the elderly: Normal doses may cause dehydration.

Unspecified adult initial antihypertensive dose for comparison:
5–20 mg daily.

BENZTHIAZIDE   (Aquatag, Exna, Hydrex, Marazide, Proaqua)

Recommended initial oral dose in the elderly: Normal doses may cause dehydration.

Unspecified adult initial antihypertensive dose for comparison:
50–100 mg daily in two divided doses.

CHLORTHALIDONE   (Hygroton, Hylidone, Thalitone, generic)

Recommended initial oral dose in the elderly: Normal doses may cause dehydration.

Unspecified adult initial antihypertensive dose for comparison:
25 mg once daily.

CHLORTHIAZIDE   (Diuril, Diachlor, Diurigen, generic)

Recommended initial oral dose in the elderly: Normal doses may cause dehydration.

Unspecified adult initial antihypertensive dose for comparison:
0.5–2 g/day in one or two divided administrations.

CYCLOTHIAZIDE   (Anhydron)

Recommended initial oral dose in the elderly: Normal doses may cause dehydration.

Unspecified adult initial antihypertensive dose for comparison: 2 mg once daily.

HYDROCHLORTHIAZIDE   (Diaqua, Esidrix, Hydro-Chlor, Hydromal, Hydro-T, HydroDIURIL, Oretic, Thiuretic, generic)

Recommended initial oral dose in the elderly: Normal doses may cause dehydration or potentially fatal hypokalemia or hypomagnesemia. Dose should be less than 50 mg/day.

Unspecified adult initial antihypertensive dose for comparison: 50–100 mg/day in one or two divided administrations.

HYDROFLUMETHIAZIDE   (Diucardin, Saluron, generic)

Recommended initial oral dose in the elderly: Normal doses may cause dehydration.

Unspecified adult initial antihypertensive dose for comparison: 50 mg twice daily.

INDAPAMIDE   (Lozol)

Recommended initial oral dose in the elderly: Normal doses may cause dehydration.

Unspecified adult initial antihypertensive dose for comparison: 2.5 mg once daily.

METHYCLOTHIAZIDE   (Aquatensen, Enduron, Ethon, generic)

Recommended initial oral dose in the elderly: Normal doses may cause dehydration.

Unspecified adult initial antihypertensive dose for comparison: 2.5–5 mg once daily.

METOLAZONE   (Diulo, Microx, Zaroxolyn)

Recommended initial oral dose in the elderly: Normal doses may cause dehydration.

Unspecified adult initial antihypertensive dose for comparison: 2.5–5.0 mg once daily for Diulo or Zaroxolyn; 0.5 mg once daily in the morning for Microx.

POLYTHIAZIDE   (Renese)

Recommended initial oral dose in the elderly: Normal doses may cause dehydration.

Unspecified adult initial antihypertensive dose for comparison: 2–4 mg daily.

QUINETHAZONE   (Hydromox)

Recommended initial oral dose in the elderly: Normal doses may cause dehydration.

Unspecified adult initial antihypertensive dose for comparison: 50–100 mg once daily.

TRICHLORMETHIAZIDE   (Diurese, Metahydrin, Naqua, Niazide, Trichlorex, generic)

Recommended initial oral dose in the elderly: Normal doses may cause dehydration.

Unspecified adult initial antihypertensive dose for comparison: 2–4 mg daily.

High-Ceiling Diuretics

BUMETANIDE   (Bumex)

Recommended initial oral dose in the elderly: Normal doses may cause dehydration.

Unspecified adult initial antihypertensive dose for comparison: 0.5–2 mg/day as a single dose; if response is not adequate, give a second or third dose at 5-hour intervals

ETHACRYNIC ACID (Edecrin)

Recommended initial oral dose in the elderly: Normal doses may cause dehydration.

Unspecified adult initial antihypertensive dose for comparison: 50–200 mg daily.

FUROSEMIDE (Fumide, Lasix, Luramide, generic)

Recommended initial oral dose in the elderly: Normal doses may cause dehydration.

Unspecified adult initial antihypertensive dose for comparison: 40 mg twice daily.

Potassium-Sparing Diuretics

AMILORIDE (Midamor, generic)

Recommended initial oral dose in the elderly: No specific recommendation.

Unspecified adult initial antihypertensive dose for comparison: 5 mg/day; increase to 10 mg/day if necessary.

SPIRONOLACTONE (Alatone, Aldactone, generic)

Recommended initial oral dose in the elderly: No specific recommendation.

Unspecified adult initial antihypertensive dose for comparison: 50–100 mg/day.

TRIAMTERENE (Alazide, Aldactazide, Maxzide, Moduretic, generic, combinations with thiazide diuretics)

Recommended initial oral dose in the elderly: No specific recommendation.

Unspecified adult initial antihypertensive dose for comparison: 100 mg twice daily after meals when used alone.

ANGIOTENSIN-CONVERTING ENZYME (ACE) INHIBITOR USE IN THE ELDERLY

One of the factors that contributes to essential hypertension in most cases is excess activity of the renin-angiotensin-aldosterone system that controls salt retention by the kidneys. ACE inhibitors provide the most direct way of suppressing the activity of this system. They inhibit the activation of the middle component of the system, angiotensin, by converting enzyme. The end effect of these drugs is a lot like that of diuretics: salt elimination and volume depletion.

Clinical Indications in the Elderly.   ACE inhibitors are indicated for hypertension. They are effective alone, but are usually not used as a first approach to management of hypertension because of serious side effects. They are usually combined with a thiazide diuretic and provide additive volume depletion and hypotension with diuretics. Captopril and enalapril are also approved for achieving elimination of excess body fluid in congestive heart failure.

Altered Pharmacokinetics or Pharmacodynamics in the Elderly.
ACE-inhibitors are rapidly absorbed after oral administration. Five of the eight available drugs in this family produce active metabolites. Renal excretion provides the main route of inactivation for captopril, enalapril, enalaprilat, and lisinopril. Fosinopril, quinapril, and ramipril are 50–60% inactivated by renal excretion, with the remainder excreted in the feces. Therefore, decreases in renal function that occur with aging can be expected to prolong the half-life of these compounds, and prolongations have in fact been reported for all seven of them that have been tested. Elderly patients will therefore develop a higher plasma concentration to any given dose than younger patients.

Adverse Effects and Contraindications in the Elderly.   Adverse effects common among the ACE inhibitors are neurological symptoms, hematological toxicity, cardiovascular problems, gastrointestinal irritation, cough and dyspnea, and skin reactions. Neurological symptoms can include headache, dizziness, fatigue, insomnia, paresthesias, and diminished taste sensitivity, but each of these occurs in less than 1% of clients receiving these drugs. Hematological effects have included neutropenia (with captopril, ramipril, benazepril, and quinapril) and decreased hemoglobin (with enalapril, lisinopril, ramipril, fosinopril, and benazepril). Cardiovascular side effects occur in less than 1% of clients but can include excess hypotension, tachycardia, claudication, angina, myocardial infarction, or congestive heart failure. Gastrointestinal problems are relatively uncommon with ACE-inhibitors and typically take the form of nausea, vomiting, or diarrhea. Enalapril and lisinopril can cause upper respiratory problems including pneumonia, hoarseness, sore throat, or cough. Skin rash is most likely with captopril (7-10% of treated individuals). The incidence with the other drugs is less than 1%.

Like the potassium-sparing diuretics, ACE-inhibitors can cause hyperkalemia. Clients taking ACE-inhibitors need to be taught to avoid potassium-rich foods and to recognize the warning symptoms (fatigue and weakness) of hyperkalemia.

Interactions in the Elderly.   Hyperkalemic effects of ACE-inhibitors are potentially additive with those of potassium-sparing diuretics and concurrent use of the two classes is not recommended. Use of potassium supplements along with an ACE-inhibitor could likewise lead to dangerous hyperkalemia.

Administration in the Elderly.   Most ACE inhibitors are administered once daily. Captopril is administered 2 or 3 times daily with meals.

BENAZEPRIL   (Lotensin)

Recommended initial oral dose in the elderly: No specific recommendation.

Unspecified adult initial dose for comparison: 10 mg once daily.

CAPTOPRIL   (Capoten)

Recommended initial oral dose in the elderly: No specific recommendation.

Unspecified adult initial antihypertensive dose for comparison: 25 mg 2 or 3 times daily, 1 hour before meals.

ENALAPRIL   (Vasotec)

Recommended initial oral dose in the elderly: No specific recommendation.

Unspecified adult initial antihypertensive dose for comparison: 5 mg once daily; 2.5 mg once daily in moderate to severe renal impairment.

FOSINOPRIL   (Monopril)

Recommended initial oral dose in the elderly: No specific recommendation.

Unspecified adult initial dose for comparison: 10 mg once daily.

LISINOPRIL   (Prinivil, Zestril)

Recommended initial oral dose in the elderly: Blood pressure responses and adverse effects are similar in older and younger adults given the same dose, but maximum blood levels and bioavailability is double in older clients.

Unspecified adult initial dose for comparison: 10 mg once daily.

QUINAPRIL   (Accurpril)

Recommended initial oral dose in the elderly: No specific recommendation.

Unspecified adult initial dose for comparison: 10 mg once daily.

RAMIPRIL   (Altace)

Recommended initial oral dose in the elderly: No specific recommendation.

Unspecified adult initial dose for comparison: 2.5 mg once daily.

BETA-BLOCKER USE IN THE ELDERLY

Beta-blockers available for medical practice all have two properties in common—inhibition of renin secretion and ability to block beta-1 receptors, including those in the heart that provide the primary sympathetic control over such cardiac parameters as force of contraction, conductance, and rate. Together, these two actions provide the therapeutic action in hypertension with the inhibition of renin probably the more important of the two contributions. Clients with high renin levels respond to low doses of beta-blockers, while those with low levels of renin respond only at higher doses.

The various drugs differ, however, in the extent of five additional properties: blockade of beta-2 receptors, blockade of alpha-1 receptors, intrinsic sympathomimetic activity, a local anesthetic action resembling that of the antidysrhythmic drug, quinidine, and lipid solubility (see Table 13.3). Each of these additional properties affects side effects, contraindications, and clinical uses for the particular drug.

Beta-blockers that do not block beta-2 receptors are characterized as **cardioselective,** because the primary locus of beta-1 receptors is the heart. These drugs have a distinct advantage, in most applications and especially

Table 13.3 Comparative Properties of Beta-Blockers

Property	Acebutolol	Atenolol	Bisoprolol	Betaxolol	Labetalol	Metoprolol	Nadolol	Penbutolol	Pindolol	Propranolol	Timolol
Pharmacological Actions											
Beta-1 Blockade	Yes	Yes	Yes	Yes	Yes	Yes	Yes	Yes	Yes	Yes	Yes
Beta-2 Blockade	No	No	No	No	Yes	No	Yes	Yes	Yes	Yes	Yes
Alpha-1 Blockade	No	No	No	No	Yes	No	No	No	No	No	No
Local Anesthetic Activity	0	0	0	+	+	+/-	0	+	+	++	0
Intrinsic Sympathetic Activity	+	0	0	0	0	0	0	+	+++	0	0
Pharmacokinetic Properties											
Equivalent Dose Propranolol = 1	8.0	1.0	0.06	0.1	2.0	1.5	0.5	0.25	0.25	1.0	0.5
Half-Life (Hrs)	3–4	6–8	9–12	14–22	6–8	3–4	20	5	3–4	3–5	4–5
Absolute Bioavailability	40	40	80	90	25	50	30	100	90	30	50
Lipid Solubility	Low	Low	Low	Low	Moderate	Moderate	Low	High	Moderate	High	Low
Approved Applications											
Hypertension	Yes	Yes	Yes	Yes	Yes	Yes	Yes	Yes	Yes	Yes	Yes
Antiarrhythmic	Yes									Yes	
Angina Pectoris							Yes			Yes	
Hypertrophic Subaortic Stenosis										Yes	
Pheochromocytoma										Yes	
Migraine Prophylaxis										Yes	
After Myocardial Infarct										Yes	Yes
Glaucoma											Yes

in the elderly, because several important adverse effects are attributable to beta-2 blockade. Diabetes mellitus, which is common among the elderly, is aggravated by nonselective beta-blockers, because beta-2 receptors contribute to insulin secretion. Asthma is likewise aggravated by nonselective beta-blockers, because beta-2 receptors also promote bronchodilation. Beta-1 receptors also contribute slightly to bronchodilation, but much less so than beta-2 receptors. The cardioselective beta-blockers are acebutolol, atenolol, betaxolol, bisoprolol, esmolol, and metoprolol.

Labetalol, uniquely among the beta-blockers, also blocks alpha-1 adrenergic receptors. This property adds to the antihypertensive benefit of this drug and makes it useful for some clients who do not respond to other beta-blockers. However, alpha-1 blockade also adds an additional set of side effects.

Intrinsic sympathomimetic activity occurs with pindolol, oxprenolol, carteolol and, to a lesser extent, with acebutolol and penbutolol. These drugs will provide a bit less antihypertensive action and more cardiac stimulation than other beta-blockers, and can be useful for clients with bradycardia or compromised pulmonary function. They are also a useful intermediate step in weaning clients from beta-blocker therapy.

The quinidine-like local anesthetic action is a property mainly of propranolol and, to a lesser extent, acebutolol, betaxolol, oxprenolol, and pindolol. This property can be an advantage when beta-blockers are used for treating cardiac dysrhythmias, but is mostly a disadvantage in other applications. Two of the three beta-blockers approved for use as antidysrhythmics have this property. Lipid solubility of various beta-blockers is mainly important in dictating their pharmacokinetics (see below).

Clinical Indications in the Elderly. Beta-blockers are among the most versatile drugs in medicine, with many approved clinical applications. A dozen or so of the beta-blockers are approved for treatment of hypertension, where they may be used as the sole drug in the regimen or in drug combinations with diuretics and/or vasodilators. Other applications are approved only for specific drugs based mainly on whether clinical testing has been conducted for the particular drug in the particular application (see Table 13.3).

Propranolol, the oldest beta-blocker, has the widest array of approved applications, including hypertension, dysrhythmias, angina pectoris, hypertrophic subaortic stenosis, pheochromocytoma, migraine prophylaxis, glaucoma, essential tremor, and secondary prevention after a myocardial infarction.

Altered Pharmacokinetics or Pharmacodynamics in the Elderly.
Beta-blockers are well-absorbed after oral administration, but those that have high lipid solubility are subject to a high degree of **first-pass extraction.** What this means is that a large part of the administered dose is taken up by the liver as the newly absorbed drug makes its way past the liver via the portal vein in its passage from the intestinal mucosa to the systemic circulation. With propranolol, for example, only about 30–40% of a dose administered to a young adult even reaches the systemic circulation, even

though most of the administered dose is absorbed. First-pass extraction is a complicating pharmacokinetic factor, because individuals vary in the extent of this effect, first-pass extraction is proportionately less at high doses, and because first-pass extraction decreases with aging. Those beta-blockers subject to considerable first-pass extraction, including propranolol, penbutolol, metoprolol, latebalol, and oxyprenolol, will have greater bioavailability at any given dose in older persons than in younger ones. First-pass extraction is reduced by concurrent administration of the antiulcer drug, cimetidine.

Lipid solubility also determines the major route of inactivation for beta-blockers. Propranolol, labetalol, metoprolol, and pindolol are mainly metabolized in the liver before excretion. Their half-lives will be significantly prolonged by liver disease. Age-related decreases in hepatic extraction and consequent increases in half-life have been reported for propranolol, labetalol, and metoprolol. For example, the half-life of propranolol increases from an average of 3 hours in young adults to 6–8 hours in the elderly.

Beta-blockers such as nadolol and atenolol have poor lipid solubility and are excreted largely unchanged by the kidneys. Their half-lives and peak plasma concentrations will be increased in proportion to diminished renal function. For example, the half-life of atenolol increases from 6–9 hours for young adults to 16–27 hours for the elderly. Doses of these drugs must be decreased in the elderly to the extent that declines in renal function are evident.

The concentration of beta-receptors in at least one target tissue, lymphocyte membranes, has been shown to decrease as a function of age. The extent of cardiac response to a given plasma level of propranolol has been reported to decrease with age. These observations suggest that pharmacodynamic sensitivity to beta-blockers may decrease somewhat with age.

Adverse Effects and Contraindications in the Elderly. Adverse effects of beta-blockers are more common among the elderly and increase with age, renal insufficiency (for beta-blockers inactivated to a significant extent by renal excretion), intravenous administration, and length of hospitalization. The higher liabilities for the elderly derive from the presence of preexisting diseases (e.g., cardiovascular problems or diabetes mellitus), a higher incidence of drug interactions, and altered pharmacokinetics.

Beta-blockers depress contractility of the heart (a negative inotropic effect) and can thereby aggravate or even precipitate congestive heart failure. Beta-blockers are contraindicated for use in clients with preexisting serious congestive heart failure. Decreased cardiac output and lowered blood pressure serve to decrease glomerular filtration, which can paradoxically increase sodium and water retention in the absence of concurrent diuretic therapy. Labetalol is more likely than other beta-blockers to cause congestive heart failure or bradycardia, because of its unique additional blocking effect at alpha-1 receptors, and it causes side effects specifically related to alpha-1 receptors, including sexual dysfunction, urinary retention, and nasal stuffiness.

Beta-blockers also decrease conductance in cardiac tissue and can aggravate existing heart block or add to that caused by other drugs, including quinidine, procainamide, calcium-channel blockers, or digoxin. Beta-blockers are contraindicated for clients with preexisting second- or third-degree block.

Beta-blockers prevent mobilization of fats and glucose by epinephine via beta-receptors in response to stress or fasting. As a result, beta-blockers tend to increase low-density lipoproteins (LDL) and very low-density lipoproteins (VLDL), substances that correlate with rates of development of atherosclerosis. Clients receiving beta-blockers need to be especially attentive to maintaining dietary restrictions on intake of cholesterol and saturated fats.

Beta-blockers inhibit stimulation of insulin secretion by epinephrine, but also prevent the epinephrine-mediated compensatory reaction to excess insulin. Therefore, diabetic clients may need increased doses of insulin, but are also more susceptible to insulin-induced hypoglycemic shock. Even nondiabetic clients on beta-blockers can suffer extreme hypoglycemia if they undertake crash diets or prolonged fasting.

Beta-blockers aggravate asthma because beta-receptors normally help maintain bronchodilation. Beta-2 receptors contribute much more to this activity than do the beta-1 receptors, so cardioselective drugs are much less prone to this problem. Nevertheless, selective beta-1 drugs are not entirely free of potential for aggravating severe asthma when used in high doses. Bronchospasm occurs more frequently in response to beta-blockers for elderly clients than for younger adults. Beta-blockers are contraindicated for individuals with severe asthma or chronic obstructive pulmonary disease.

Since gastrointestinal activity is normally suppressed by sympathetic tone, partly through beta-receptors, beta-blockers sometimes cause gastrointestinal hyperactivity, manifested potentially as nausea, vomiting, diarrhea, cramps, or constipation.

The elderly are particularly prone to psychiatric symptoms of beta-blockers, which can include depression, drowsiness, fatigue, lethargy, bad dreams, and confusion. Preference should be given to the drugs with low lipid solubility, such as atenolol, because these do not cross the blood-brain barrier to an appreciable extent, especially if the client has existing problems with depression, tiredness, or cognitive impairment. Drowsiness caused by beta-blockers can render such activities as driving quite hazardous. Clients who experience this side effect should be advised to refrain from activities requiring mental alertness during peak drug action.

Rapid discontinuation of beta-blockers is often associated with dangerous withdrawal symptoms. Blood pressure may rebound to a dangerous extent. Angina, myocardial infarction, and dysrhythmias may occur. Sweating, trepidation, and palpitations can be early signs of an imminent anginal attack. Since withdrawal effects can develop in as little as a few hours after a missed dose, regular adherence to beta-blocker regimens is of utmost importance. Clients should be instructed not to abruptly discontinue their beta-blocker without consultation with the prescribing physician. Withdrawal effects can be minimized by tapering the drug dosage or by transitional use of a beta-blocker with intrinsic sympathomimetic activity.

Interactions in the Elderly.   The hypotensive action of beta-blockers is additive with that of diuretics and vasodilators, for better or for worse. Combination drug therapy is commonplace for hypertension and makes positive use of this interaction, but other times such interactions can lead to excess hypotension. Hypotension can cause fainting or dizziness to occur with rapid shifts in body position from prone or sitting to standing, and the elderly are more likely to suffer hazardous falls as a result.

The contribution of beta-blockers to heart failure is additive with that of other cardiac depressants, including antidysrhythmic drugs, local anesthetics, and general anesthetics. Beta-blockers potentiate the pressor action of sympathomimetic amines that might be employed in clinical settings to raise dangerously low blood pressure. However, beta-blockers prevent the beneficial effect that epinephrine would otherwise have in anaphylaxis via beta-receptor stimulation.

Beta-blockers are not a particularly good choice for managing digoxin-induced dysrhythmias. Although they do serve to alleviate ectopic beats, they also enhance the conduction block that cardiac glycosides produce at the AV node.

Beta-blockers, particularly the nonselective ones, aggravate asthma. Moreover, they prevent the beneficial effect of bronchodilators that act as beta-agonists and even reduce the bronchodilating action of theophylline.

The efficacy of beta-blockers for hypertension is diminished by smoking tobacco, use of salicylates, or indomethacin. Activity of beta-blockers is enhanced by phenothiazines and oral contraceptives.

Administration in the Elderly.   Beta-blocker therapy should be initiated at lower doses for elderly clients. Maintenance doses must be individualized based on blood pressure monitoring. Gastrointestinal hyperactivity caused by beta-blockers can be minimized by taking these medications 1 hour before meals. Inderal, Lopressor, and Tenormin rank among the most widely used prescription drugs.

ACEBUTOLOL   (Sectral)

Recommended initial oral dose in the elderly: May require lower maintenance doses, because bioavailability increases about two-fold. Avoid doses greater than 800 mg/day.

Unspecified adult initial dose for comparison: 400 mg/day in one or two divided doses.

ATENOLOL   (Tenormin, generic)

Recommended initial oral dose in the elderly: 25 mg once daily. Dosage adjustment is required in renal impairment if creatinine clearance falls below 35 ml/min/1.73 m^2.

Unspecified adult initial dose for comparison: 50 mg once daily.

BETAXOLOL   (Kerlone)

Recommended initial oral dose in the elderly: 5 mg once daily.

Unspecified adult initial dose for comparison: 10 mg once daily.

BISOPROLOL   (Zebeta)

Recommended initial oral dose in the elderly: Dose adjustment is not necessary.

Unspecified adult initial dose for comparison: 5 mg once daily.

CARTEOLOL   (Cartrol)

Recommended initial oral dose in the elderly: No specific recommendation.

Unspecified adult initial dose for comparison: 2.5 mg once daily.

ESMOLOL   (Brevibloc)

A rapid-acting beta-blocker used only for in-hospital, intravenous control of dysrhythmias.

LABETALOL   (Normodyne, Trandate)

Recommended initial oral dose in the elderly: No specific recommendation.

Unspecified adult initial dose for comparison: 100 mg twice daily.

METOPROLOL   (Lopressor, Toprol)

Recommended initial oral dose in the elderly: 25 mg twice daily.

Unspecified adult initial dose for comparison: 50–100 mg/day in a single dose.

NADOLOL   (Corgard)

Recommended initial oral dose in the elderly: 20 mg once daily.

Unspecified adult initial dose for comparison: 40 mg once daily.

PENBUTOLOL   (Levatol)

Recommended initial oral dose in the elderly: No specific recommendation.

Unspecified adult initial dose for comparison: 20 mg once daily.

PINDOLOL   (Visken, generic)

Recommended initial oral dose in the elderly: No specific recommendation.

Unspecified adult initial dose for comparison: 5 mg twice daily.

PROPRANOLOL   (Inderal, generic)

Recommended initial oral dose in the elderly: 10 mg one to four times daily.

Unspecified adult initial dose for comparison: 40 mg twice daily or 80 mg once daily.

SOTALOL   (Betapace)

Used for life-threatening ventricular dysrhythmias only. Dosing interval must be modified in conditions of renal impairment.

TIMOLOL   (Blocadren, generic)

Recommended initial oral dose in the elderly: 5 mg twice daily.

Unspecified adult initial dose for comparison: 10 mg twice daily.

USE OF OTHER SYMPATHOLYTICS IN THE ELDERLY

Sympatholytic drugs work in hypertension by reducing sympathetic tone and thereby decreasing peripheral vascular resistance. However, sympatholytics other than beta-blockers have lost much of their previous favor in treatments for hypertension. They are seldom used as the exclusive intervention, because concurrent use of diuretics both improves the benefit of sympatholytics and decreases the risk of fluid accumulation that they confer. Among the sympatholytics, methyldopa, guanabenz, guanfacine, and clonidine act centrally, at the level of the vasomotor center of the medulla, while reserpine, guanethidine, and guanadrel act peripherally at the level of the sympathetic nerve terminals.

Clinical Indications in the Elderly.   Sympatholytics are indicated for use in multi-drug regimens for hypertension.

Altered Pharmacokinetics or Pharmacodynamics in the Elderly.
Methyldopa is not well absorbed, with only about 25% bioavailability after oral administration. Its peak effect occurs in about 4–6 hours. Clonidine and guanfacine are better absorbed—about 75%. Guanfacine is completely absorbed.

Methyldopa is inactivated mainly by renal excretion, necessitating dosage adjustment in those with impaired renal function. Clonidine is inactivated about 60% by renal excretion and 40% by liver metabolism and also requires dosage adjustment in renal impairment. Guanfacine is inactivated 30% by renal excretion and 70% by liver metabolism.

Adverse Effects and Contraindications in the Elderly.   All of the sympatholytic drugs produce a set of adverse effects known as anti-adrenergic side effects (see Table 13.4), although they will vary with respect to the likelihood of the particular problems. Antiadrenergic side effects include ones related to both the peripheral and the central roles of the adrenergic hormones, norepinephrine and epinephrine. Peripheral anti-adrenergic effects are much less severe with methyldopa, clonidine, guanabenz, or guanfacine than with guanethidine or reserpine.

Table 13.4 Antiadrenergic Side Effects

Peripheral	Central
Excess hypotension	Sedation
Orthostatic hypotension	Sleep disturbances
Vascular headaches	Weakness
Excess Gastrointestinal activity	Extrapyramidal reactions
Nausea	Weight gain
Diarrhea	Galactorrhea
Ulcers	
Impotence	
Bladder and eye control problems	
Aggravation of asthma	

Orthostatic hypotension can occur with any of these drugs and is essentially an exaggeration of the effect for which the drug is being employed. It may result in a tendency toward vertigo or syncope when body position is abruptly shifted from prone or sitting to a standing position. The elderly are often more susceptible to this problem, because of diminished control of balance and poorer motor control. Elderly also often pay a higher price for accidental falls that may follow from orthostatic hypotension. Like the beta-blockers, these sympatholytics can cause salt and water retention due to diminished renal filtration pressure and vasodilation.

Bladder and eye control problems, especially common with reserpine and methyldopa, occur more frequently among the elderly because they are often superimposed on visual impairments of aging and bladder control problems secondary to urinary retention, incontinence, or, in males, prostatic hypertrophy. Inhibition of ejaculation is a common problem for males taking these drugs, especially the peripherally acting agents.

Central antiadrenergic side effects are especially problematic with methyldopa, reserpine, clonidine, guanabenz, and guanfacine. The central nervous system depressants may cause sedation, depression, or cognitive impairments and are especially likely to exacerbate existing mental alterations that often accompany aging. Clients receiving centrally active sympatholytics need to be advised to avoid hazardous tasks, such as driving during the peak sedative action. If the drug is given as a single daily dose, taking the drug at bedtime will minimize daytime sedation. Nightmares, vivid dreams, anxiety, restlessness, and extrapyramidal reactions are other possibilities with methyldopa, clonidine, and other centrally acting sympatholytics.

Allergic reactions occur more frequently to methyldopa among the elderly and those with arteriosclerotic vascular disease.

Withdrawal hypertension is a particular problem with clonidine and occasionally a problem for guanabenz and guanfacine. Associated symptoms may include nervousness, anxiety, insomnia, headaches, tremor, nausea, or abdominal cramps. Whenever possible, sympatholytics in this subgroup should have doses tapered (over a 2- to-4-day period) rather than being abruptly withdrawn. Guanethidine is so long-acting that it may complicate control of blood pressure during surgical procedures. Therefore, clients are typically switched to shorter acting antihypertensive medications two weeks prior to elective surgery.

Interactions in the Elderly.   Depressive influences of centrally acting sympatholytics are additive with those of other central nervous system depressants, including hypnotics, anxiolytics, antiepileptics, antihistamines, narcotics, and neuroleptics. Tricyclic antidepressants interfere with the action of clonidine and guanethidine, so the two kinds of drug should not be used concurrently. Guanethedine causes supersensitivity of noradrenergic receptors that can dangerously potentiate the pressor effect of sympathomimetic amines. Reserpine can cause cardiac dysrhythmias in clients also receiving quinidine or digitalis.

Administration of Centrally Acting Sympatholytics.

CLONIDINE   (Catapres, generic)

Recommended initial oral dose in the elderly: Reduce for renal impairment.

Unspecified adult initial dose for comparison: 0.1 mg twice daily.

GUANABENZ   (Wytensin)

Recommended initial oral dose in the elderly: Reduce dose for renal or hepatic impairment.

Unspecified adult initial dose for comparison: 4 mg twice daily.

GUANFACINE   (Tenex)

Recommended initial oral dose in the elderly: No specific recommendation.

Unspecified adult initial dose for comparison: 1 mg/day at bedtime.

METHYLDOPA   (Aldomet, generic)

Recommended initial oral dose in the elderly: Lower doses to avoid increased sensitivity.

Unspecified adult initial dose for comparison: 250 mg 2 or 3 times daily.

Administration of Peripherally Acting Sympatholytics.

GUANADREL   (Hylorel)

Recommended initial oral dose in the elderly: No specific recommendation.

Unspecified adult initial dose for comparison: 5 mg twice daily.

GUANETHIDINE (Ismelin, generic)

Recommended initial oral dose in the elderly:
No specific recommendation.

Unspecified adult initial dose for comparison: 10 mg daily for ambulatory patients; 25–50 mg/day for hospitalized patients.

RESERPINE (Serpasil, Serpalan, generic)

Recommended initial oral dose in the elderly: Lower doses for elderly and debilitated clients.

Unspecified adult initial dose for comparison: 0.5 mg/day.

CALCIUM-CHANNEL BLOCKER (CCB) USE IN THE ELDERLY

Calcium-channel blockers have been available for clinical use since 1982, and they have rapidly gained an important place in the treatment of hypertension, angina pectoris, and cardiac dysrhythmias. These drugs, as their class name suggests, block the influx of calcium into muscle and nerve cells. When they act on vascular smooth muscle, the result is vasodilation and suppression of vasospasms. When they act on the myocardium, the result is a decrease in contractility (negative inotropism), a decrease in conductance, and a decrease in automaticity.

Clinical Indications in the Elderly. Collectively, the nine drugs currently available in this category have four approved uses and four unlabeled ones. Six of the nine are approved for angina pectoris and seven for hypertension. Verapamil is the only CCB approved for dysrhythmias, while nimodipine is uniquely approved for minimizing sequelae following subarachnoid hemorrhage. Unlabeled applications include the use of nifedipine, nimodipine, and verapamil for migraine prophylaxis, the use of diltiazem or nifedipine for Raynaud's syndrome, the use of nicardipine and nifedipine for congestive heart failure, and the use of nifedipine or verapamil for cardiomyopathy.

Altered Pharmacokinetics or Pharmacodynamics in the Elderly.
All of the CCBs are at least 90% absorbed after oral administration. Protein binding in the plasma is greater than 90% for all but verapamil (83–92%) and diltiazem (70–80%). All are inactivated mainly by hepatic metabolism and significant increases in peak plasma concentrations and half-life prolongation have thus far been demonstrated for clients with hepatic dysfunction for two of the drugs, verapamil and nifedipine. Moreover, an increase in

the area under the plasma concentration versus time curve has been reported for nicardipine. Odds are that all CCBs have impaired inactivation in proportion to hepatic dysfunction. The elderly exhibit on average a greater hypotensive response to verapamil, nifedipine, and felodipine than younger patients, most likely due to reduced hepatic clearance. Significant alterations in relation to renal impairments have not been reported.

Adverse Effects and Contraindications in the Elderly. Adverse effects of CCBs occur mainly in three categories:

1. excess peripheral vasodilation,
2. negative inotropism, and
3. depression of nodal conductance.

Symptoms of excess vasodilation can include dizziness, vertigo, syncope, facial flushing or warmth, vascular (migraine-like) headache, edema, and fatigue. The elderly are especially prone to such effects and to falls occurring as a consequence of dizziness or syncope.

Negative inotropism, when it occurs, contributes to congestive heart failure. Although it occurs in only about 1% of those receiving CCBs, the likelihood is elevated in those with preexisting congestive heart failure. Conduction blocks are most likely to occur with verapamil and diltiazem. Administration of calcium salts will reverse cardiac toxicities of verapamil.

Interactions in the Elderly. Hypotension caused by CCBs is additive with that produced by diuretics, sympatholytics, and other vasodilators. Negative inotropic effects of CCBs are additive with those of beta-blockers. Depression of conductance by CCBs is additive with conductance effects of quinidine, local anesthetics, and other antidysrhythmic drugs. It is best not to use quinidine and CCBs concurrently. Verapamil and nifedipine have been reported to increase plasma concentrations of digoxin. Dosage adjustments for digoxin are required. Inducers of liver enzymes, such as barbiturates and hydantoins, decrease plasma concentrations of felodipine and verapamil.

Administration in the Elderly. Doses should be individualized on the basis of blood pressure monitoring when CCBs are used for hypertension.

AMLODIPINE (Norvasc)

Recommended initial oral dose in the elderly: 5 mg once daily.

Unspecified adult initial antihypertensive dose for comparison: 5 mg once daily.

Unspecified adult initial antianginal dose for comparison: 5–10 mg once daily.

BEPRIDIL   (Vascor)

Recommended initial oral dose in the elderly: Starting dose does not differ, but elderly may require more frequent monitoring.

Unspecified adult initial antianginal dose for comparison: 200 mg/day.

DILTIAZEM   (Cardizem)

Recommended initial oral dose in the elderly: Use caution in titrating doses for clients with impaired renal or hepatic function, as dosage requirements are not available.

Unspecified adult initial antihypertensive dose for comparison: 60–120 mg twice daily of the sustained release product.

Unspecified adult initial antianginal dose for comparison: 30 mg 4 times daily; for the sustained release product, 60–120 mg twice daily.

FELODIPINE   (Plendil)

Recommended initial oral dose in the elderly: Reduce for hepatic dysfunction.

Unspecified adult initial antihypertensive dose for comparison: 5 mg once daily.

ISRADIPINE

Recommended initial oral dose in the elderly: No specific recommendation.

Unspecified adult initial antihypertensive dose for comparison:
2.5 mg twice daily.

NICARDIPINE   (Cardene)

Recommended initial oral dose in the elderly: Reduce for hepatic impairment to 20 mg twice daily.

Unspecified adult initial antihypertensive or antianginal dose for comparison: 20 mg 3 times daily.

NIFEDIPINE   (Adalat, Procardia, generic)

Recommended initial oral dose in the elderly: Reduce for hepatic dysfunction.

Unspecified adult initial antihypertensive dose for comparison: 30 or 60 mg once daily of the sustained release product.

Unspecified adult initial antianginal dose for comparison: 10mg 3 times daily.

NIMODIPINE   (Nimotop)

Used only to improve neurologic deficits due to spasm following subarachnoid hemorrhage.

VERAPAMIL   (Calan, Isoptin, generic)

Recommended initial oral dose in the elderly: 40 mg 3 times daily; for sustained release product, 120 mg/day in morning. For antidysrhythmic applications, give IV bolus over at least 3 minutes to minimize risks.

Unspecified adult initial antihypertensive dose for comparison: 80 mg 3 times daily; for sustained release product, 240 mg/day in morning.

Unspecified adult initial antianginal dose for comparison: 80–120 mg 3 times daily.

Unspecified adult initial antidysrhythmic dose for comparison: 5–10 mg as IV bolus over 2 minutes.

USE OF OTHER VASODILATORS IN THE ELDERLY

Vasodilators used for chronic hypertension include alpha-1 blocking drugs (prazosin, terazosin, and doxazosin), hydralazine, and minoxidil. Their mechanism is a reduction in peripheral resistance to blood flow by relaxing vascular smooth muscle. The alpha-blockers do this by interfering with the influence exerted by the sympathetic nervous system on vascular tone, while the remaining drugs produce the same effect by a direct action on the smooth muscle itself. These drugs are usually added in the third step of treatment for hypertension to a regimen that already includes a diuretic and a beta-blocker. They work better in combination with other antihypertensives than alone, because diuretics help prevent the tendency of vasodilators to cause fluid retention, while beta-blockers protect the heart from reflex cardiac stimulation that would otherwise tend to occur with vasodilators. Vasodilators are less viable for use with elderly clients because of the high risk of excess hypotension.

Clinical Indications in the Elderly.   Severe hypertension not adequately controlled by salt-restrictions, weight loss, diuretics, and beta-blockers.

Altered Pharmacokinetics or Pharmacodynamics in the Elderly.
Prazosin is subject to extensive first-pass extraction with only 5% of an administered dose reaching the systemic circulation. In the presence of heart failure or hepatic dysfunction, first-pass extraction and hepatic inactivation of the bioavailable fraction is reduced, prolonging the half-life of prazosin. Terazosin, by contrast, is well-absorbed orally (about 90%), while doxazosin provides approximately 65% bioavailability. All three of the alpha-1 blocking vasodilators are highly bound to plasma proteins. Prazocin and doxazosin are mainly metabolized by the liver and excreted in the bile, while terazosin depends 40% on renal elimination. There is no evident difference in blood pressure responses to doxazosin in clients above or below 65 years of age.

Hydralazine is well-absorbed but subject to extensive and variable first-pass extraction. It is acetylated in the liver. Its metabolism provides a classic example of idiosyncratic reaction, because some people are rapid acetylators (a genetically determined characteristic), while others are slow acetylators. Hydralazine is only 30% bioavailable in rapid acetylators, but 50% bioavailable in slow acetylators. Slow acetylators develop higher plasma concentrations to a given dose and require dosage reduction.

Minoxidil is 90% absorbed after oral administration and 90% inactivated by hepatic metabolism before renal excretion. Smaller doses may be required when renal function is impaired.

Adverse Effects and Contraindications in the Elderly.   Orthostatic hypotension is always a potential with vasodilators and can be severe. Fainting may occur upon standing and result in injury to elderly clients. Alpha-1 blocking vasodilators are especially likely to cause a severe **first-dose effect,** with marked orthostatic hypotension and loss of consciousness. This problem can be circumvented by instituting therapy slowly, with small doses, and by giving the first dose at bedtime. Other signs of excess vasodilation include vascular headaches and facial flushing. Preexisting salt depletion increases the likelihood of a first-dose effect when therapy with an alpha-1 blocking vasodilator is initiated.

Fluid retention is a definite problem with vasodilators, because of the expanded capacitance of the vasculature. For that reason, vasodilators should only be used as add-ons to a regimen already including a diuretic, especially for elderly clients.

Vasodilators will cause reflex cardiac stimulation and even dangerous tachydysrhythmias without the protective effect of concurrent beta-blocker medication. Therefore, vasodilators are best reserved for regimens that already include a beta-blocker.

The alpha-blocking vasodilators may produce side-effects specifically associated with alpha-blockade, including drowsiness, fatigue, dry mouth, urinary incontinence, and impotence.

Hydralazine presents additional problems and its use can seldom be justified, especially for elderly clients. Gastrointestinal bleeding may occur, for example. A particularly problematic aspect of hydralazine's activity is the likelihood of a drug-induced lupus-like syndrome. It occurs in 10–20% of clients receiving doses of hydralazine in excess of 400 mg/day and is a definite threat to any client receiving more than 200 mg/day or who is a slow acetylator. If hydralazine therapy is being considered, determination should be made of the client's hepatic acetylator status.

Minoxidil has the unique potential for causing generalized hypertrichosis, or excess hair growth, especially over the shoulders, back, forearms, temples, and cheeks. Indeed, a second use for this drug is treatment of male-pattern baldness. Needless to say, women may be particularly troubled by this side effect of minoxidil.

Interactions in the Elderly.   The main interaction of vasodilators is the potential for additive hypotensive effects with other antihypertensive drugs. This can be put to good effect in multi-drug regimens for hypertension, but can also result in symptoms of orthostatic hypotension, fluid retention and edema, or dangerous reflex cardiac stimulation. Beneficial interactions with vasodilators include the ability of diuretics to protect against fluid retention and the ability of beta-blockers to protect the heart from reflex tachycardia that would otherwise be routine with vasodilators.

Administration in the Elderly.   Dosage adjustments should be made on the basis of a regular program of blood pressure monitoring. Tolerance may develop to the action of hydralazine with chronic administration, necessitating upward dosage adjustment. Vasodilator therapy should be discontinued gradually to avoid a sudden rebound hypertension.

Alpha-1 Blocking Vasodilators

DOXAZOSIN   (Cardura)

Recommended initial oral dose in the elderly: No specific recommendation.

Unspecified adult initial dose for comparison: 1 mg once daily.

PRAZOSIN   (Minipress)

Recommended initial oral dose in the elderly: No specific recommendation.

Unspecified adult initial dose for comparison: 1 mg 2 or 3 times daily.

TERAZOSIN   (Hytrin)

Recommended initial oral dose in the elderly: No specific recommendation.

Unspecified adult initial dose for comparison: 1 mg at bedtime.

Other Vasodilators

HYDRALAZINE   (Alazine, Apresoline, generic)

Recommended initial oral dose in the elderly: No specific recommendation; reduce for slow acetylators.

Unspecified adult initial dose for comparison: 10 mg 4 times daily.

MINOXIDIL   (Loniten, Minodyl, and generic)

Recommended initial oral dose in the elderly: No specific recommendation.

Unspecified adult initial dose for comparison: 5 mg/day in a single dose.

CONGESTIVE HEART FAILURE AND CARDIAC GLYCOSIDES IN ELDERLY CLIENTS

Basically, congestive heart failure (CHF) is a failure of the cardiac muscle (or myocardium) to pump enough blood to meet the requirements of the various bodily tissues. When the flow of blood declines, the peripheral vasculature becomes congested with blood; hence the term *congestive* is the name of the disorder. The defect may be intrinsic to the cardiac muscle itself (e.g., myocardial disease from myocarditis, myocardial infarction, or cardiomyopathy), but the single most frequent cause of CHF, particularly among the elderly, is essential hypertension. Serum cholesterol level is a major risk factor for hypertension and therefore also for CHF. There is an increase in risk of approximately 6 per 1000 for occurrence of congestive heart failure for each 50 mg/dl increase in serum cholesterol. The heart itself might function adequately for additional years were it not for the fact that the increase in afterload associated with hypertension reduces what the heart is able to accomplish with a given amount of work. Other causes of CHF extrinsic to the heart itself are thyrotoxicosis, anemia, acidosis, pulmonary embolism, or drugs with negative inotropic effects (e.g., beta-blockers).

In the early stages of the disease, overt clinical symptoms may be averted by the ability of the heart to compensate for changing requirements. For example, the cardiac muscle is stretched further as filling pressure (**preload**) increases and then responds with a greater contraction. The heart may enlarge to meet the added workload. These compensations will not suffice indefinitely, if the circumstances continue to grow worse.

As the condition progresses, it tends to perpetuate and exacerbate itself. Renal output declines in response to decreased cardiac output, resulting in further fluid retention, further increase in afterload, and further declines in cardiac output. The sympathetic nervous system fights to maintain arterial pressure, but thereby adds to the declines in tissue perfusion. The ultimate consequence of progressing CHF is cardiogenic shock, with severe drop in vascular tone and perfusion and high mortality rates.

Treatment objectives for CHF are

1. Improve cardiac output by increasing contractility.
2. Reduce cardiac workload.
3. Correct impairments of tissue function or fluid balance that have developed as a result of CHF.

The first objective, improving cardiac output, is undertaken with drugs called **cardiotonics.** The most familiar drugs in this category are a family called the **cardiac glycosides,** which occur naturally in the squill, or sea onion, and, most importantly, the foxglove plant. The squill was used in early Egyptian civilization and the leaves of the foxglove from at least AD 1250. There are synthetic cardiotonics available today, but the natural drugs, especially digoxin, continue to enjoy greatest popularity. Cardiotonics are discussed in detail in the following section.

Reducing cardiac workload, the second objective, should be given high priority, since it can provide significant benefit in management of CHF without the need for pushing the heart to more vigorous levels of output than it can sustain in the long run. Sometimes, cardiac workload can be significantly reduced by adjustments in lifestyle. Reductions in physical activity (especially short, high-energy burst activities), more frequent rest periods throughout the day, weight loss, and stress reduction can all provide benefit and help to preserve limited cardiac output for the client's most important activities. Salt and fluid retention is a frequent factor in CHF, for the elderly especially. Salt restriction is a good starting point. The average American diet provides 6–15 g/day of salt. Eliminating salt from the table and cooking can reduce salt intake by 3–4 g/day, while the elimination of salty foods (and drugs) can provide even greater reductions. If salt restriction fails to provide an adequate reduction in afterload and preload, diuretics are the next step and a routine means of treating congestive heart failure. Thiazide diuretics are most often used, but high-ceiling diuretics might be selected when fluid retention is great. A recent development in the protocol for reducing cardiac workload is the addition of a vasodilator, especially if the condition is not adequately responsive to salt restriction, diuretics, and cardiac glycoside combinations. Vasodilators (such as nitroprusside, isosorbide, prazosin, or calcium channel blockers) help to reduce cardiac workload by lowering both preload and afterload.

USE OF DIGOXIN IN THE ELDERLY

Age-dependent pharmacokinetics and other effects of aging are especially relevant for drugs that have a low therapeutic index, or safety margin, and that most certainly characterizes the cardiac glycosides. The two major cardiac glycosides are digoxin and digitoxin. These drugs have the same pharmacology, but differ significantly in pharmacokinetic parameters, such as route of inactivation and half-life. Digoxin is used far more frequently than digitoxin or other cardiotonics and is one of the most widely used of all drugs in elderly clients. As a result, adverse reactions and adverse drug interactions involving digoxin occur with great frequency. On the other hand, this drug has life-extending capabilities that justify its careful use.

Clinical Indications in the Elderly. As in other adults, cardiac glycosides have two indications for the elderly: congestive heart failure and reducing ventricular response rates in atrial tachydysrhythmias. Approximately 80% of individuals taking digoxin are over 60 years of age, and about 60% are over 70, so digoxin use is characteristically among the elderly. Cardiac glycoside treatment for CHF should be reserved for those cases not adequately responsive to dietary adjustments, activity adjustments, and treatment with a diuretic, because of the significant potential for adverse effects and uncertain benefits. Cardiac glycosides are most effective in heart failure related to chronic overload caused by hypertension, atherosclerosis, or valve lesions. These drugs are less likely to provide benefit in CHF secondary to thyrotoxicosis, hypoxia, advanced cardiomyopathy, or myocarditis due to infections or toxic drug effects.

Digoxin is indicated for reduction of ventricular response rates in most kinds of atrial tachydysrhythmias, including atrial fibrillation, atrial flutter, and atrial paroxysmal tachycardia. An appropriate antidysrhythmic drug (e.g., a calcium-channel blocker) may be used concurrently for further reduction of ventricular response rate and stabilization of the atrial rhythm itself. Digoxin used for reducing ventricular response rate should be reevaluated at approximately 3-month intervals and discontinued if the cause of the atrial dysrhythmia has resolved or if the client remains symptom-free at serum concentrations of digoxin below 0.8 ng/ml.

Altered Pharmacokinetics or Pharmacodynamics in the Elderly.
Digoxin is absorbed from the upper part of the small intestines, usually 70–75% (range 40–90%). Absorption of digoxin is reduced by malabsorption syndrome and, in great measure by jejunal-ileal bypass or major small bowel resections. Absorption of digoxin can be significantly altered, however, by time of administration in relation to meals or other factors that alter gastric emptying time and product formulation. Delays in gastric emptying time delay but do not alter ultimate extent of absorption of digoxin, but clients should be encouraged to maintain consistency in the times they take their medication in relation to mealtimes. Tablets of digoxin manufactured by different pharmaceutical companies vary widely in both rate and extent of absorption provided and, for this particular drug, clients should be urged not to switch brands without consultation with the prescribing physician.

One factor that decreases dosage requirements for digoxin in the elderly is a decrease in lean body mass and, hence, volume of distribution for drugs, like digoxin, with mainly aqueous solubility. Also, binding of digoxin by plasma proteins is diminished for elderly persons, so the fraction of digoxin in the plasma that is free and pharmacologically active is greater.

Digoxin is inactivated mainly by renal excretion, although hepatobiliary clearance accounts for approximately 25% of digoxin elimination normally. The decrease in renal function that occurs inevitably with aging will decrease dosage requirement for digoxin, both with respect to loading dose requirements and maintenance doses. **Decreased clearance of digoxin in proportion to decreased renal function is the single most important age-related change influencing dosage requirements for this drug.** Creatinine clearance, the clinical test most often used to assess changes in glomerular filtration rate, can be misleading in the elderly (because of changes in volume of distribution of creatinine in the elderly) and therefore cannot be relied upon as a basis for making the necessary dosage adjustments for digoxin. When renal clearance declines with aging, hepatobiliary clearance becomes proportionally more important, but it is not known whether it too is subject to age-related declines.

Together, these changes in renal clearance, volume of distribution, and plasma protein binding mean that an elderly person will have, on average, blood levels near **twice** those of a young adult in response to any given dose of digoxin. The half-life of digoxin increases from an average of 36 hours for young adults to 70 hours for the elderly. This also means that the time required to reach steady-state concentrations of digoxin in the plasma after initiating treatment will be much longer. The usual assumption is that steady-state levels are reached after approximately 4 to 5 half-lives, so for an elderly person, this might require as long as two weeks—twice as long as for a younger person.

While it is true that renal digoxin clearance decreases and half-life increases with aging, variability in these parameters also increases. Some clients exhibit changes in digoxin kinetics with aging to a much greater extent than others. Therefore, the need to individualize doses and to closely monitor plasma level, therapeutic response, and adverse effects is all the more evident when the client is elderly.

Digitoxin, in contrast to the more widely used digoxin, is primarily inactivated by hepatic metabolism. Its kinetics are therefore less influenced by renal impairment and more by hepatic dysfunction. The drug should be avoided in those with hepatitis, liver cirrhosis, or other hepatic difficulties.

Pharmacodynamic responses to digoxin are more likely to be altered in the elderly, as well, because the elderly more often experience the requisite conditions. Sensitivity to digoxin, particularly for the deleterious effects in the heart and brain, is increased for those with hypothyroidism, hypokalemia, ischemic heart disease, or chronic pulmonary disease—all conditions common among the elderly.

Adverse Effects and Contraindications in the Elderly.   Adverse reactions to digoxin are among the most common drug side effects in the elderly. The reported incidence of such reactions among hospitalized geriatric patients is 10–20% of such individuals. Adverse effects of cardiac glycosides are often more severe and more frequent and even manifest differently among the elderly. The problems can be grouped into five categories:

1. cardiac toxicity
2. gastrointestinal problems
3. neurologic side effects
4. psychiatric changes
5. other side effects.

Potential cardiac toxicities include the whole gamut of cardiac dysrhythmias. For younger people, cardiac dysrhythmias seldom occur without prior extracardiac symptoms of digoxin toxicity; in the elderly, life-threatening dysrhythmias may occur without any such prior warning. One-quarter of those with EKG evidence of digoxin-induced cardiac dysrhythmias are asymptomatic and can be identified only by EKG monitoring. Bradycardia frequently occurs as a result of the effect of a cardiac glycoside on the SA node. First-degree block is a commonplace action of digoxin on the AV node with higher degrees of block a possibility. Ectopic foci often develop in response to digoxin, resulting in ventricular tachydysrhythmias ranging from isolated premature ventribular beats to life-threatening ventricular fibrillation. Bigemini or trigemini rhythms are common signs of intermediate toxicity, these being rhythms where normal beats alternate with one or two ectopic beats. Patients requiring digoxin are often those also at liability for dysrhythmias related to cardiac ailments, so it is often difficult to know when the dysrhythmias are drug-induced and when not. The EKG provides the best basis for differentiation. EKG characteristics of digoxin toxicity include a prolongation of the PR interval, depression and shortening of the ST segment, bradycardia, and premature ventricular beats. Fortunately, digoxin-induced dysrhythmias will respond to appropriate treatment if treatment is undertaken soon enough. Phenytoin and lidocaine are the most useful antidysrhythmic drugs for digoxin-induced tachydysrhythmias. Atropine can be used for digoxin-induced bradycardia. Potassium salts provide direct antagonism, but need to be administered with great caution, especially if AV block is present. Quinidine and calcium-channel blockers should not be given, and beta-blockers should be reserved for last resort.

Gastrointestinal side effects are very common in response to digoxin and can include nausea, vomiting, anorexia (loss of appetite), and gastrointestinal discomfort. Nausea and vomiting are less frequent complaints among elderly clients, but anorexia and gastrointestinal discomfort are more frequent. Diarrhea can sometimes occur.

Neurological symptoms, such as headache, fatigue, drowsiness, and general malaise are common complaints. The elderly are more likely to experience fatigue or, conversely, restlessness than their younger counterparts. Alterations in visual perception are common for the elderly as for younger patients, but are more likely to take the form of hazy vision than the alterations in color vision that occur in younger people. Psychiatric symptoms such as depression, disorientation, and delirium, are particularly common and problematic for the elderly, because they are more likely than younger adults to be suffering already from major depression or organic brain syndrome. Psychiatric side effects of digoxin are quite common among the elderly and should always be considered when mental status changes in an elderly person. Measurement of serum levels will help to identify when symptoms are due to digoxin toxicity, but psychiatric side effects do sometimes occur even when digoxin levels lie within the normal limits. Other side effects of digoxin, such as skin rash and eosinophilia, have similar expression in the elderly as in younger people.

Interactions in the Elderly. A variety of drugs used by the elderly decrease absorption of digoxin from the intestines, including magnesium-containing antacids, antidiarrheal suspensions containing kaolin-pectin, steroid-binding resins (such as cholestyramine and colestipol), sulfasalazine, aminosalicylic acid, and antibiotics (especially oral aminoglycosides). Dietary fiber, which the elderly often utilize to maintain good motility, can also have this effect.

Drugs that induce liver enzymes, such as barbiturates, antiepileptics, antihistamines, phenylbutazone, and rifampin, can increase digoxin metabolism and dosage requirements. Hyperthyroidism also increases digoxin metabolism.

Cardiac glycosides interact with any drug or circumstance that alters levels of potassium in bodily fluids. Potassium and cardiac glycosides have a basically antagonistic relationship, so hyperkalemia can decrease both benefits and side effects of digoxin, while hypokalemia increases both positive and negative effects. Drugs that most often alter potassium levels are diuretics, which cause hypokalemia, and angiotensin-converting enzyme inhibitors and potassium-sparing diuretics, which cause hyperkalemia. The antibiotic, amphotericin B, also promotes hypokalemia. Potassium salts can be used to alleviate digoxin toxicity. Phenytoin and digoxin-immune antigen-binding fragments (Digibind) are alternatives for that purpose.

One of the usually disadvantageous effects of digoxin on the heart is that it decreases conductance, thereby increasing conduction delays and possibly inducing heart block. Many antidysrhythmic drugs also have this action and will add to the blocking action of digoxin. Additive potential for block has been reported with quinidine, procainamide, beta-blockers, and calcium-channel blockers, for example.

Digoxin increases the risk of the various kinds of tachydysrhythmias, including premature beats, paroxysmal tachycardia, tachycardia, flutter, and fibrillation. This liability is additive with that of sympathomimetics such as epinephrine.

Administration in the Elderly.   Digoxin is derived from the white fox-glove, while digitoxin is derived from the purple foxglove. Digoxin is used far more often than digitoxin because its shorter half-life makes it safer for use than digitoxin. It also provides a more rapid onset. Plasma levels are, however, less stable for digoxin if adherence to the regimen by the client is sporadic. If treatment with a cardiac glycoside is begun without urgency for a quick response, maintenance doses can be given from the beginning with the expectation that steady-state concentrations will be reached after approximately four half-lives, about 1 week for digoxin or a month for digitoxin for a young or middle-aged adult or about twice those time periods in the elderly. If more rapid response is required, a one-time loading dose (also called **digitalizing doses**) can be administered intravenously.

DIGITOXIN   (Crystodigin, De-Tone, Purodigin)

Recommended intravenous loading dose in the elderly: No specific recommendation. Dosage reductions required if hepatic dysfunction is present.

Unspecified adult intravenous loading dose for comparison: 1.2–1.6 mg IV.

Recommended oral maintenance dose in the elderly: No specific recommendation. Dosage reduction required if hepatic dysfunction is present.

Unspecified adult oral maintenance dose for comparison: 0.05–0.3 mg daily.

DIGOXIN   (Lanoxin)

Recommended intravenous loading dose in the elderly: 5–10 mcg/kg in two or three divided intravenous injections each given over 10 to 20 minutes over a 24-hour period.

Unspecified adult intravenous loading dose for comparison: 8–12 mcg/kg in one or two divided intravenous injections each given over 10 to 20 minutes 3–4 hours apart.

Recommended oral maintenance dose in the elderly: 0.125–0.25 mg orally once daily. Adjust dosage downward in proportion to decreased renal function.*

Unspecified adult oral maintenance dose for comparison:
0.125–0.5 mg orally once daily.*

*Exact dosage is calculated based on loading dose, lean body weight, and creatinine clearance as follows: Maintenance dose = loading dose × (14 + creatinine clearance/5)/100 × lean body weight (Kg)/70.

ISCHEMIC HEART DISEASE IN ELDERLY CLIENTS

Ischemia is a condition of inadequate blood flow to a tissue, usually related to pathological changes in small blood vessels that perfuse that tissue. Ischemic heart disease is usually a result of atherosclerosis of coronary blood vessels. The healthy heart extracts oxygen from the blood with great efficiency—near optimum efficiency. Therefore, when oxygen requirements are higher than normal for a period of time, the major mechanism for meeting increased oxygen requirements is dilation of coronary vessels. When coronary vessels become sclerotic, they provide less flow, less efficient oxygen transit, and diminished ability to dilate to meet extra demand requirements. By the time clinical symptoms occur, 50–75% of blood supply has been lost after several decades of atherosclerotic plaque formation. Angina pectoris is a subacute, intermittent ischemia, probably brought on by exercise and usually alleviated by rest. Myocardial infarction arises from the same predisposing conditions, but is an abrupt reduction in blood supply to a region of the myocardium that is so sharp and severe that the cells affected are at risk of damage or death. Thus, atherosclerotic changes in coronary vessels are the prelude to both of the classic manifestations of ischemic heart disease.

Androgens increase atherosclerotic processes, while estrogens reduce these events, so prior to climacteric, the incidence of ischemic heart disease is higher for men than women. The gender difference decreases thereafter. Some of the other factors known to contribute to risk of atherosclerosis are race, family history of the problem, diabetes mellitus, hyperlipemia, diets rich in cholesterol or saturated fats, obesity, lack of exercise, stress, hypertension, alcohol consumption, and smoking tobacco.

Myocardial Infarction and Its Management in the Elderly

Myocardial infarction is an abruptly developing ischemia caused by a sharp drop in blood flow to a part of the myocardium, with development of necrosis (cell death) unless the flow is restored promptly. The telltale clinical symptom is severe chest pain, often described as heavy or crushing. The pain is often experienced as radiating through the arms, back, and jaw. The pain resembles that of angina, but fails to respond to antianginal medications (such as nitroglycerin). If severe, the myocardial infarction (which clients usually refer to as a "heart attack") may lead to complications, including dysrhythmias, congestive heart failure, thromboembolism, pericarditis, or other difficulties. Fifty percent of victims of myocardial infarction die from dysrhythmia before receiving medical attention, and half of deaths occur within 2.5 hours of pain onset.

The five short-term objectives in treating a client who has just experienced a myocardial infarction are

1. reduce the workload of the heart;
2. minimize the peri-infarction zone (that is, keep the permanent cell damage to the smallest extent possible);
3. prevent complications;
4. treat complications;
5. provide comfort and support.

The early phase of treatment is critically important to ultimate survival. Morphine is given to alleviate pain, but unfortunately also causes orthostatic hypotension. Elevation of the legs helps to minimize the consequences of hypotension. Lidocaine is sometimes given routinely before transport to a clinical facility; if not it may be given in the emergency room, if EKG monitoring indicates dysrhythmia. Atropine or digoxin might be given, if the dysrhythmia is atrial, to reduce ventricular response rate. If serious hypotension develops, dopamine (Intropin) or dobutamine (Dobutrex) are likely to be given intravenously.

Once the immediately life-threatening concerns have been dealt with, the next concern is for minimizing the peri-infarction zone. Interventions taken early on can reduce the ultimate extent of permanent damage. If hypotension is not already evident, blood pressure might be judiciously reduced to decrease the work requirements on the heart. Tranquilizers and analgesics may be given to calm the patient and control pain. A major new development in management of this phase of therapy for myocardial infarction is the use of thrombolytic drugs. Although expensive, thrombolytic drugs (such as streptokinase, alteplase, and anistreplase) have the unique capacity to break down clots. Administered within a few hours after an infarction, a thrombolytic drug can destroy a thrombus (the substance of the clot in approximately 80% of infarcts), improve ventricular function, and reduce the likelihood of subsequent congestive heart failure.

Long-term management is also important after myocardial infarction. Beta-blockers reduce subsequent mortality, but it is not certain whether this has to do with preventing dysrhythmias or reducing cardiac work. Aspirin also has an accepted role in preventing secondary infarctions. (It has also been touted for prophylactic use, or primary prevention, in the high risk group for myocardial infarction, middle age men, but this application is controversial.) Clients who smoke tobacco or who have diabetes mellitus, elevated cholesterol levels, or atherosclerosis are at greater risk than others of second attacks and so should be given special consideration for aspirin and/or propranolol therapy. When the beta-blocker is ultimately discontinued, the drug should be tapered rather than withdrawn abruptly, to minimize rebound increase in adverse cardiac events.

The drugs that provide the main basis for management of myocardial infarction (beta-blockers, antidysrhythmics, vasodilators, analgesics, aspirin) all have other more characteristic uses discussed in this chapter or other chapters, therefore, no additional discussion of them is provided here.

Angina Pectoris and Its Management in the Elderly

Angina pectoris means literally a choking of the chest. It manifests as episodes of wrenching substernal pain with sensations of tightness. It is usually brought on by exertion and alleviated after a few minutes of rest. The pain is often felt as radiating through the left arm, neck, jaws, or even the right arm. The pain derives from the action of metabolites of anaerobic metabolism, such as lactic acid, that the heart is obliged to produce when its oxygen supply is unable to keep up with its oxygen demand. Relief occurs only when provision of oxygen to the heart by coronary perfusion once again catches up with demand. Since cardiac oxygen consumption is a function of heart rate, preload, contractility, and afterload, a change in any one of these factors can alleviate or intensify anginal episodes.

Some of the factors that often contribute to triggering individual episodes are physical exertion, eating a heavy meal, exposure to cold, and emotional crisis. These are basically circumstances that create demand on the heart and competition for limited blood flow. Smoking tobacco, consumption of alcoholic beverages, excess intake of caffeine, and sympathomimetic drugs can also contribute to onset of attacks of angina. The frequency of attacks can vary from rare, isolated attacks to several per day. Any sudden increase in the incidence indicates **unstable angina,** which is a high-risk situation that typically culminates in myocardial infarction.

Though most cases of angina pectoris are a consequence of coronary arteriosclerosis, as previously discussed, one exception is **variant angina,** also known as **Prinzmetal's angina** or **vasospastic angina.** The last of these names characterizes the cause of this condition. Spasms occur periodically in one or another coronary vessel to cause the attacks, not unlike the spasms that can develop in peripheral blood vessels to cause peripheral vascular disorders such as Raynaud's disease or migraine headaches.

Treatment of angina pectoris aims to achieve five objectives:

1. eliminating factors that advance the sclerotic process;
2. eliminating trigger factors for anginal attacks;
3. alleviating attacks quickly when they occur;
4. reducing the frequency of attacks;
5. preventing life-threatening sequelae of angina pectoris, namely, myocardial infarction and sudden death.

The first objective depends on clients' education and their willingness to discontinue smoking, alcohol consumption, overeating, overconsumption of coffee, and to increase exercise. The second objective centers on identification of trigger factors and their avoidance. Overeating, going out on cold nights, and overly intensive exercise can all be avoided. Use of an antianginal drug immediately before scheduled periods of vigorous exercise can be helpful. The third objective is accomplished with the help of medications designed for acute action at the time of an attack. These are drugs with a rapid action and quick delivery to the site of action, for example, nitroglycerin. The fourth objective is accomplished with the help of drugs that provide chronic prophylaxis: the nitrates, calcium-channel blockers, and the beta-blockers. Although the fifth objective is met only incompletely by current therapeutic approaches, carefully implemented measures together with client education usually provide the individual with about 5 years of healthy life before the first episode of myocardial infarction.

The use of calcium-channel blockers and beta-blockers in the elderly was discussed earlier as regards their application in hypertension. The only point that might be added here relating expressly to treatment of angina is that while many of the drugs provide benefit in classic, effort-induced angina, only certain of the calcium-channel blockers have the spasmolytic activity necessary to confer benefit in vasospastic angina. Only amlodipine, diltiazem, nifedipine, and verapamil are approved for vasospastic angina, while these plus nicardipine and bepridil are approved for classic angina. Beta-blockers are effective only for classic angina. The approved beta-blockers for this application are atenolol, metoprolol, nadolol, and propranolol, but angina is also an unlabeled use of bisoprolol, carteolol, and esmolol. The following section discusses the use of nitroglycerin for angina.

Nitrogylcerin Use in the Elderly for Angina Pectoris

Nitroglycerin has been recognized for its extraordinary vasodilating properties ever since its synthesis in 1846. Nitrates such as nitroglycerin are more universal in their action on the vasculature than are other vasodilators, acting on both the arterioles and the venules, while other vasodilators act only on the arterial side. As a result, nitroglycerin and similar drugs reduce both preload and afterload. Although nitroglycerin does not increase total coronary blood flow, it does increase flow to the part of the myocardium most susceptible to ischemia—the subendocardium. Moreover, nitroglycerin and other nitrates provide a spasmolytic action that suppresses coronary vasospasms that are the basis for Prinzmetal's angina. Nitroglycerin also decreases myocardial oxygen requirements.

Clinical Indications in the Elderly. Nitroglycerin is used in a rapid acting dosage form (sublingual tablets) for rapid relief from anginal attacks that are in progress. Sublingual tablets can also be used for periodic prophylaxis before exercise, sexual intercourse, or events anticipated to be stressful. However, clients need to be discouraged from use of nitroglycerin for aches and pains not reasonably attributable to angina.

The sustained release oral formulation and the transdermal patch are indicated for chronic prophylaxis in effort-induced angina. Clients will be best able to adjust doses used for prophylaxis if they maintain careful records of the frequency of attacks.

Altered Pharmacokinetics of Pharmacodynamics in the Elderly.
After sublingual administration, nitroglycerin normally appears in the blood within 2 minutes and reaches peak levels within four. Little effect

remains after 30 minutes. Sustained-release oral formulations of nitroglycerin can maintain effective serum concentrations for 8–12 hours. The transdermal patch provides sustained release over approximately 24 hours. The patch needs to be placed over a non-hairy part of the chest so that the drug is absorbed into the systemic circulation where it can reach the target tissue before being metabolized by the liver. Age-dependent pharmacokinetic alterations have not been reported for nitroglycerin.

Adverse Effects and Contraindications in the Elderly. The main side effects of nitroglycerin derive from excess vasodilation. Dizziness, fainting, weakness, or other signs of orthostatic hypotension may occur. Vascular headaches are a common response. Persons using nitroglycerin need to be warned that concurrent use of alcohol intensifies the risk of excess hypotension.

Tolerance can occur to nitrates with chronic exposure, a fact first observed for munitions workers subject to chronic environmental exposure to these chemicals. Although tolerance can be a problem with chronic oral use for prophylaxis, it does not occur with infrequent sublingual use of nitroglycerin for acute relief of attacks. If they have heard stories regarding nitrate dependence, some clients may require reassurance that occasional sublingual or topical administrations do not carry this risk. If dependence does occur after chronic oral use, there is a risk of withdrawal syndrome if discontinuation is abrupt. During withdrawal, clients can experience increased blood pressure, anginal attacks, anxiety, and even myocardial infarction. If nitroglycerin treatment is to be terminated, doses should be tapered over a 4-to-6-week period to prevent dangerous withdrawal reactions.

Interactions in the Elderly. The hypotensive action of nitroglycerin is increased by concomitant consumption of alcoholic beverages or simultaneous use of aspirin or calcium-channel blockers. Dihydroergotamine, a vasoconstrictor used for acute relief of migraine headaches, antagonizes nitroglycerin and vice versa.

Administration in the Elderly. Nitroglycerin deteriorates easily and clients need to be reminded to store this drug only in airtight, amber containers in a cool location. All but a small amount on hand for easy access should be refrigerated. Any supply not used before 3 months of age should be discarded and replaced, if there is a continuing need for it. Plastic containers should not be used for nitroglycerin, because this material may absorb the drug. The site of application for the transdermal patch needs to be rotated to minimize skin irritation.

NITROGLYCERIN (Nitrostat)

Recommended sublingual dose in the elderly: 0.15–0.3 mg as needed.

Unspecified adult sublingual dose for comparison: 0.15–0.6 mg as needed.

> ***Recommended transdermal patch dose for the elderly:***   0.2 mg/hr.
>
> ***Unspecified adult transdermal patch dose for comparison:***
> 0.2–0.4 mg/hr.
>
> ***Recommended oral sustained release dose in the elderly:***   No specific recommendation.
>
> ***Unspecified adult oral sustained release dose for comparison:***
> 2.5–2.6 mg 3 or 4 times daily.

CARDIAC DYSRHYTHMIAS IN THE ELDERLY

Dysrhythmias are disturbances of the cardiac electrical rhythm. They can be grouped into five broad categories:

1. abnormal pacemaker rhythms
2. ectopic foci
3. reentrant cycles
4. conduction blocks
5. ventricular preexcitation.

The pacemaker for the normal heart beat is the sinoatrial (SA) node. For the healthy adult at rest, it normally generates beats at approximately 70 beats per minute. Abnormal pacemaker rhythms are dysrhythmias that arise from the pacemaker itself, when it establishes a rhythm that is either abnormally slow or abnormally fast. An abnormally slow rhythm is called **bradycardia.** It is defined as an atrial rhythm less than 60 beats per minute. Young people who are in exceptional physical condition because of training for athletic competition may exhibit an unusually slow heart rate during rest that, though technically bradycardia, is quite normal and healthy. **Tachycardia,** an abnormally rapid beat, is a heart rate in excess of 100 beats per minute. Hyperthyroidism, hypotension, anemia, hemorrhage, and use of tobacco, caffeine, or marihuana are common causes of tachycardia.

Ectopic foci are abnormal pacemakers that develop in parts of the heart other than the normal site of pacemaker activity. All cardiac cells exhibit a kind of pacemaker activity, called automaticity, but in the healthy heart, the cells in the SA node have the fastest rate. When the SA node initiates a beat, the beat spreads throughout the heart before the other cells have a chance to initiate a beat on their own. However, any circumstances that increase the rate of automaticity for a group of cells outside the SA node can turn those cells into an extra pacemaker. The term *ectopic foci* means literally displaced pacemakers; i.e., pacemakers outside the SA node. Ectopic foci can cause three types of abnormal rhythms, depending on the severity of the problem. The mildest and least significant possibility are occasional ***premature beats.*** Most healthy people have isolated premature beats, with little health significance. Frequent premature beats are, however, an indication that more serious problems are likely in the future. At the second level of severity, ectopic foci can cause tachycardia. This could be **atrial tachycardia** if the foci are located in the atrium, or **ventricular tachycardia** if the foci are located in the conductile system or ventricles. Ventricular dysrhythmias are more immediately life-threatening than atrial dysrhythmias. When tachycardia occurs in brief episodes interrupted by long periods of normal rhythm it is called **paroxysmal tachycardia** and it too can be atrial (supraventricular) or ventricular. The third level of severity of dysrhythmias that can arise from ectopic foci is fibrillation. **Ventricular fibrillation** is a life-threatening emergency.

Reentry dysrhythmias are cyclical patterns that develop around scar tissue. They are the usual cause of **atrial flutter** (240 to 400 beats per minute) or **atrial fibrillation** (300 to 600 beats per minute). Reentry phenomena can also be a cause of ventricular fibrillation.

Conduction blocks occur when the heart beat is unable to complete its normal passage along the full length of the conductile system. The most common site of block is at the atrioventricular node, where some delay in conductance of the beat is supposed to occur under normal circumstances. Conduction blocks can also develop in the SA node. Blocks can be first, second, or third degree. In first degree block, beats are slow to pass, but each beat ultimately completes its cycle. In second degree block, only some beats get past the site of blockage. Second degree block can actually be desirable and serve a protective role if the atria are in flutter or fibrillation by protecting the more critical ventricular function from the overly rapid beat of the atria. Second degree block that occurs under this protective circumstance is also known as a **slow ventricular response rate.** In third degree block, none of the normal beats get past the block causing the parts of the heart on the two sides of the block to operate essentially independently. For example, in third degree AV block, the atria and the ventricles develop independent rhythms.

Ventricular preexcitation occurs when there is an abnormal conduction pathway between one of the atria and a ventricle in addition to the pathway across the AV node. The excitation of the ventricles will then occur in a less coordinated manner, as some parts of the ventricle respond to one pathway of conductance, while other parts respond to the other.

Cardiac dysrhythmias are common among the elderly. Even elderly persons without symptoms often show evidence upon EKG monitoring of complex atrial and ventricular dysrhythmias. Yet there is no solid evidence that treatment of unusual rhythms that are not accompanied by clinical symptoms provides any protection against sudden death. Moreover, antidysrhythmic drugs have potentially serious side effects and can themselves cause mortality. Therefore, dysrhythmias should be treated with antidysrhythmic drugs only if a clear relationship exists between the abnormality of rhythm and clinical symptoms. Since a given antidysrhythmic drug will have effectiveness in only certain types of dysrhythmias and will indeed exacerbate other types, treatment with an antidysrhythmic drug should not be commenced until the nature of the dysrhythmia is fully characterized, except in emergency situations where death is imminent in the absence of quick response based on best preliminary judgment.

Antidysrhythmic Drug Use in the Elderly

Antidysrhythmic drugs are used to prevent or control the various kinds of abnormalities of the cardiac rhythm. The drugs might act to alter conduction velocity, suppress excitability of cardiac cells, shorten or lengthen refractory period, or modify autonomic control of the heart. Antidysrhythmic drugs currently available are divided into four main groups, although the first of these groups is further subdivided.

- Group 1 drugs are drugs with local anesthetic properties that decrease excitability of cardiac cells and slow conductance.
- Group 2 drugs, the beta-blockers, slow conductance and block the sympathetic influence on the heart.
- Group 3 drugs act to prolong refractory period by slowing repolarization of cardiac cells. (Group 3 drugs are reserved for use in life-threatening dysrhythmias when other measures fail.)
- Group 4 drugs, the calcium-channel blockers, increase refractory period in the AV node, thereby reducing ventricular response rate in atrial dysrhythmias.

Use of both beta-blockers and calcium-channel blockers in the elderly was fully discussed in relation to their more prevalent application for hypertension above. In this section these drugs will be discussed only in regard to their specific application for cardiac dysrhythmias. In the main, this section will deal with the Group 1 antidysrhythmics. Prominent Group 1A drugs are quinidine, procainamide, and disopyramide. Group 1B and Group 1C drugs are local anesthetics, including lidocaine, tocainide, flecainide, and encainide.

Clinical Indications in the Elderly.   No one drug is effective for all kinds of dysrhythmias; rather, each one has specific clinical indications. Ventricular tachydysrhythmias are managed most often with Group 1 antidysrhythmics, including drugs from all three subgroups. Supraventricular tachydysrhythmias are usually managed with Group 2, Group 4, or Group 1A drugs. Quinidine is used both acutely and chronically for supraventricular dysrhythmias and to suppress ventricular premature beats. Procainamide is reserved largely for acute use for conversion of ventricular dysrhythmias because of the severity of adverse reactions with long-term administration. Disopyramide is used for the same applications as quinidine, although in the United States it is mainly utilized for suppression of ventricular dysrhythmias.

Lidocaine was for many years the only local anesthetic type of antidysrhythmic available. It remains a very useful drug, but is limited by its lack of oral effectiveness. Consequently, it is used only for acute management of ventricular dysrhythmias, where its benefit is often life-saving. The orally effective Group 1B drugs, tocainide and mexiletine, are used for chronic prophylaxis against documented ventricular dysrhythmias. Group 1C drugs pose a higher risk for clients and are reserved for chronic prophylaxis against documented life-threatening dysrhythmias.

The only beta-blockers (Group 2 drugs) approved for use in dysrhythmias are propranolol, acebutolol, and esmolol. Each of these provides distinct values. Esmolol is unusually rapid acting and provides quick response by intravenous injection for supraventricular tachycardia. Acebutolol is a cardioselective beta-blocker indicated only for management of ventricular premature beats. Propranolol is a nonselective beta-blocker with an additional quinidine-like effect not fully shared by other beta-blockers. It is effective mainly for reducing ventricular response rate in supraventricular tachydysrhythmias.

Group 3 drugs, bretylium and amiodarone, are indicated only for emergency use in ventricular dysrhythmias not responsive to other drugs. The only Group 4 drug, or calcium-channel blocker, approved for use in dysrhythmias is verapamil. It is the calcium-channel blocker with the strongest effects on the heart. It reduces ventricular response rate during atrial tachydysrhythmias and often provides the additional benefit of terminating and preventing recurrences of supraventricular tachycardia.

Altered Pharmacokinetics or Pharmacodynamics in the Elderly.
Quinidine is normally given orally, after which it is rapidly absorbed, with onset in 0.5 hours and peak action between 1 and 1.5 hours. The gluconate and polygalacturonate salts of quinidine are absorbed more slowly, achieving peak plasma concentrations only after 3 to 4 hours. Quinidine is 60–80% bound to plasma proteins while in the blood. Elderly individuals and those with liver disease often have reduced serum proteins. These individuals will have a higher free fraction of quinidine, will require lower serum concentrations for efficacy, and will therefore require dosage reduction. Quinidine penetrates most tissues freely with the exception of the brain. Quinidine is 60–85% inactivated by liver metabolism and otherwise is excreted unchanged in the urine. Urinary excretion plays a proportionately larger role in the inactivation of quinidine if the urine is acidified. The half-life of quinidine in young adults is 6 to 7 hours, but is prolonged in the elderly to 10 hours. This increase is the combined effect of decreased hepatic clearance and decreased renal clearance. Elderly individuals with hepatic dysfunction or greater than typical declines in renal function will be especially likely to develop higher plasma concentrations of quinidine due to prolonged half-life. Clients with heart failure will likewise have a longer quinidine half-life due to impaired clearance and a decreased volume of distribution.

Procainamide is well-absorbed from the small intestine with an onset of action in about 0.5 hours and peak action between 45–75 minutes for the capsule formulation. Absorption is a bit slower when tablets are used. Absorption is significantly slower in clients with heart failure to the extent that perfusion of the intestinal mucosa is diminished. Procainamide is inactivated 50–60% by renal excretion and the remainder by acetylation in the liver. Liver acetylator activity varies as a result of heredity, with some individuals classified as rapid acetylators and others as slow acetylators. The half-life of procainamide will vary accordingly. Procainamide has a half-life of 2.5–4.5 hours in young adults, but this can be significantly increased for elderly clients who have renal insufficiency or congestive heart failure, because of reduced clearance and a smaller volume of distribution. These clients will develop higher steady-state serum concentrations of procainamide. Measurement of plasma concentrations of procainamide and its active metabolite, N-acetyl procainamide (NAPA), provide a basis for guarding against age-dependent pharmacokinetic changes. Serum concentrations of these substances in the range of 4–8 mcg/ml provide therapeutic response, while levels about 16 mcg/ml are associated with toxicity. Procainamide has a narrow therapeutic index and therefore caution needs to be exercised in the use of this drug for the elderly. Elderly clients with renal impairments will require not only dosage reduction for procainamide, but a lengthened interval between doses. Factors that need to be considered in dosage adjustments include renal function, acetylator status, and the drug formulation.

Disopyramide is 90% absorbed after oral administration with an onset in approximately 0.5 hours and peak action at 1–2 hours. Inactivation of disopyramide is a balanced 50% by hepatic metabolism and 50% by renal excretion. Elderly clients with renal insufficiency or congestive heart failure will experience higher plasma concentrations at any given dose, because of reduced clearance and smaller volume of distribution. Smaller doses need to be employed in proportion to reductions in renal clearance.

Tocainide is 60% inactivated by conjugation in the liver and 40% excreted unchanged. Its half-life is significantly increased by renal dysfunction. Mexiletine is 90% metabolized by the liver. Its dosage requirements are unchanged in renal failure, but may need to be reduced in severe liver dysfunction.

Encainide and propafenone are metabolized in the liver to active metabolites and two distinct genetic patterns of metabolism have been noted. However, these differences were not associated with altered dosage requirements. The active metabolites are inactivated mainly by renal excretion, so dosage reduction needs to be effected for encainide in clients with renal creatinine clearance less than 20 ml/min.

Flecainide is inactivated 30% by renal excretion and 70% by hepatic metabolism. Either renal or hepatic impairment extends the half-life of flecainide. Flecainide inactivation is somewhat slower for elderly individuals.

The pharmacokinetics and age-related changes for beta-blockers and calcium-channel blockers was previously discussed in the section relating to hypertension.

Adverse Effects and Contraindications in the Elderly.   Whenever drug or DC shock therapy is undertaken for atrial flutter or fibrillation, one related risk is arterial embolism. Thrombi often form in a fibrillating atrium and may be dislodged after conversion of the dysrhythmia to a normal sinus rhythm. Nevertheless, the sooner the conversion is undertaken, the lower the risk. Administration of oral anticoagulants for a week or two prior to cardioversion provides a safeguard against arterial embolism.

Adverse effects of quinidine are of six kinds:

1. cinchonism
2. neurological symptoms
3. hypotension
4. cardiotoxicity
5. arterial embolism
6. hypersensitivity reactions.

Cinchonism is a set of symptoms resembling those caused by aspirin overdose; headache, fever, facial flushing, apprehensiveness, excitement, confusion, delirium, ringing of the ears or other auditory or vestibular impairments, visual problems such as double vision or night blindness, gastrointestinal symptoms such as nausea or diarrhea, and potential hematological problems of thrombocytopenia, hemolytic anemia, or hypoprothrombinemia. Clients on long-term quinidine therapy should receive periodic visual and auditory evaluation and inspection of the mouth for signs of bleeding. Depression is the most frequent neurological side effect of quinidine. Orthostatic hypotension can be severe. Elderly clients are at risk of syncope (fainting) or dizziness when they stand abruptly from a prone or sitting position. Paradoxically, quinidine can trigger idiosyncratic ventricular tachycardia due to reflex cardiac stimulation as the body tries to compensate for extreme hypotension. This problem occurs in as many as 4% of patients treated with quinidine. Other cardiac toxicities of quinidine include heart block and cardiac arrest. Quinidine is contraindicated in clients with preexisting conduction defects. EKG monitoring during initiation of quinidine therapy provides the best means of detecting developing cardiotoxicity.

Procainamide has side effects in five categories:

1. cardiotoxicity
2. hypotension
3. gastrointestinal symptoms
4. neurological symptoms
5. allergic reactions.

Cardiotoxicity resembles that produced by quinidine but idiosyncratic ventricular tachycardia is a less common event with procainamide. Gastrointestinal problems include nausea, vomiting, diarrhea, and anorexia. Neurological symptoms may include depression, irritability, confusion, hallucinations, or nightmares. The major problem with procainamide is an alarming incidence of drug-induced systemic lupus erythematosus–like syndrome. Symptoms of this condition include arthralgia, pericarditis, pleuritic pain, fever, hepatomegaly, and insomnia. A butterfly shaped rash on the face is a telltale indicator of this condition. Procainamide is largely limited to acute applications today mainly because as many as 25% of those on extended procainamide therapy develop the lupus-like syndrome and as many of 70% develop elevated antinuclear antibodies indicative of early stages of the condition.

Disopyramide is less likely to cause cardiotoxicity than quinidine or procainamide, but has similar risk of orthostatic hypotension. Disopyramide has much greater anticholinergic properties than quinidine and procainamide, resulting in anticholinergic side effects such as dry mouth, urinary retention, constipation, blurred vision, and aggravation of glaucoma. All of these problems are greater difficulties for the elderly, on average, than for younger clients, because these side effects are superimposed on conditions such as constipation, glaucoma, prostatic hypertrophy, or visual impairments that render the elderly person less tolerant to the drug's side effects. Consequently, disopyramide is seldom an appropriate drug selection for use in elderly clients.

Adverse effects of antidysrhythmic drugs in Groups 1B and 1C are the result of excess depression of the central nervous system or the heart. CNS disturbances can include somnolence, respiratory depression, agitation, confusion, dizziness, tremor, or even seizures. Visual changes or tinnitus might occur. Cardiotoxicity can include block or arrest.

Adverse effects in the elderly for beta-blockers and calcium-channel blockers were previously discussed in the section on hypertension.

Interactions in the Elderly. Metabolism of quinidine in the liver is hastened by inducers of liver enzymes, such as barbiturates, many antihistamines, and most antiepileptics. Many elderly people take hypnotics for sleep problems and, if the drug selected induces liver enzymes, will require an increase in the quinidine dose. Acidification of the urine hastens renal excretion of quinidine, but alkalinization (by drugs such as thiazide diuretics, sodium bicarbonate, or antacids, and foods such as milk or citrus fruits) slows excretion of quinidine. Hypoprothrombinemia induced by quinidine is additive with anticoagulant effects of other drugs, such as warfarin or aspirin.

Hypotensive effects of antidysrhythmic drugs are additive with those of vasodilators, sympatholytics, diuretics, or CNS depressants. Depressive effects of antidysrhythmic drugs on conductance are additive with block-promoting effects of other drugs, such as digoxin, other antidysrhythmic drugs, phenothiazines, reserpine, or cocaine. Anticholinergic effects of quinidine and, especially, disopyramide are additive with those of other anticholinergic medications. Quinidine and procainamide have weak curare-like neuromuscular blocking actions, which are additive with that of neuromuscular blockers, used as adjuncts to anesthesia, or aminoglycoside antibiotics. This action of quinidine will also serve to aggravate myasthenia gravis.

Quinidine elevates serum concentrations of digoxin, necessitating a dosage reduction of the latter. Although the mechanism of this interaction is not known, it is one of the most frequent and significant interactions in elderly patients. Quinidine promotes hyperkalemia, which adds to the same tendency of potassium-sparing diuretics or angiotensin converting enzyme inhibitors.

Procainamide competes for renal secretion with certain other drugs, notably cimetidine. If these drugs are used concurrently, plasma levels of each will be elevated.

Administration in the Elderly. EKG monitoring should always be conducted before and during initiation of antidysrhythmic drug therapy.

Group 1A Antidysrhythmics

DISOPYRAMIDE (Norpace)

Recommended initial oral dose in the elderly: 100 mg orally 4 times daily.

Unspecified adult initial dose for comparison: 100 or 150 mg orally 4 times daily.

PROCAINAMIDE (Pronestyl)

Recommended initial oral dose in the elderly: 250 mg orally every 6 hours.

Unspecified adult initial dose for comparison: 375 mg orally every 3 hours.

QUINIDINE SULFATE (Cin-Quin, Quinora, Quinidex)
QUINIDINE GLUCONATE (Quinaglute, Duraquin)
QUINIDINE POLYGALACTURONATE (Cardioquin)

Recommended initial oral dose in the elderly: 200 mg every 8 to 12 hours for the sulfate formulation.

Unspecified adult initial dose for comparison: 300–500 mg PO 4 times daily of the sulfate formulation. (268 mg of the gluconate salt or 275 mg of the polygalacturonate salt are equivalent to 200 mg of quinidine sulfate.)

Group 1B Antidysrhythmics

LIDOCAINE

Recommended initial oral dose in the elderly: IV infusion at 0.5–1.0 mg/min.

Unspecified adult initial dose for comparison: IV infusion at 1–5 mg/min.

MEXILETINE (Mexitil)

Recommended initial oral dose in the elderly: Reduce in severe hepatic dysfunction.

Unspecified adult initial dose for comparison: 200 mg orally every 8 hours.

TOCAINIDE (Tonocard)

Recommended initial oral dose in the elderly: Reduce for renal insufficiency.

Unspecified adult initial dose for comparison: 400 mg orally every 8 hours.

Group 1C Antidysrhythmics

ENCAINIDE (Enkaid)

Recommended initial oral dose in the elderly: Reduce for renal impairment (creatinine clearance less than 20 mg/min) to 25 mg once daily. Consider reduction for severe hepatic dysfunction.

Unspecified adult initial dose for comparison: 25 mg orally every 8 hours.

FLECAINIDE (Tambocor)

Recommended initial oral dose in the elderly: Reduce for severe renal impairment to 50 mg twice daily.

Unspecified adult initial dose for comparison: 100 mg orally every 12 hours.

INDECAINIDE (Decabid)

Investigational.

LORCAINIDE

Investigational.

PROPAFENONE (Rythmol)

Recommended initial oral dose in the elderly: The effective dose may be lower if renal or hepatic impairment is present.

Unspecified adult initial dose for comparison: 150 mg orally every 8 hours.

Group 2 Antidysrhythmics

ACEBUTOLOL (Sectral)

Recommended initial oral antidysrhythmic dose in the elderly: Bioavailability increased two-fold in older patients. Lower doses may be required. Do not use more than 800 mg/day.

Unspecified adult initial antidysrhythmic dose for comparison: 400 mg orally in 2 divided doses.

ESMOLOL (Brevibloc)

Recommended initial oral antidysrhythmic dose in the elderly:
No specific recommendation.

*Unspecified adult initial antidysrhythmic dose for
comparison:* 50–200 mcg/kg/min by infusion.

PROPRANOLOL (Inderal)

Recommended initial oral antidysrhythmic dose in the elderly:
Lower doses because of increased bioavailability.

*Unspecified adult initial antidysrhythmic dose for
comparison:* 10–30 mg orally 3 or 4 times daily.

Group 3 Antidysrhythmics

AMIODARONE (Cordarone)

Recommended initial oral dose in the elderly: No specific
recommendation.

Unspecified adult initial dose for comparison: 800–1600 mg/
day orally.

BRETYLIUM (Bretylol)

Recommended initial oral dose in the elderly: Increase dosage
interval for patients with impaired renal function.

Unspecified adult initial dose for comparison: 5–10 mg/kg
infused over 10 to 30 minutes.

Group 4 Antidysrhythmics

VERAPAMIL (Calan, Isoptin, generic)

Recommended initial oral antidysrhythmic dose in the elderly:
Give slow IV injection over at least 3 minutes to minimize untoward
drug effects.

*Unspecified adult initial antidysrhythmic dose for
comparison:* 10 mg IV by slow injection over 2 minutes or more.

THROMBOEMBOLIC DISORDERS IN THE ELDERLY

Thromboembolism is the sudden occlusion of a blood vessel by a thrombus (clot), calcium plaque, atherosclerotic plaque, tissue mass, or a foreign body. Thromboembolism can be triggered by changes in blood constituents (e.g., a dislodged mass or particle), changes in vessel walls (e.g., progressing atherosclerosis), or blood stasis (e.g., likely in congestive heart failure). Occlusions occurring on the venous side of the circulation are called thromboembolism or, if associated with inflammation, thrombophlebitis. Occlusions on the arterial side cause ischemia in the corresponding tissue. Arterial occlusions affect mainly the lungs (pulmonary embolism), the heart (coronary artery disease), and the brain (cerebrovascular disease). Coronary artery disease is the usual cause of ischemic heart disease, which was discussed earlier in this chapter. Cerebrovascular disease is a contributing factor in many cases of organic brain syndrome, which is discussed in Chapter 8. Although age by itself may not increase risk of thromboembolic disorders, many of the changes that typically accompany aging are known risk factors (see Table 13.5).

Pulmonary embolism occurs when a thrombus lodges in a pulmonary artery, interfering with perfusion of the lung parenchyma. The origin of the clot is usually the leg or pelvis, but less frequently can be a tissue fragment or a particle contained in an intravenous infusion fluid. Annual deaths in the United States from pulmonary embolism are estimated at 50,000–100,000, with approximately 75% of these occurring in persons over 50 years of age. Complications of pulmonary embolism can include tachypnea, dyspnea, pulmonary hypertension, which can lead to right heart failure, or pulmonary infarction, which can lead to pulmonary hemorrhage and necrosis. Respiratory symptoms together with presence of risk factors provide the first clue while chest x-ray, serum enzymes, blood cell counts, and an EKG provide the basis for definitive diagnosis. In difficult cases, radioisotope perfusion with ventilation scans or a pulmonary angiogram may be required for conclusive diagnosis.

Coronary artery disease is initially manifested as angina pectoris and later may lead to myocardial infarction as discussed in previous sections of this chapter. Cerebrovascular disease occurs when a thrombus forms in the cerebral vasculature, resulting in stroke (also called a cerebrovascular acci-

Table 13.5 Risk Factors for Thromboembolism Common among the Elderly

Atherosclerosis
Atrial fibrillation
Cancer
Congestive heart failure
Hip surgery
Immobilization due to myocardial infarction, stroke, surgical
  procedures, or vertebral collapse
Obesity
Previous thrombophlebitis
Varicose veins

dent) or less acute neurological deficits. Multiple small infarcts in the cerebrovasculature are the basis for multi-infarct dementia, one of the types of organic brain syndrome.

Thrombophlebitis (or deep venous thrombus) is the most common venous disease and accounts for more than 300,000 hospitalizations annually in the United States. It typically develops over a period of a few hours or up to a day or two. Major risk factors for occurrence of thrombophlebitis are trauma caused by cannulas, needles, drugs, or infection; hypercoagulability due to estrogen (from pregnancy or birth control pills), carcinomas, or blood dyscrasias; or stasis due to immobility, congestive heart failure, stroke, or myocardial infarction. Leg exercises, early ambulation, and frequent changes of position can help reduce likelihood of thrombophlebitis associated with confinement to bed. Symptoms of thrombophlebitis include pain, swelling, and tenderness in the region of the embolism. Venography provides the basis for definitive diagnosis. Thrombophlebitis is not only a major problem in its own right, but is also the major cause of pulmonary embolism. Clients may be tempted to rub the area of soreness, but this poses a serious risk of promoting dislodgement of a clot, which can then next appear in the pulmonary vasculature as an embolism or the cerebral vasculature as a stroke. Compression stockings often help to alleviate symptoms.

Anticoagulants play an important part in management of thromboembolic disorders. Anticoagulants are used as primary prophylaxis for prevention of venous thromboembolism for clients undergoing surgical procedures and for secondary prevention of complications or expansion in thrombophlebitis, pulmonary embolism, stroke, and, sometimes, myocardial infarction.

Anticoagulant Drug Use in the Elderly

The hemostatic system provides for the clotting that seals minor damage to blood vessel walls by the combined effort of a platelet phase and the coagulation cascade. Antithrombotic drugs, such as aspirin, suppress the platelet phase, while anticoagulant drugs, the subject of this section, suppress the coagulation phase. The end-point of the coagulation cascade is the formation of fibrin, a tough protein strand that binds together the platelet masses formed in the platelet phase. Anticoagulants inhibit formation of fibrin, reducing coagulability of the blood. This is sometimes referred to loosely as "thinning the blood." Anticoagulants do not dissolve existing clots, which, however, is a recent possibility for clinical medicine with the advent of thrombolytic drugs, such as streptokinase, urokinase, and alteplase.

There are two distinct types of anticoagulants: heparin and the oral anticoagulants. Heparin provides a rapid, safe means of controlling coagulability, but is largely limited to clinical settings because it lacks oral effectiveness. Oral anticoagulants provide the main basis for extended anticoagulant action for outpatients, but are fraught with great potential for interactions with other drugs. Oral anticoagulants act by inhibiting the vitamin K dependent synthesis of several clotting factors by the liver. As a result, their action occurs only *in vivo* (within the body, not in a test tube) and develops only after the supply of the related clotting factors already in the serum is exhausted, usually after 1.5–3 days.

Clinical Indications in the Elderly.   Anticoagulants are used as prophylaxis against pulmonary embolism during periods of elevated risk—after a leg or hip fracture, for example. Anticoagulants are also used to prevent clot expansion and for secondary prevention of additional embolisms. Anticoagulants may be used electively after a myocardial infarction to reduce the likelihood of secondary complications, such as pulmonary embolism or thrombophlebitis. Anticoagulants are indicated for stabilization of stroke in progress, but are contraindicated for completed stroke due to risk that hemorrhage might be precipitated. Anticoagulants are used in thrombophlebitis, not to alleviate the disorder itself, but to reduce the risk of secondary pulmonary embolism, myocardial infarction, or further thromboembolism.

Altered Pharmacokinetics or Pharmacodynamics in the Elderly.
Heparin is used only by parenteral administration, usually intravenously, and therefore only in clinical settings. It has an immediate onset of action and lasts about 4–6 hours. It can be used safely during pregnancy or in women who are breast feeding, because of inability to distribute across the placental barrier or into breast milk. Enoxaparin, a low-molecular-weight form of heparin, exhibits delayed elimination in the elderly and others with renal impairment. Heparin likewise needs to be employed cautiously in clients with renal insufficiency.

Oral anticoagulants are rapidly absorbed after oral administration. Warfarin, for example, works almost as quickly after oral administration as after intravenous injection. Warfarin is the quickest acting of the oral anticoagulants, achieving peak effect after 1.5–3 days. Anisindione achieves peak action in 2 to 3 days. Both drugs are metabolized by the liver to inactive metabolites that are then excreted mainly in the urine. Both drugs need to be used with caution in clients with impaired renal or hepatic function. Effects of warfarin last 2–5 days, while those of anisindione last 1–3 days.

Both warfarin and anisindione are more than 97% bound to plasma proteins during circulation in the blood. This is a crucial issue for this class of drugs because it is the basis for the most important kind of interaction between these drugs and others and one of the most important of all drug interactions for elderly persons.

Adverse Effects and Contraindications in the Elderly.   The main adverse effect with both heparin and the oral anticoagulants is hemorrhage, which is a toxic extension of the therapeutic effect. Minor bleeding occurs in 4% of clients receiving heparin and serious hemorrhaging in 2%. Minor bleeding is likely to be occult, from the nose, gastrointestinal tract, or genitourinary tract. Cerebral hemorrhage can occur and may be fatal. Monitoring coagulability is crucial for either type of anticoagulant to ensure adequate benefit while minimizing risk of hemorrhage. Usually the object of therapy with oral anticoagulants is an increase in prothrombin time from the normal value of 11–12 seconds to a therapeutic value of 20–25 seconds. Heparin doses are adjusted based on Lee-White whole blood clotting time (WBCT) (normally 9–14 minutes) and activated partial thromboplastin time (APTT) (normally 25–38 seconds). The goal of heparin therapy is to increase WBCT by 2.5- to 3-fold and APTT by 1.5- to 2-fold.

The elderly are more susceptible to the risk of hemorrhage. Elderly persons are more sensitive to oral anticoagulants. Preexisting liver dysfunction may have resulted in already depressed formation of clotting factors. Hyperthyroidism will also increase responsiveness to oral anticoagulants. A higher incidence of bleeding has been reported for women over 60 receiving heparin.

When hemorrhage occurs, heparin can be antagonized on a one-to-one molar basis with protamine sulfate, a drug that complexes with heparin. Oral anticoagulants can be rapidly antagonized only by administration of fresh whole plasma, which replaces clotting factors that are depressed by oral anticoagulants. If antagonism is less urgent, vitamin K given orally or by injection provides some reversal in a few hours and complete reversal in approximately 24 hours.

Other side effects are rare with anticoagulants. Either heparin or an oral anticoagulant can cause allergic reactions, such as skin eruptions. Long-term use of heparin can result in osteoporosis, alopecia, or hypoaldosteronism. The later effect can result in potassium depletion. As a result, heparin needs to be used cautiously in clients with renal impairments or diabetes.

Interactions in the Elderly. Drug interactions involving oral anticoagulants are numerous, among the most common kinds of interactions for elderly clients, and a likely cause of occult bleeding or hemorrhage. Doses of oral anticoagulants must be carefully titrated against prothrombin time, and relatively small changes in free plasma concentrations of the drug can have serious consequences, resulting in hemorrhage or, conversely, loss of protection against thromboembolism.

Many drugs potentiate the effect of oral anticoagulants, a smaller number antagonize their action (see Table 13.6). Elderly clients are far more likely to experience such interactions for the simple reason that they take, on average, many more drugs. Antagonism can occur when drugs interfere with absorption of warfarin, increase coagulation factors (notably vitamin K or estrogens), or speed the metabolism or warfarin by induction of liver enzymes. The interaction with vitamin K leads secondarily to dietary interactions, since vitamin K is abundant in yellow and dark green vegetables.

The more common kinds of interactions with warfarin are those that potentiate its effect, causing occult bleeding or hemorrhage. There are at least seven mechanisms by which this can occur. Three of these mechanisms have in common that the interacting drug itself decreases the capacity of the blood for clotting, one way or another. This includes drugs like aspirin that have an antithrombotic effect, drugs like quinidine and aspirin that inhibit synthesis of coagulation factors, and many drugs that each rarely causes thrombocytopenia by bone marrow suppression.

Table 13.6 Drug Interaction of Oral Warfarin

Antagonism

Impaired absorption of warfarin
  Cholestyramine
  Cholestipol
  Griseofulvin
Increase in coagulation factors
  Estrogens
  Vitamin K

Induction of liver metabolism
  of warfarin
  Antiepileptics
  Antihistamines
  Barbiturates
  Griseofulvin
  Nafcillin
  Nonbarbiturate nonbenzodiazepine
    hypnotics
  Rifampin

Potentiation

Displacement of warfarin from
    albumin binding sites
  Aspirin
  Chloral derivatives
  Clofibrate
  Diazepam
  Diazoxide
  Nonsteroidal anti-inflammatory
    drugs
  Phenytoin
  Sulfonamides
  Sulfonylureas
Decreased vitamin K availability
  Broad-spectrum antibiotics
  Anabolic steroids
  Clofibrate
  Thyroid hormones
Inhibition of warfarin metabolism
  Alcohol
  Allopurinol
  Chloramphenicol
  Cimetidine
  Disulfiram
  Methylphenidate
  Metronidazole
  Oxyphenbutazone
  Phenylbutazone
  Sulfinpyrazone
  Sulfonamides

Antithrombotic effect
  Aspirin
  Clofibrate
  Dipyridamole
  Indomethacin
  Oxyphenbutazone
  Phenylbutazone
  Sulfinpyrazone
Inhibition of coagulation factors
  Antimetabolites
  Quinidine
  Quinine
  Salicylates
Possible drug-induced
    thrombocytopenia

Acetazolamide	Lincomycin
Amitriptyline	Mefenamic acid
Barbiturates	Methyldopa
Benzodiazepines	Nalidixic acid
Bromocriptine	Neuroleptics
Carbamazepine	Nitrofurans
Cardiac glycosides	Penicillins
Cephalosporins	Procainamide
Chloramphenicol	Quinacrine
Cimetidine	Quinidine
Doxepin	Quinine
Estrogens	Rifampin
Furosemide	Succinimides
Gentamicin	Sulfonamides
Gold compounds	Tetracycline
Hydantoins	Thiazides
Ibuprofen	Thiouracil
Levodopa	Valproate
Lidocaine	

Probably the single most important type of interaction with oral anti-coagulants involves drugs that displace them from albumin protein binding sites. Displacement may be caused by any other highly bound drug, including notably aspirin, diazepam, nonsteroidal anti-inflammatory drugs, antiepileptic drugs, oral hypoglycemic drugs, and sulfonamides—in short, several of the most widely used classes of drugs for elderly people. Some drugs, notably alcohol, cimetidine, disulfiram, and sulfonamides, inhibit the hepatic metabolism of oral anticoagulants.

Oral anticoagulants act as competitive inhibitors of vitamin K, thus any factor that diminishes supplies of vitamin K will potentiate the effect of oral anticoagulants. Vitamin K is only partly an essential dietary constituent because some vitamin K, though not generally enough, is produced by commensal flora of the intestines and then absorbed across the intestinal mucosa into the blood. Broad-spectrum antibiotics often severely disturb the commensal flora of the intestines and can virtually eliminate endogenous vitamin K production for a period of time. Other drugs can inhibit absorption of dietary vitamin K (clofibrate) or speed its metabolism (anabolic steroids or thyroid hormones).

Interactions with heparin are less an issue, because it is employed almost exclusively in controlled clinical settings. Penicillins and cephalosporins have each been reported to sometimes cause deficits in platelet aggregation and coagulation, and this action could be additive with that of heparin. Salicylates and other drugs with an antiplatelet or anticoagulant effect of their own increase the risk of bleeding when heparin is being used.

Administration in the Elderly. Different brands of warfarin are sometimes not bioequivalent. Brand interchange is not recommended. Clients should take oral anticoagulants at the same time each day. Clients receiving oral anticoagulants need to wear an identification bracelet which states that they are taking an anticoagulant and otherwise advise all medical personnel with whom they deal of their drug regimen.

Intravenous Anticoagulant

HEPARIN

Recommended dose in the elderly: No specific recommendation.

Unspecified adult dose for comparison: Individualize based on WBCT and APTT taken 4–6 hours after SC injections, every 4 hours with continuous IV infusion, or immediately before each dose and at appropriate intervals thereafter with intermittent IV infusion. Recommended initial SC dose is 10,000–20,000 units followed by 8,000–10,000 units every 8 hours or 15,000–20,000 units every 12 hours. Recommended initial intermittent IV dose is 10,000 units followed by 5,000–10,000 units every 4–6 hours. Recommended initial IV infusion rate is 20,000–40,000 units/day.

Oral Anticoagulants

ANISINDIONE (Maradon)

Recommended oral dose in the elderly: Lower doses recommended.

> ***Unspecified adult dose for comparison:*** 300 mg PO on the first day, 200 mg on the second day, 100 mg on the third day, and 25–250 mg daily for maintenance.

WARFARIN (Coumadin, Panwarfarin)

Recommended oral dose in the elderly: Lower maintenance doses will maintain therapeutic anticoagulant action in elderly clients, but the same protocol can be used for introduction of therapy as for younger clients.

Unspecified adult dose for comparison: 10–15 mg PO initially. Maintenance therapy requires 2–15 mg and continued weekly or monthly prothrombin determinations.

REFERENCES AND RECOMMENDED READINGS

Abrams M: Nitroglycerine and long-acting nitrates. *N. Engl. J. Med.* 1980; 302:1234–1236.

Akhtar M: Management of ventricular tachyarrhythmias. *JAMA.* 1982; 247:671–674.

Albeit, S, et al.: Recognizing digitalis toxicity. *Am. J. Nurs.* 1977; 77:1935–1943.

Bigger JT Jr, et al.: Quinidine and digoxin: an important drug interaction. *Drugs.* 1982; 24:229–239.

Braunwald E: Mechanisms of action of calcium-channel blocking agents. *N. Engl. J. Med.* 1982; 307:1618–1627.

Brignoli ETB (ed): Using the antithrombotic agents. *Patient Care.* 1980; 14:62.

Buhler FR et al.: Age and antihypertensive response to calcium antagonists. *J. Hypertens.* (Suppl) 1987; 5(4):S111–114.

Butler JD, Harrison BL: Keeping pace with calcium channel blockers. *Nurs.* 1983; 13:38–43.

Cavanaugh AL, Manconi RE: Drug interactions with digitalis toxicity. *Am. J. Nurs.* 1980; 80:2170–2171.

Chalmers CT, et al.: Evidence favoring the use of anticoagulants in the hospital phase of acute myocardial infarction. *N. Engl. J. Med.* 1977; 297:1091–1096.

Chamberlain SL: Low-dose heparin therapy. *Am. J. Nurs.* 1980; 80:1115–1117.

Chatterjee K, Parmley WW: Vasodilator treatment for acute and chronic heart failure. *Br. Heart J.* 1977; 39:706–720.

Chatterjee K, Rouleau, JL, Parmley WW: Medical management of patients with angina. *JAMA.* 1984; 252(9):1170–1176.

Crumpley L: An overview of antiarrhythmic drugs. *Crit. Care Nurse.* 1983; 3(4):57–64.

Daniels LL: What influences adherence to hypertensive therapy. *Nurs. Forum* 1979; 18:231–245.

Farah AE, et al.: Positive inotropic agents. *Annu. Rev. Pharmacol. Toxicol.* 1984; 24:275–328.

Federman J, Vlietstra RE: Antiarrhythmic drug therapy. *Mayo Clin. Proc.* 1979; 54:531–542.

Fleg JL, Lakatta EG: *Cardiovascular disease in old age,* in Rossman: *Clin. Geriatr.* Philadelphia, Lippincott, 1986, pp. 169–196.

Frishman WH: *Clinical pharmacology of the beta-adrenoceptor blocking drugs.* New York, Appleton-Century-Crofts, 1980.

Goldberg PB: How do digitalis tolerance and toxicity change with age? *Geriatr. Nurs.* 1980; 1:142–144.

Hanson MS, Woods SL: Nitroglycerin ointment. *Am. J. Nurs.* 1980; 80:1122–1124.

Hansson L, Werko L: Beta adrenergic blockade in hypertension. *Am. Heart J.* 1977; 93:394–402.

Hirsh J, et al.: Using the antithrombitic agents. *Patient Care.* 1980; 14:62.

Hoffman W: The behavioral side effects of the antihypertensive agents. *Am. Fam. Physician.* 1981; 23(2):213–216.

Hovrath PT, DePew CC: Towards preventing digitalis toxicity. *Nurs. Drug Alert* 1980; 4:25.

Hutchins LN: Drug treatment of high blood pressure. *Nurs. Clin. North Am.* 1981; 16:365–377.

Jones LN: Hypertension: Medical and nursing implications. *Nurs. Clin. North Am.* 1976; 11(2):283–295.

Kelly JG et al.: Nitrates in the elderly: Pharmacological considerations. *Drugs Aging* 1992; 2(1):14–19.

Kirschembaum M: Digitalis. *RN.* 1981; 81(11):69–71.

Klein DM, Cook D: Angina, physiology signs, and symptoms. *Nursing.* 1984; 14(2):44–46.

Laffel GL, Braunwald E: Thrombolytic therapy—a new strategy for the treatment of acute myocardial infarction. *N. Engl. J. Med.* 1984; 311(11):710–717, 311(12):770–776.

Leonard RG, Talbert RL: Calcium-channel blocking agents. *Clin. Pharm.* 1982; 1:17–33.

Lewis HD Jr, et al.: Protective effects of aspirin against acute myocardial infarction and death in men with unstable angina: results of a Veterans' Administration study. *N. Engl. J. Med.* 1983; 309:396–403.

Lowther NB, Carter VD: How to increase compliance in hypertensives. *Am. J. Nurs.* 1981; 81(5):963.

Lute E: Calcium blockers: the important difference. *RN.* 1984; 84(6):36–39.

Marcinek MB: Hypertension: what it does to the body. *Am. J. Nurs.* 1980; 80:928–932.

Martin A, Camm AJ: *The management of cardiac arrhythmias in the elderly,* in *K. O'Malley and JL Waddington (eds): Therapeutics in the elderly.* New York, Elsevier Sci. Publ., 1985, pp. 201–212.

Marx JL: Hypertension: a complex disease with complex causes. *Science.* 1980; 194:821–825.

McCauley K, Burke K: Your detailed guide to drugs for congestive heart failure. *Nursing.* 1984; 14(5):47–50.

McKenney JM: Methods for modifying compliance behavior in hypertensive patients. *Drug Intell. Clin. Pharm.* 1981; 15:8–14.

Meissner JE, Gever LN: Reducing the risks of digitalis toxicity. *Nursing.* 1980; 10:32–38.

Michaelson CR (ed): *Congestive Heart Failure.* St. Louis, C.V. Mosby Co., 1983.

Moore K, Maschak B: How patient education can reduce the risk of anticoagulation. *Nursing.* 1977; 7(9):24–29.

Moore LC: An on-the-spot guide to antihypertensive drugs. *Nursing.* 1986; 16(1):54–57.

Moser M: Hypertension: how therapy works. *Am. J. Nurs.* 1980; 80:937–941.

O'Brien E: *The management of hypertension in the elderly,* in K. O'Malley and JL Waddington (eds): *Therapeutics in the elderly,* New York, Elsevier Sci. Publ., 1985, pp. 213–222.

Pas DA, Lawlor MC: Beta-blocker agents: an update. *J. Emerg. Nurs.* 1986; 12(1):18–22.

Pepper GA: New antiarrhythmic drugs. *Nurse Pract.* 1986; 11(7):62–70.

Rosenberg JM, Kirschenbaum JL: What to watch for with heparin. *RN* 1981; 44(9):50–52.

Rossi LP, Antman EM: Calcium-channel blockers—new treatment. *Am. J. Nurs.* 1983; 83:382–387.

Sabanathan K, Castleden CM, Adam HK, Ryan S, Fitzsimons TJ: A comparative study of the pharmacokinetics and pharmacodynamics of atenolol, hydrochlorthiazide, and amiloride in normal young and elderly subjects and elderly hypertensive patients. *Eur. J. Clin. Pharmacol.* 1987; 32:53–60.

Shan ZS, Neild GH: Enalapril in elderly hypertensive patients with moderate to severe renal dysfunction. *J. Clin. Exp. Gerontol.* 1992; 14(2):131–143.

Shashaty GG: *Thromboembolism in the elderly,* in Reichel: *Clinical Aspects of Aging,* 3rd ed., Baltimore, Williams & Wilkins, 1989, pp. 93–98.

Singh BN: Beta-adrenoreceptor blocking drugs and acute myocardial infarction. *Drugs.* 1978; 15:218–225.

Sloan RW: Digitalis glycosides. *Am. Fam. Physician.* 1983; 28(5):206–216.

Stowe HO: Review of calcium-channel blockers. *Nurs. Pract.* 1986; 11(4):57–65.

Talman CL: Drugs used to treat angina pectoris. *Nurs. Drug Alert.* 1981; 5:28–30.

Taylor SH, Silke B, Lee PS: Intravenous beta-blockade in coronary heart disease. Is cardioselectivity or intrinsic sympathomimetic activity hemodynamically useful? *N. Engl. J. Med.* 1982; 306:631–635.

Thompson DA: Teaching the client about anticoagulants. *Am. J. Nurs.* 1982; 82:278–281.

Vedin JA, Wilhelmsson CE: Beta receptor blocking agents in the secondary prevention of coronary heart disease. *Annu. Rev. Pharmacol. Toxicol.* 1983; 23:29–44.

Walton C, Hammond B: Angina: teaching your patient to prevent recurring attacks. *Nursing.* 1978; 8(2):32–38.

Ward GW, Bundy P, Fink JW: Treating and counseling the hypertensive patient. *Am. J. Nurs.* 1978; 78:824–828.

Winslow EH: Digitalis. *Am. J. Nurs.* 1974; 74:1062–1065.

Williams BO: Treatment of congestive cardiac failure in the elderly, in K. O'Malley and JL Waddington (eds): *Therapeutics in the elderly.* New York, Elsevier Sci. Publ. 1985, pp. 189–200.

CHAPTER 14

Antidiabetic Drug Therapy for the Elderly

Diabetes mellitus has been recognized as a disease for at least 3000 years. The name, provided by a first-century Greek physician, means literally a "melting down of the flesh into urine," a description that bears some accuracy. In diabetes mellitus, the body is unable to take up ingested glucose into tissue cells, forcing those cells to burn off their own structural elements and alternative caloric stores—protein and fat. Meanwhile, glucose is wasted in the urine.

GLUCOSE HOMEOSTASIS

In the healthy person, glucose homeostasis is maintained by the interaction of several hormones, most notably insulin and glucagon, with lesser contributions from growth hormone and glucocorticoids. Insulin is the real workhorse of these hormones and the one at risk of not being able to keep up with its responsibilities when the system is overtaxed by disease or obesity. Insulin is formed in the beta cells of the endocrine part of the pancreas, called the Islets of Langerhans. It is a subunit of a larger protein and is split off and released into the blood when required. Insulin acts on receptors located on the surface membrane of most tissue cells, promoting uptake of glucose to furnish the target cells with energy. The secondary result is that blood levels of glucose are drawn down as the glucose moves from the blood into tissue cells.

Most tissue cells need insulin to obtain adequate glucose for their energy requirements, the main exceptions being the brain cells, red and white blood cells, parenchymal cells of the kidney, and cells of the intestinal mucosa. The action of insulin in the liver is quite exceptional as well. Liver cells do not require insulin for uptake of glucose, but provide a major storage site for glucose reserves in the form of glycogen. In these cells, insulin promotes formation of glycogen, which can later be mobilized during fasting or bursts of activity, by the action of the hormone glucagon.

Under normal circumstances, blood glucose levels are carefully controlled by the body to prevent undue losses in the urine while ensuring adequate supply to tissue cells. Blood glucose values in adults are normally about 80–90 mg/dl in the fasting state. Immediately after ingestion of food, blood glucose levels begin to rise as glucose is absorbed out of the gastrointestinal system into the blood, up to about 120–140 mg/dl in the healthy person. These increased serum glucose levels immediately after eating are called **postprandial** (after-eating) **values.**

In response to the postprandial rise in blood glucose, insulin is secreted by beta cells of the pancreas into the bloodstream. Insulin then stimulates uptake of glucose into tissue cells until blood levels return to the normal fasting value. Blood glucose levels are the primary impetus for insulin secretion, but insulin secretion is also activated by sympathetic impulses through beta-2 adrenergic receptors and by parasympathetic impulses through muscarinic receptors. Alpha-adrenergic receptors, on the other hand, inhibit insulin secretion. After eating, insulin secretion begins even before blood glucose levels start to rise, anticipating the rise, in effect, because insulin secretion can be activated by gastrointestinal hormones (secretin, gastrin, gastric-inhibiting peptide, and pancreozymin cholecystokinin) released during digestive activity.

DIABETES MELLITUS IN THE ELDERLY

There are currently about 12 million persons in the United States with diabetes mellitus and that number is increasing for reasons unknown. Diabetic patients occupy 5–7% of all hospital beds in the United States. The prevalence of diabetes increases with age, at least up to age 75, after which it appears to level off. At age 60, 10% of Americans have diabetes, but by age 80 the fraction has increased to 16–20%. Diabetes is twice as common in women as in men in the United States, but in some countries it is more common in men than women. Among older Americans, diabetes is more prevalent among blacks than whites.

The classification of diabetes mellitus generated by the National Diabetes Data Group specifies five types:

- Type I or insulin dependent diabetes mellitus (IDDM)
- Type II or noninsulin dependent diabetes mellitus (NIDDM)
- Impaired glucose tolerance (IGT)
- Gestational diabetes
- Diabetes secondary to other medical problems

This discussion of diabetes mellitus will relate mainly to the first three of those categories: Type I, Type II, and IGT.

Diabetes mellitus (Type I or II) is defined as a fasting blood sugar level above 140 mg/dl (on two occasions) or greater than 200 mg/dl at 2 hours and one other time point after a standard glucose load (75 g). IGT is defined as a blood sugar level between 140 and 200 mg/dl at 2 hours after a standard glucose load and one other point greater than 200 mg/dl prior to 2 hours.

About 10% of clients with primary diabetes have Type I, but among the elderly, only 5% have Type I. The reason for the decline in prevalence of Type I diabetes among the elderly is, sadly, that these individuals are prone to periodic episodes of ketoacidosis or hyperosmolar coma. The mortality rate from these episodes increases with age from just 6% for individuals under age 50 to 43% for those over 50. This, together with the longterm complications of diabetes mellitus, means that many people with Type I diabetes mellitus fail to survive into old age.

Ninety-five percent of elderly persons with diabetes have the noninsulin dependent type of diabetes mellitus. Type II diabetes is usually associated with obesity. Approximately 20% of all elderly people have Type II diabetes and another 20% have IGT, which is basically a less severe form of the same alterations that lead to Type II diabetes. Impaired glucose tolerance can also be viewed simply as an exaggeration of changes inherent with aging in the body's ability to manage blood glucose, because glucose tolerance declines with age even in the absence of overt diabetes. Fasting blood glucose values rise after the fourth decade of life at a rate of 1–2 mg/dl per decade. However, many elderly diabetic clients continue to be able to normalize fasting blood sugar levels, but develop extreme hyperglycemia following meals. Postprandial blood glucose values rise 8–20 mg/dl per decade after the fourth decade of life. It may not be so much that aging itself is diabetogenic as the fact that aging is associated with increased obesity and decreased exercise, which are known diabetogenic factors.

Type II diabetes and its lesser form, IGT, are not due to a failure of insulin production as in Type I. Instead, the disorder results from a gradual loss of responsiveness on the part of tissue cells to insulin. The defect is said to be postreceptor, meaning that it is not a reduction in the number of insulin receptors, but a problem with the events that are supposed to occur within the target cell after receptor occupation by insulin. Insulin actually increases in Type II diabetes and IGT, but not enough to overcome the resistance of target tissue cells. Overweight elderly people who are not diabetic have even higher increases in serum insulin levels and are thus able to overcome the loss of cell sensitivity to insulin.

Elderly clients with IGT or Type II diabetes may be undiagnosed until the condition is revealed by testing during routine evaluation, evaluation for another disorder, or a complication of the diabetes. Renal clearance of glucose declines in older people, so that urine glucose is sometimes not elevated until plasma sugar levels exceed 300 mg/dl. Often the development of a peripheral neuropathy is the first indication in an otherwise asymptomatic elderly diabetic. Sometimes the condition is temporarily exacerbated by infections, stress, or diabetogenic drugs, bringing it to clinical attention. Diabetogenic drugs include thiazide and high-ceiling diuretics, glucocorticoids, catecholamines, thyroid hormone, oral contraceptives, neuroleptics, antidepressants, lithium, beta-blockers, phenytoin, and anticancer drugs.

Some elderly people, of course, carry long-standing diabetes mellitus with them into old age. These clients will already be experienced in managing their condition, but may require changes in their treatment plan as they age. Doses of medications or dietary protocols may need to be altered.

COMPLICATIONS OF DIABETES MELLITUS

People with diabetes have increased mortality rates due to its various complications, which include macrovascular disease and three types specific for diabetes: retinopathy, neuropathy, and nephropathy. Macrovascular complications of diabetes often add to cardiovascular problems developing in elderly people due to independent causes, such as heart disease, atherosclerosis, and hypertension. Coronary atherosclerosis is five times more frequent for diabetic individuals; and myocardial infarction is a common cause of death for these individuals. Cerebrovascular accidents are likewise more common. Peripheral vascular disorders are 50 to 100 times more common for people with diabetes. Ischemic lesions and gangrene may occur in the feet and lower extremities. More than 20,000 leg and foot amputations are performed annually in the United States because of this problem alone. Most of the increased mortality rates for those with diabetes are directly attributable to the macrovascular complications. Even those with IGT have somewhat higher mortality rates associated with macrovascular complications. Studies have shown unequivocally that the hyperinsulinemia that accompanies IGT or Type II diabetes is a risk factor for cardiovascular disease.

On the other hand, the complications specific for diabetes are a risk only for those with frank diabetes, not for those with IGT. Neuropathies can result in sensory loss, paresthesias, pain, muscle weakness and atrophy, movement problems, or erectile impotence for males. Diabetic retinopathy occurs as a result of thickening of the microvasculature, microaneurysms, and micorangiopathies. It is responsible for 5000 new cases of blindness annually in the United States. More than 92% of instances of blindness caused by diabetes occur after age 50. Cataracts are another common problem for diabetics. Nephropathy is another major contributor to increased mortality for diabetic individuals.

The tissues prone to complications of diabetes—the retina, lens, kidneys, and nerves—are those that take up glucose without dependence on insulin. These tissues take up excess glucose whenever hyperglycemia occurs and convert that glucose to sorbitol using an enzyme called aldose reductase. Accumulations of sorbitol cause tissue cells to swell and sometimes burst. Two inhibitors of aldose reductase, sorbinil and tolrestat, are currently undergoing clinical trials as possible means of preventing or reducing the complications of diabetes mellitus.

Ketoacidosis is less likely to occur among elderly people with diabetes mellitus than their younger counterparts simply because fewer elderly diabetics have Type I diabetes mellitus, which is the type most often associated with ketotic coma. Elderly clients are, however, more likely to suffer nonketotic hyperosmolar coma, another serious metabolic complication of diabetes. These individuals will typically present with central nervous system symptoms such as seizures, depressed consciousness, or coma. Mortality rates from this problem are high.

Skin infections occur commonly for persons with diabetes. Candidal infections will occur and persist on the skin and, for women, vaginally. Bacterial infections may occur, as well.

TREATMENT OF DIABETES MELLITUS IN THE ELDERLY

If there is good news with respect to this difficult disorder, it is that the evidence is overwhelming that treatment does make a difference. A large part of the increased risk of mortality can be eliminated by aggressive, preventive treatment. The more carefully blood glucose levels are regulated, the slower the development of complications.

The basic principles for management of diabetes are not different for elderly than younger individuals. The goals are control of blood glucose levels, management of acute metabolic imbalances, and prevention of long-term complications. Specifics need to be tailored to the individual's circumstances. The older the client, the less attention needs to be paid to the risk of long-term complications, and control of blood glucose can therefore be less rigid. However, given the longer life expectancies of today, one must be careful not to apply that reasoning to clients in the 50–75 age range who are otherwise healthy excepting the diabetes. Elderly clients are often less willing to comply with rigorous protocols. Dietary adjustments may be harder to accomplish if the individual subsists on institutional or restaurant foods or simply because of long-standing dietary preferences. Individuals living alone may be poorly motivated toward meal preparation. Frequent monitoring of blood glucose levels may be intolerable to the elderly person or made more difficult because of impaired dexterity. Some allowances may need to be made.

Dietary adjustments and weight reduction should be all that is required for the majority of elderly diabetics, because mild Type II diabetes and IGT predominate. Intake of simple sugars, such as sucrose, should be restricted with meals otherwise balanced to provide adequate protein, carbohydrate, and fat. Cereals, breads, rice, vegetables, and noodles should be used as the primary source of carbohydrates. Added dietary fiber may also be helpful. Regular exercise up to the comfort level of the individual will help with weight reduction and well-being, but vigorous exercise regimens are not required. For clients with mild or asymptomatic diabetes, these nondrug measures should be given a one-month trial, at least, before resorting to drug therapy.

When diet and exercise fail to reduce fasting blood sugar to less than 200 mg/dl or postprandial glucose to less than 200–250 at the 2 hour point, an oral hypoglycemic drug should be added to the regimen. The combination of an oral hypoglycemic drug with dietary and exercise regimens will adequately control blood glucose for 85% of elderly diabetics. Severe cases not otherwise manageable will require insulin.

Self-monitoring of blood glucose is an essential part of management of diabetes mellitus. Urine tests are not an adequate alternative, especially for elderly clients, because renal clearance of glucose declines with aging and is more erratic. Fortunately, blood glucose testing has become a good deal more practical in recent years with the development of meters and automatic finger pricking devices, but it is not an inexpensive proposition. Frequency of tests can be reduced once good control is achieved.

USE OF ORAL HYPOGLYCEMIC DRUGS BY ELDERLY CLIENTS

The six available oral hypoglycemic drugs are sulfonylureas. They are divided into two subgroups called first-generation and second-generation, based on their sequence of development. The first-generation drugs are tolbutamide, acetohexamide, tolazamide, and chlorpropamide. The second-generation drugs are glyburide and glipizide. When a sulfonylurea is first given to a client, it stimulates the beta-cells of the pancreas, increasing basal output of insulin as well as the response to nonglucose stimuli. With continued use, however, serum levels of glucose decline without increased insulin levels, indicating improved sensitivity of target cells to insulin. The improvement, like the defect of Type II diabetes, appears to be a postreceptor phenomenon.

Clinical Indications in the Elderly. There is considerable controversy regarding the appropriate place for sulfonylureas in management of diabetes. The main points of agreement are that sulfonylureas are never appropriate as the sole basis of therapy for Type I diabetes, they are not needed for mild Type II diabetes that can be controlled by dietary adjustments and weight loss, and they are not adequate for severe Type II diabetes. What that leaves for appropriate use of sulfonylureas is a middle group of individuals with Type II conditions that are not severe enough to require insulin but not responsive to diet and exercise, whether because of noncompliance or severity of the problem. One controversial study even suggested that dietary adjustments plus tolbutamide performed no better than dietary adjustments alone and actually increased the risk of cardiovascular complications. There were questions, however, as to whether the group receiving tolbutamide was starting from a greater severity of disorder. At the least, treatment failures are commonplace with sulfonylureas and there is no hard evidence that sulfonylureas succeed in reducing the risk of complications from diabetes. Clients who do respond favorably to sulfonylureas may nevertheless require insulin during periods of illness or unusual stress.

Altered Pharmacokinetics or Pharmacodynamics in the Elderly.
The six available drugs vary somewhat in pharmacokinetic parameters (see Table 14.1). Tolbutamide, acetahexamide, chlorpropamide, and glipizide are well-absorbed after oral administration. Tolazamide absorption is slow, and glyburide absorption is incomplete (24%). All can be taken with food except glipizide, which is best taken 30 minutes before meals, because food delays its absorption.

A major difference between the first- and second-generation drugs is that all of the first-generation drugs are highly bound to plasma proteins. Protein binding for second-generation drugs is low, eliminating one category of troublesome interactions between oral hypoglycemics and other drugs.

All of the sulfonylureas are metabolized in the liver, but two, acetahexamide and tolazamide, produce active metabolites. The metabolites, active

Table 14.1 Comparisons among the Oral Hypoglycemic Drugs

Characteristic	Drug					
	Tolbutamide	Acetahexamide	Tolazamide	Chlorpropamide	Glyburide	Glipizide
Generation	First	First	First	First	Second	Second
Preparations	Orinase	Dymelor	Tolinase	Diabinase	DiaBeta	Glucotrol
Potency	+	++	+	+++	+++++	+++++
Typical Daily Dose	0.5–3 g	0.25–1.5 g	0.1–1.0 g	0.1–0.75 g	2.5–30 mg	2.5–40 mg
Number of Doses Daily	2 or 3	1 or 2	1 or 2	1	1 or 2	1 or 2
Onset (hr)	1	1	4–6	1	2–4	1–1.5
Half-Life (hr)	5–6	1.6 parent compound; 5.3 active metabolite	7	30–36	biphasic 3.2 & 10	3–4
Duration (hr)	6–12	10–24	10–20	30–72	10–24	6–24
Absorption	Rapid, complete	Rapid, complete	Slow	Well-absorbed	Only 24%	Well-absorbed
Metabolism in Liver	100%	100%	100%	80%	100%	100%
Activity of Metabolite	Inactive	More active	Less active	Inactive	Inactive	Inactive
Excreted via	Urine	Urine	Urine	Urine	Urine and bile	Urine
Protein Binding	High	High	High	High	Low	Low

and inactive, are excreted entirely by the kidneys except that glyburide is excreted slightly in the bile. Tolbutamide's short half-life necessitates administration 2–3 times per day; chlorpropamide can be given just once per day, while the others are given once or twice per day. The hypoglycemic effect of sulfonylureas can be prolonged by severe hepatic dysfunction and even by renal failure because of drug accumulation. Care must be taken with the drugs having a long half-life (e.g., chlorpropamide) that accumulation does not occur even in the absence of significant hepatic dysfunction.

Adverse Effects and Contraindications in the Elderly.   Oral hypoglycemic drugs are relatively free of serious adverse effects. The most important potential problem is hypoglycemia. The risk is especially great for elderly clients with impaired hepatic or renal function or who have erratic food intake. The elderly are more susceptible to dangerously severe hypoglycemia because of diminished ability to maintain glucose homeostasis. Mental impairment associated with hypoglycemia may be added to whatever neurologic or psychiatric problems may already exist. Hypoglycemia increases risk of angina or myocardial infarction and can induce seizure. Moreover, hypoglycemia is more difficult to recognize in elderly clients because the compensatory massive release of epinephrine that occurs in young people, causing tremulousness, nervousness, palpitations, sweating, flushing, and faintness, is much less evident for elderly persons. Elderly people may lose consciousness due to severe hypoglycemia without any warning symptoms whatsoever. Even when warning symptoms do occur, such as bizarre behavior, disorientation, confusion, somnolence, or slurred speech, they may be attributed to advancing cerebral arteriosclerosis. Frequent blood glucose determinations, especially during the period of dosage adjustment, will help to minimize the risk of severe hypoglycemia. Clients with diabetes mellitus should be taught to recognize the symptoms of hypoglycemia to aid in early detection.

Other uncommon adverse responses to oral hypoglycemics include hematological reactions (in less than 1% of clients), skin reactions (less than 1%), neurological problems (less than 0.5%), and gastrointestinal disturbances (approximately 1.5%). Some elderly clients will experience fluid retention.

Interactions in the Elderly.   Sulfonylureas participate in five categories of drug interactions:

1. additive hypoglycemia with other drugs with hypoglycemic actions;
2. decreased hypoglycemic benefit with drugs having opposing hyperglycemic actions;
3. potentiation of the sulfonylurea by drugs that inhibit their metabolism;
4. potentiation of first-generation sulfonylureas by displacement from plasma protein binding sites;
5. disulfiram-like interactions with alcohol.

The hypoglycemic effect of sulfonylureas is additive with hypoglycemic influences of alcohol, salicylates, haloperidol, chlorpromazine, propoxyphene, beta-blockers, MAO inhibitors, warfarin, guanethidine, probenecid, anabolic steroids, and of course, insulin. Drugs that have opposing hyperglycemic influences that counter the therapeutic benefit of sulfonylureas include thiazide and high-ceiling diuretics, triamterene, estrogens, phenytoin, thyroid hormones, epinephrine, glucagon, diazoxide, and L-asparaginase.

Drugs that inhibit metabolism of sulfonylureas, increasing the risk of hypoglycemic reactions, include sulfonamides, chloramphenicol, phenylbutazone, and clofibrate. Drugs that potentiate effects of first-generation sulfonylureas by competing for plasma protein binding sites include warfarin, salicylates, phenytoin, diazepam, and a host of other drugs.

Some of the sulfonylureas inhibit metabolism of alcohol, in the manner of the drug disulfiram that is used in certain alcohol-treatment programs. Chlorpropamide is most likely to cause this problem, but it has occurred also with other first-generation sulfonylureas. Persons with diabetes should be advised to discontinue even moderate consumption of alcoholic beverages because of the disulfiram-like effect of sulfonylureas, and also because the hypoglycemic effect of alcohol complicates effective management of blood glucose levels.

Administration in the Elderly.   Oral hypoglycemics are best taken at the same time each day to improve stability of response. Oral hypoglycemics should not be taken at bedtime to avoid the risk of nocturnal hypoglycemia. Once-a-day oral hypoglycemics are best taken in the morning, while those taken twice or three times per day are best taken with meals.

ACETOHEXAMIDE   (Dymelor, generic)

Recommended initial oral dose in the elderly: Start with a lower initial dose before breakfast and check blood and urine glucose during the first 24 hours. Continue or gradually increase the dose if control is satisfactory. Lower the dose or discontinue the drug if there is any tendency toward hypoglycemia.

Unspecified adult initial dose for comparison: 250 mg to 1.5 g/day.

CHLORPROPAMIDE   (Diabinese, generic)

Recommended initial oral dose in the elderly: 100–125 mg/day in the morning. See also acetohexamide.

Middle-aged adult initial dose for comparison: 250 mg/day in the morning.

GLIPIZIDE   (Glucotrol)

Recommended initial oral dose in the elderly: 2.5 mg 30 minutes before breakfast. See also acetohexamide.

Unspecified adult initial dose for comparison: 5 mg 30 minutes before breakfast.

GLYBURIDE   (DiaBeta, Glynase, Micronase)

Recommended initial oral dose in the elderly: 0.75 mg/day for patients who may be more sensitive to hypoglycemic drugs. See also acetohexamide.

Unspecified adult initial dose for comparison: 1.5–3 mg/day with breakfast or in 2 divided doses.

TOLAZAMIDE   (Tolinase, generic)

Recommended initial oral dose in the elderly:
See acetohexamide.

Unspecified adult initial dose for comparison: 100–250 mg/day with breakfast or the first main meal.

TOLBUTAMIDE   (Orinase, generic)

Recommended initial oral dose in the elderly:
See acetohexamide.

Unspecified adult initial dose for comparison: 1–2 g/day in 1–3 divided doses.

USE OF INSULIN BY ELDERLY CLIENTS

Insulin discovery in 1920, its introduction into clinical practice in 1922, and the identification of its exact peptide sequence between 1945 and 1955 are all milestones in the history of medicine. Insulin is a life-saving medication, particularly for those individuals with Type I diabetes mellitus.

The insulin products available today are derived from five sources: pork pancreas, beef pancreas, pork-beef mixtures, human insulin derived by conversion of pork insulin, and human insulin produced by recombinant DNA technology. Differences between the five sources relate to likelihood of allergic reactions and cost, but do not impact on potential therapeutic benefits. Even the least pure of the products on the market today are much purer than just a few years ago.

Clinical Indications in the Elderly. Insulin preparations are indicated for treatment of all clients with Type I diabetes mellitus and those with severe Type II diabetes not manageable by other measures. Insulin is indicated for acute control during temporary exacerbations of mild Type II diabetes. Intermediate- and long-acting preparations provide for daily maintenance, while short-acting preparations are useful for fine-tuning therapy or rapid treatment of ketoacidosis. Most elderly clients have Type II diabetes and produce some insulin endogenously, especially in response to food intake. Therefore, blood glucose can be effectively managed for most elderly clients with a single morning dose of an intermediate-acting insulin preparation to raise basal insulin levels, allowing the client's own endogenous production to respond to increases in glucose that follow meals. Long-acting preparations are usually inappropriate for elderly clients because of excessive risk of nocturnal hypoglycemia. If adequate control is not achieved with a single daily dose of an intermediate-acting insulin, clients may benefit from a second small dose of the same drug at dinner or bedtime or from one or two doses of a short-acting insulin taken premixed with the intermediate-acting drug. The goal of therapy is to maintain fasting blood glucose levels between 120 and 180 mg/dl and postprandial values between 200 and 250 mg/dl.

Altered Pharmacokinetics or Pharmacodynamics in the Elderly.
Insulin is given by injection only because oral administration does not provide any significant bioavailability. The major difference between various insulin preparations is duration of action (see Table 14.2). Insulin preparations are categorized as short, intermediate, or long. Duration determines the most likely time when hypoglycemia will be a risk (namely, at peak effect) as well as the most likely time of hyperglycemia due to inadequate effect (at the end of duration).

Adverse Effects and Contraindications in the Elderly. The principal risk of insulin is the same as that for oral hypoglycemic drugs: excess hypoglycemia. In the extreme, this culminates in coma or shock. As previously discussed (see Adverse Effects of Oral Hypoglycemics in the Elderly), the elderly are more prone to hypoglycemic extremes, more likely to have conditions exacerbated by hypoglycemia, and more likely to have no warning signs before hypoglycemia reaches extreme proportions. The risk of hypoglycemic reactions is increased during exercise and by concurrent use of alcohol or other drugs with hypoglycemic actions of their own. Diabetic clients prone to such reactions need to carry a carbohydrate source with them at all times. In clinical settings, hypoglycemia is treated with a soluble carbohydrate source, such as orange juice or a sugar cube or, if the client is unconscious, intravenous dextrose.

Some clients will have allergic reactions to insulins derived from animal sources. Human insulin produced by recombinant DNA technology is least likely to cause such problems, but is somewhat more expensive than alternative products. Converted pork insulin is next lowest in frequency of allergic reactions and beef-pork insulin is highest. Those clients who require insulin only during intermittent exacerbations of their condition should always receive human insulin so that the risk of antibody formation and

Table 14.2 Preparations of Insulin

Characteristic	Insulin Preparations					
	Rapid		Intermediate		Long	
Type						
Preparation	Regular or crystalline zinc (insulin injection)	Prompt insulin zinc suspension (semilente, semitard)	Isophane insulin suspension (NPH insulin)	Slow insulin zinc suspension (Lente, Monotard, Lentard)	Protamine zinc insulin	Extended insulin zinc suspension suspension (Ultralente, Ultratard)
Source	Beef, pork, beef-pork, human (converted pork), human (recombinant DNA)	Beef, pork, or beef-pork	Beef, pork, beef-pork, human (recombinant DNA)	Beef, pork, beef-pork, human (converted pork)	Beef, pork, or beef-pork	Beef or beef-pork
Protein Modifier	None	None	Protamine	None	Protamine	None
Appearance	Clear solution	Cloudy suspension	Cloudy suspension	Cloudy suspension	Cloudy suspension	Cloudy suspension
Time of Administration	15–20 min before meal (SC); any time for ketoacidosis (IV)	30–45 min before breakfast	1 hr before breakfast	1 hr before breakfast	1 hr before breakfast	1 hr before breakfast
Latency to Onset	1 hr	1–3 hr	3–4 hr	2–4 hr	4–6 hr	8 hr
Peak Effect	2–3 hr	2–8 hr	4–12 hr	6.5–14.5 hr	14–20 hr	16–18 hr
Time When Hypoglycemia is Most Likely	Before lunch	Before lunch	Before dinner	Before dinner	Late night	Late night or early morning
Duration	5–7 hr	12–16 hr	24–28 hr	24–28 hr	30–36 hr	36+ hr
Time When Glycosuria Is Most Likely	At night	At night	Before lunch	Before lunch	At bedtime	At bedtime

resistance will be minimized; also cost is less a factor when use is infrequent. Otherwise, it comes down to an issue of cost versus the advantage of lower risk of allergic reactions. Typical allergic reactions are pruritus, urticaria, and redness at the site of injection. Antihistamines provide some relief.

Interactions in the Elderly.   Many drugs have additive hypoglycemic effects with those of insulin, including alcohol, anabolic steroids, salicylates, fenfluramine, propoxyphene, guanethidine, beta-blockers, monoamine oxidase inhibitors, haloperidol, chlorpromazine, and of course, oral hypoglycemic drugs. On the other hand, drugs with opposing hyperglycemic influences include thiazide and high-ceiling diuretics, triamterene, glucocorticoids, epinephrine, glucagon, antidepressants, lithium, levodopa, phenytoin, indomethacin, isoniazid, niacin, alloxan, streptozocin, and *L*-asparaginase.

Insulin tends to lower serum potassium levels by increasing its cellular uptake. The resultant hypokalemia increases toxicity of cardiac glycosides and potassium-wasting diuretics.

Administration in the Elderly.   As in younger clients, sites of injection need to be rotated to reduce local irritation and accumulation of fat. It is best to rotate sites within one general locale so that absorption will not vary unduly.

INSULIN

Recommended dose in the elderly: 10–15 units in obese elderly persons; 6–10 units in thin elderly persons. Adjust doses to achieve fasting glucose levels of 120–180 mg/dl and postprandial values of 200–250 mg/dl.

Dose for unspecified adults for comparison: 0.5–1 unit/kg/day. Adjust doses to achieve premeal and bedtime blood glucose levels of 80–140 mg/dl.

Rapid Preparations

- Insulin injection (Regular insulin, Regular Iletin, Velosulin, Novolin R, Humulin R)
- Insulin zinc suspension prompt (Semilente Iletin)

Intermediate Preparations

- Isophane insulin suspension (NPH) (NPH insulin, NPH Iletin, Insulatard NPH, Humulin N, Novolin N)
- Insulin zinc suspension (Lente Iletin, Humulin L, Novolin L)

Mixed Rapid and Intermediate Preparations

- Isophane insulin suspension and insulin injection (Mixtard, Novolin 70/30, Humulin 70/30)

Long Preparations

- Protamine zinc insulin suspension (Protamine, Zinc & Iletin)
- Insulin zinc suspension extended (Ultralente Iletin, Humulin Ultralente)

REFERENCES AND RECOMMENDED READINGS

Blankenship GW, Skyler JS: Diabetic retinopathy: a general survey. *Diabetes Care* 1978; 1(2):127–137.

Blevins DR: *The Diabetic and Nursing Care.* New York, McGraw-Hill, 1979.

Bliss M: *The Discovery of Insulin.* Chicago, University of Chicago Press, 1983.

Boyden TW: The proper place of oral hypoglycemics in diabetes management. *Drug Therapy* 1978; 8:66–77.

Bressler R, Galloway JA: The insulins: pharmacology and uses. *Drug Therapy* 1978; 8:43–61.

Chambers JK: Save your diabetic patient from early kidney damage. *Nursing* 1983; 13(5):58–63.

Dardick L, Rodney WM, Sakiyama R: Human insulin. *Am. Fam. Physician* 1984; 29(6):204–206.

DeFronzo RA, Ferrannini E, Koivisto V: New concepts in the pathogenesis and treatment of noninsulin-dependent diabetes mellitus. *Am. J. Med.* 1983; 74(1A):52–81.

Drury MI, Drury RM, Keenan P, Gayer EPM: The management of newly diagnosed diabetes mellitus in the elderly, in K. O'Malley and JL Waddington (eds): *Therapeutics in the elderly,* Elsevier Sci. Publ, 1985, pp. 143–152.

Galloway JA, Bressler R: Insulin treatment in diabetes. *Med. Clin. North Am.* 1978; 62(4):663–680.

Guthrie D: Helping the diabetic manage his self-care. *Nursing* 1980; 10(2):57–64.

Haire-Joshu D: Diabetes: controlling the insulin balance. *Am. J. Nurs.* 1986; 86(11):1239–1258.

Hayter J: Fine points in diabetic care. *Am. J. Nurs.* 1976; 76:594–599.

Herget M: For visually impaired diabetics. *Am. J. Nurs.* 1983; 83:1557–1560.

Home PD, Alberti, KG: The new insulins: their characteristics and clinical indications. *Drugs* 1982; 24(5):401–413.

Kolterman DG, Prince MJ, Olefsky JM: Insulin resistance in noninsulin-dependent diabetes mellitus: impact of sulfonylurea agents in vivo and in vitro. *Am. J. Med.* 1982; 74(1A):82–101.

Nemchick R: Diabetes today (part 6): the new insulin pumps: tight control at a price. *RN* 1983; 46:52–54.

Page M, et al.: Treatment of diabetic ketoacidosis. *N. Engl. J. Med.* 1976; 294:1183.

Pelczynski L, Reilly A: Helping your diabetic patients help themselves: a plan for inpatient education. *Nursing* 1981: 11(5):24–29.

Pendergast B: Glyburide and glipizide, second-generation oral sulfonylurea hypo-glycemic agents. *Clin. Pharmacy* 1984; 3:473–485.

Poole D: Type II diabetes mellitus update: diagnosis and management. *Nurse Pract.* 1986; 11(8):26–41.

Price MJ: Insulin and oral hypoglycemic agents. *Nurs. Clin. North Am.* 1983; 18(4):687–706.

Rancilio H: When a pregnant woman is diabetic: postpartal care. *Am. J. Nurs.* 1979; 79(3):453–456.

Renshaw DC: Impotence in diabetics. *Dis. Nerv. System* 1975; 36(7):369–371.

Rodman M: Glyburide. *RN* 1984; 84(8):76–78.

Schuler K: When a pregnant woman is diabetic: antepartal care. *Am. J. Nurs.* 1979; 79(3):448–450.

Shen SW, Bressler R: Clinical pharmacology of oral antidiabetic agents. *N. Engl. J. Med.* 1977; 296:493–497, 787–793.

Surr C: Teaching patients to use the new blood glucose monitoring products. *Nursing* 1983; 13:42–45.

Rizza RA, et al.: Control of blood sugar in insulin-dependent diabetes: compari-son of an artificial endocrine pancreas, continuous subcutaneous insulin infu-sion, and intensified conventional insulin therapy. *N. Engl. J. Med.* 1980; 303:1313–1318.

Slater NL: Insulin reactions vs. ketoacidosis: guidelines for diagnosis and inter-vention. *Am. J. Nurs.* 1978; 78(5):875–877.

Walesky ME: Diabetic Ketoacidosis. *Am. J. Nurs.* 1978; 78(5):772–874.

Wilson DE: Excessive insulin therapy: biochemical effects and clinical repercus-sions: current concepts of counterregulation in type I diabetes. *Ann. Intern. Med.* 1983; 98(2):219.

Witty KT (ed): Retinopathy: eye care for your diabetic patients. *Patient Care* 1978; 12:174–196.

CHAPTER 15

Pain Management
for the Elderly

The physiological basis for pain is not much different for the elderly person than younger adults. Pain receptors are relatively unchanged with aging and are activated by the same kind of mechanical and chemical stimuli to trigger impulses that then travel along the pain pathways to the brain. Yet pain is, in many ways, as much a matter of the spirit as of the flesh. Support and understanding can go a long distance, if not always an entirely sufficient distance, in increasing a person's tolerance for minor aches and pains. If there is a part of the management of pain that is different for elderly than younger people, it is that elderly people are more likely to be isolated, lonely, deprived of the normal complement of support, hurting, and in need of understanding, contact, and sympathy. Clinicians sometimes tend to treat pain too much with medications and too little with care and understanding. If medications provide somewhat more maximum analgesic potential, their actions also entail risks, which is seldom the case with care and understanding.

Attending to matters of physical comfort, even if not directly related to the source of pain, can be helpful. Ensuring proper body position and alignment, reducing sources of stress, and providing appropriate environmental control (temperature, lighting, noise reduction) can be important. Massage or applications of hot or cold can help alleviate some kinds of pain or provide compensating comfort. These kinds of measures do no harm and often reduce the need for and reliance on drugs for pain relief.

Some kinds of pain have been helped by biofeedback techniques. Clients can be taught to identify mental adjustments that promote a decrease in sympathetic tone by providing them with biofeedback based on measurement of finger temperature. When blood vessels dilate due to reduced sympathetic tone, finger temperature goes up. This technique has worked for some clients who suffer migraine headaches. Feedback from EMG measurement taken from a cranial muscle has been helpful for some clients who suffer tension headaches.

There have been many opportunities in this book to discuss circumstances where elderly clients need to be treated differently with drugs than younger persons, because of altered pharmacokinetics, pharmacodynamics, or interacting disease states. Perhaps here, in the management of pain, we have the foremost example of a circumstance where elderly people should probably be treated less differently from their younger counterparts than is often the case in current medical practice. Too often clinicians will exempt elderly people from the usual standards of caution that they exercise in the prescription of pain relievers, thinking to themselves that if the client is elderly, potential dependence is less an issue. This attitude has been dubbed the "old-age write off" and should not be condoned. There may be validity in less discriminant use of pain-killers for the terminally ill near the time of death, but never for elderly people with an indefinite life expectancy ahead of them.

Assessment of pain is an important prelude to its appropriate management. Accurate assessment depends on close attention to the client's description and explanation of the pain. The person should be encouraged to describe the pain in his or her own words, but sometimes it will be helpful if the client is furnished with a selection of descriptive terms for pain, such as burning, aching, stabbing, cramping, dull, sharp, penetrating, or radiating. Attention needs to be paid to whether the pain is indeed the client's central issue or whether the voicing of the complaint is an expression of need for support and sympathy.

TYPES OF PAIN

There are many different forms of pain; often the form dictates the most appropriate method of management, drug or nondrug measures, or even the drug selection. Pain may be superficial or deep. **Superficial pain** is usually sharp and localized and seems to emanate from surface tissues. Nonnarcotic analgesics often provide relief of superficial pain that compares favorably with the ability of even the strongest narcotics. **Deep pain** arises from deep tissues, usually the viscera. It is usually perceived as a poorly localized, dull ache. Narcotic analgesics may be required and generally outperform nonnarcotic analgesics for relief of deep pain. Sometimes pain is experienced in a location other than the one from which it actually arises. If so, it is **referred pain.** The pain of angina pectoris may be referred to the left arm or the jaw. Pain from problems in the eyes or ears is sometimes referred to the head, being experienced as a general headache rather than localized to the tissues of origin.

A critically important issue both for the client's mental state and for clinical pain management is whether pain is acute or chronic. **Acute pain** is pain that develops suddenly and, though it may be sharp and unrelenting while it lasts, ultimately subsides. The drugs currently available for clinical use in pain management provide all that is really necessary for managing acute pains, from mild to severe, in doses that vary relatively little from person to person.

Chronic pain persists or recurs for long periods of time and resists treatment. It is chronic pain that poses the ultimate challenge to the moral fortitude of clients and the skills of clinicians. The analgesics available for medical practice today cannot always provide what is needed in the way of relief without significant adverse effects. Nonnarcotic analgesics can be used for long periods of time without tolerance or dependence, but the upper limit of their analgesic potential is often inadequate and even these drugs produce significant side effects with long term use. An appropriately selected narcotic analgesic can provide all the pain relief that is required for acute pain of any level of severity, but tolerance and dependence develop inevitably with chronic use. When pain is chronic and if the person needs to get on with life activities despite the pain, the depressant effect of narcotics is often a drawback. The dose of the narcotic will need to be minimized to slow the rate at which tolerance develops. This means also that the dose will need to be individualized taking into account the individual's tolerance for pain and potential for misusing the medication. To allow the use of the lowest dose possible, the action of the narcotic may need to be augmented with drugs that potentiate narcotic action (a tricyclic antidepressant or amphetamine) or a nonnarcotic analgesic for additive pain relief. Management of chronic pain is thus a greatly more difficult task.

NONNARCOTIC ANALGESIC USE FOR THE ELDERLY

Nonnarcotic analgesics are generally equivalent to weak narcotics, such as propoxyphen, in their analgesic potential. Yet, for certain types of pain nonnarcotic analgesics compare favorably with potent narcotics, such as morphine. Nonnarcotics work especially well for superficial pain triggered by chemical mediators but less well for deep visceral pain or pain caused by pressure or mechanical activation of pain receptors. Nonnarcotics work better for dull, throbbing pain than for sharp stabbing pain.

Aspirin is the prototype nonnarcotic analgesic and so familiar that the family of nonnarcotics is often referred to simply as aspirin-like drugs. This is a group of drugs with unusual pharmacological versatility, providing several clinical values. Aspirin-like drugs not only provide relatively safe, low-level analgesia but also furnish the best antipyretic (fever-reducing) action known. Many aspirin-like drugs have impressive anti-inflammatory activity and this group is referred to as nonsteroidal anti-inflammatory drugs (see Chapter 16). Aspirin itself enjoys some additional values not substantially shared by other members of the family. It is an antithrombotic drug and as such can reduce risk of secondary infarctions after an initial myocardial infarction. It is sometimes used prophylactically against a variety of thromboembolic problems, such as second strokes after a completed first stroke. Aspirin was once an important part of treatment of gout (hyperuricemia), but has lost favor in this condition in deference to newer antigout drugs.

The antipyretic effect of aspirin-like drugs is an action on the hypothalamus of the brain but the analgesic effect is peripheral—a decrease in the sensitivity of pain receptors to chemical mediators of pain. When cells are damaged, they release chemicals that activate pain receptors to signal the brain that injury has occurred. One chemical released by damaged cells is bradykinin, a potent activator of pain receptors. Another family of chemicals released by cells is the prostaglandins, which sensitize pain receptors to bradykinin. The prostaglandins are the group affected by nonnarcotic analgesics. Aspirin-like drugs are inhibitors of the enzyme sequence responsible for production of the prostaglandins. Aspirin-like drugs thereby prevent sensitization of pain receptors.

The aspirin-like drugs approved for use as analgesics include aspirin, seven other salicylates, acetaminophen, mefenamic acid, and three propionic acid derivatives (ibuprofen, fenoprofen, and ketoprofen). Many other aspirin-like drugs are marketed exclusively for anti-inflammatory use, mainly in rheumatoid arthritis and osteoarthritis. Aspirin, choline salicylate, sodium salicylate, magnesium salicylate, acetaminophen, and ibuprofen are the nonnarcotic analgesics available without prescription.

Clinical Indications in the Elderly.   Routine relief of mild to moderate pain, particularly dull aches of superficial origin or headaches, and suppression of fever. Only aspirin is used for prevention of secondary thromboembolic events or secondary myocardial infarctions.

Altered Pharmacokinetics or Pharmacodynamics in the Elderly.
All of the aspirin-like drugs are readily absorbed after oral administration and largely unaffected by malabsorption or food, although taking aspirin, acetaminophen, or ibuprofen with a meal can delay absorption without altering extent of absorption. Aspirin in particular exhibits significant variations in formulation characteristics that may affect gastric irritation. Poorly formulated tablets disintegrate initially into clumps that can rest against the gastric mucosa and cause local irritation or erosion. Enteric-coated aspirin preparations also vary in quality, some providing reduced absorption and all providing delayed absorption if taken with meals. Liquid forms are absorbed faster. Concurrent antacid administration hastens aspirin absorption but also speeds its urinary excretion if the antacid has any appreciable systemic absorption. Ibuprofen is unaffected by antacids.

Aspirin is bound to plasma proteins usually in excess of 90%, but the percent of an administered dose that is bound declines as the dose increases. Binding to plasma proteins also diminishes with age of the client. Plasma concentrations in the range of 100–150 mcg/mL are therapeutic, while those around 200 mcg/mL cause early signs of salicylism, and those above 400 mcg/mL can be fatal. Ibuprofen and diflunisal are highly bound to plasma proteins, but acetaminophen much less so.

Aspirin undergoes a lot of first-pass extraction, but the aspirin metabolite formed in the liver is itself active, diminishing, therefore, the importance of first-pass extraction for this drug. Aspirin exhibits nonlinear kinetics, meaning that after a certain plasma concentration, further small increases in the dose of aspirin will result in large changes in its action. The reason is that normal aspirin plasma concentrations are close to the level that saturates hepatic metabolizing capacity for the drug, and increases beyond that point cannot be matched by increased hepatic metabolism. The elderly have reduced hepatic function, on average, so aspirin concentrations in the plasma are more likely to saturate liver capacity. Indeed, aspirin's half-life is significantly longer among elderly clients. Aspirin inactivation is also partly by renal excretion and the diminished renal function in elderly people contributes to the prolonged half-life. Aspirin doses need to be reduced in elderly people based on the extent of either hepatic or renal impairment.

Acetaminophen is inactivated mainly by lever metabolism. About 4% of this metabolism uses the cytochrome P-450 oxidase system, which yields an hepatotoxic product. With chronic use, acetaminophen can thereby cause hepatic necrosis.

Adverse Effects and Contraindications in the Elderly.

Some of the side effects of nonnarcotic analgesics are common to the entire group because they relate to the same prostaglandins that are involved in the therapeutic actions for this class. All drugs in this family irritate the gastrointestinal tract, although acetaminophen and ibuprofen do so a good deal less than does aspirin. Aspirin invariably increases gastrointestinal blood loss and sometimes even causes outright ulceration or hemorrhage. Elderly people are especially at risk of irritant effects of drugs on the gastrointestinal mucosa because of the involution of mucosal membranes that occurs with aging. Moreover, elderly individuals are more susceptible to anemia when blood loss occurs day after day, even in small amounts, because their blood volume is less than for young adults. Gastric irritation also contributes to nausea, vomiting, and epigastric distress. Clients receiving chronic aspirin therapy may complain of heartburn or shortness of breath. Doses of aspirin-like drugs required for analgesia or fever reduction are a good deal lower than those necessary for anti-inflammatory purposes and treatment is less likely to be chronic, so the incidence of significant gastrointestinal irritation is less. Nevertheless, ibuprofen and acetaminophen provide a better choice than aspirin for most clients, offering the same benefits with less adverse effect on the gut. Gastric irritation is also reported less with salsalate, choline salicylate, and magnesium salicylate, but the last of these is contraindicated for clients with advanced renal failure.

All aspirin-like drugs inhibit blood clotting to some extent by blocking the formation of a substance called thromboxane A2, a promoter of clotting produced by the same enzyme family responsible for synthesis of prostaglandins. Aspirin's blood thinning effect is much greater than the other drugs in the family because it inhibits platelet aggregation in addition to the shared effect on thromboxane synthesis. Nonnarcotic analgesics must be avoided for clients with a history of hemophilia or other deficits of coagulation or those receiving anticoagulant drug therapy.

Aspirin and mefenamic acid have hypoglycemic actions, at least at high doses. Acetaminophen has this effect to a lesser extent. Drug-induced hypoglycemia can complicate management of diabetes mellitus. It is best to schedule aspirin administrations at least 1 hour prior to scheduled exercise to avoid a hypoglycemic influence that could be additive with that of exercise.

Hepatotoxicity occurs rarely with acetaminophen and mainly after chronic use. The typical manifestation is jaundice, but hepatic failure, coma, and death have occurred. Individuals with a long history of alcohol abuse are at elevated risk of hepatotoxic effects from acetaminophen. Elderly persons with preexisting hepatic dysfunction should probably receive another nonnarcotic selection. Hepatotoxicity has been reported rarely with propionic acid derivatives.

Propionic acid derivatives can cause minor neurological reactions such as dizziness, drowsiness, headache, or tinnitus. More severe problems have been reported rarely, such as depression, fatigue, confusion, hallucinations, or dream disturbances. Blood dyscrasias have occurred, but uncommonly. Baseline blood cell counts provide a basis for future evaluation if long-term use of a propionic acid derivative is anticipated. Cardiovascular reactions to propionic acid derivatives are uncommon in younger clients, but somewhat more frequent for the elderly. Possible manifestations include fluid retention, edema, hypertension, or congestive heart failure. Elderly clients with a history of cardiac decompensation should not receive ibuprofen or other propionic acid derivatives.

Mefenamic acid is somewhat more toxic than other nonnarcotic analgesics and it would be difficult to justify its selection for use in an elderly person in particular. It is specifically contraindicated for use in individuals with impaired renal function, which describes most elderly people to a lesser or greater extent.

Sodium salicylate is less effective than aspirin and also provides a significant sodium load, which few elderly people can tolerate. It would seldom be an appropriate choice for elderly clients.

As with virtually all drugs, a fraction of people will be allergic to any of the nonnarcotic analgesics. Aspirin allergies are perhaps better documented than most because it has been used by such an enormous number of people over the years. Typical examples are asthma-like bronchospasm, rash, hives, or rhinitis.

Interactions in the Elderly.   Aspirin, diflunisal, and propionic acid derivatives interact with other drugs that are highly bound to plasma proteins, by mutual displacement. The result is potentiation of each drug's effect. This is perhaps most noteworthy as regards the oral anticoagulant warfarin, because warfarin's action must be carefully regulated to ensure adequate effect without risk of hemorrhage. Aspirin's potent antithrombotic action compounds its relationship with warfarin by also adding directly to the inhibition of hemostasis. Aspirin or a proprionic acid derivative could also displace drugs such as phenytoin, valproic acid, penicillin, sulfonamides, and sulfonylureas from plasma protein binding sites.

The hypoglycemic action of aspirin is additive with that of insulin or oral hypoglycemic drugs that might be required by individuals with diabetes mellitus. Doses of the antidiabetic drugs might need to be adjusted if aspirin use is to be long-term.

Although large doses of aspirin promote excretion of uric acid and were used in gout precisely for that purpose, smaller doses antagonize the action of the newer antigout drugs, such as probenecid or sulfinpyrazone. Aspirin excretion is increased by urinary alkalinizers but decreased by urinary acidifiers or organic acids, such as furosemide, that compete with aspirin for the organic acid secretory mechanism.

Oral contraceptives increase the rate of metabolism of acetaminophen and decrease its half-life by as much as 20–30%.

A useful interaction of nonnarcotic analgesics is additive analgesia with narcotic analgesics. Nonnarcotics can be used in combination with narcotics for management of chronic pain, allowing reduction in the dose of the narcotic and a delay in tolerance development. Many products combining nonnarcotic and narcotic analgesics are available for medical practice.

Administration in the Elderly.   Aspirin is available in countless formulations, as a single drug or in combinations. Following the principle of the simplest, least complicated, safest, and least expensive medication when pain relief is required, products that combine aspirin with caffeine or other unnecessary ingredients should be avoided as unnecessarily complicated and expensive. On the other hand, the cheapest aspirin might not be the cheapest in the long run if it is a poorly formulated tablet that adds to the extent of gastric irritation. Buffered products can reduce gastrointestinal irritation but also reduce duration of action by hastening urinary excretion of aspirin. Many aspirin products do not age well and clients should be discouraged from stockpiling aspirin tablets. Storage in a cool location in an airtight container will help to prolong shelf life.

Salicylates

ACETYLSALICYLIC ACID   (aspirin)

Recommended oral analgesic dose in the elderly: Reduce dose in clients with hepatic or renal dysfunction.

Unspecified adult analgesic dose for comparison: 325–650 mg every 4 hours as needed or 500 mg every 3 hours or 1000 mg every 6 hours.

CHOLINE SALICYLATE   (Arthropan)

Recommended oral analgesic dose in the elderly: No specific recommendation.

Unspecified adult analgesic dose for comparison: 870 mg PO every 3–4 hours up to 6 times daily.

DIFLUNISAL   (Dolobid)

Recommended oral analgesic dose in the elderly: Reduce dose in clients with hepatic or renal dysfunction.

Unspecified adult analgesic dose for comparison: 1000 mg PO initially, followed by 500 mg at 8–12 hour intervals as required.

MAGNESIUM SALICYLATE   (Doan's Pills, Durasal, Efficin, Magan, Mobidin)

Recommended oral analgesic dose in the elderly: No specific recommendation.

Unspecified adult analgesic dose for comparison: 500–600 mg PO, 3 or 4 times daily, up to 3.6–4.8 g/day.

SALICYLAMIDE   (Uromide, generic)

Recommended oral analgesic dose in the elderly: No specific recommendation.

Unspecified adult analgesic dose for comparison: 325–650 mg PO, 3–4 times daily.

SALSALATE   (Disalcid, Artha-G, Mono-Gesic)

Recommended oral analgesic dose in the elderly: No specific recommendation.

Unspecified adult analgesic dose for comparison: 3000 mg/day PO in divided doses.

SODIUM SALICYLATE   (Uracel 5, generic)

Recommended oral analgesic dose in the elderly: Do not use in clients with fluid retention, edema, or hypertension.

Unspecified adult analgesic dose for comparison: 325–650 mg PO every 4–8 hrs.

SODIUM THIOSALICYLATE   (numerous tradenames)

Recommended oral analgesic dose in the elderly: Do not use in clients with fluid retention, edema, or hypertension.

Unspecified adult analgesic dose for comparison: 50–100 mg IM on alternate days.

Propionic Acid Derivatives

FENOPROFEN   (Nalfon)

Recommended oral analgesic dose in the elderly: Begin with reduced doses.

Unspecified adult analgesic dose for comparison: 200 mg every 4–6 hours as needed.

IBUPROFEN   (Motrin, Nuprin, Rufen, others, generic)

Recommended oral analgesic dose in the elderly: Begin with reduced doses.

Unspecified adult analgesic dose for comparison: 400 mg every 4–6 hours as needed.

KETOPROFEN   (Orudis)

Recommended oral analgesic dose in the elderly: Begin with reduced doses; reduce doses for clients with hypoalbuminemia or impaired renal function.

Unspecified adult analgesic dose for comparison: 25–50 mg every 6–8 hours as needed.

Other Aspirin-like Drugs

ACETAMINOPHEN   (Tylenol, Valodol, Febrinol, Panadol, Datril, Tapanol, generic)

Recommended oral analgesic dose in the elderly: Do not use in clients with hepatic impairment.

Unspecified adult analgesic dose for comparison: 300–650 mg every 4 hours.

MEFENAMIC ACID   (Ponstel)

Recommended oral analgesic dose in the elderly: No specific recommendation.

Unspecified adult analgesic dose for comparison: 500 mg, then 250 mg every 6 hours as needed; use not to exceed 1 week; give with food.

NARCOTIC ANALGESIC USE FOR THE ELDERLY

Narcotics are a family of drugs that all have fundamentally similar pharmacology. The history of the original narcotic, opium, extends back into the far reaches of history, prior, at least, to 4000 BC. Opium is the sap of the poppy plant and contains two narcotic alkaloids, morphine and codeine. Morphine was purified from opium near the beginning of the nineteenth century and that event was an important landmark in the transition from the plant-based medicine that existed through most of history to the chemical-based medicine of today. Morphine and codeine are the two **natural narcotics** and derivatives of either of these two are designated **semisynthetic.** Heroin, hydromorphone, and dihydrocodeine are all examples. Some of the narcotics in use today, such as meperidine and fentanyl, are purely **synthetic.**

Morphine found use in the wars of the nineteenth century as a painkiller but, as a result, morphine dependence soon gained the nickname *soldier's disease.* Smoking opium was legal in the United States and England throughout the nineteenth century as well. The Chinese population on the American west coast frequented opium dens that existed at that time in the booming cities of California. By the turn of the century, an estimated 1% of all Americans were addicted to morphine. Much of that addiction was physician-assisted. Opiates were removed from the nonprescription market in 1914 by the Harrison Narcotic Act.

Narcotics suppress pain by an action on the pain pathways within the central nervous system rather than by any action at the pain receptor. The flow of pain signals is regulated in part by a class of peptide transmitters, called **endorphins.** One subgroup of endorphins is called **enkephalins,** a term that has become increasingly familiar to lay people in recent years. Narcotics mimic the pain-suppressing and euphoria-producing actions of endorphins, providing a higher level of pain relief than can be provided by the natural transmitters themselves. However, many of the endorphin receptors exhibit a high potential for adaptive change if narcotics are used for extended periods of time—generally anything in excess of three weeks of daily use starts the recipient down the road of tolerance and dependence.

Narcotics suppress the affective (emotional) component of pain more than the discriminative component. Individuals in pain given a narcotic will a half-hour later report that they still feel the sensations but that they are no longer bothered by them. Narcotics separate the emotional aspect of pain from the purely informational aspect, because endorphin receptors are mainly concentrated along the part of the pain pathway that directs pain signals to the limbic system—the part of the brain associated with emotions and emotional behaviors.

The term **analgesic** is reserved for drugs that suppress pain sensitivity without causing unconsciousness. Thus, although general anesthetics certainly decrease awareness of pain, they do so only by virtue of their action on the mechanism of consciousness. Narcotics do fit the definition of analgesic, but imperfectly because they do cause considerable changes in alertness, perception, and awareness. Narcotics are depressant drugs, if not as generally so as the sedative-hypnotics. They can readily contribute to symptoms of excess depression.

Clinical Indications in the Elderly.   Narcotic analgesics are indicated for pain relief whenever the combination of nondrug measures and nonnarcotic analgesics would be or proves to be inadequate or when nonnarcotic analgesics are contraindicated for one reason or another. Clinicians should be guided by the principle of the simplest, least complicated, safest, and least expensive method of pain relief possible. When narcotics are necessary, a further guideline, to minimize likelihood of tolerance and dependence, is the lowest possible frequency at the lowest possible dose. Often the objective is to reduce pain to an acceptable level rather than its complete elimination. Care must be taken, however, not to deny adequate relief from an exaggerated fear of causing addiction, especially when the period of use is anticipated to be short-term. The stress that derives from unrelieved pain can itself pose a threat to the client's psychological and even physical health.

Although certain narcotics are still used for two other applications, suppression of cough and suppression of diarrhea, neither of these applications requires use of narcotics as there are entirely adequate and suitable nonnarcotic alternatives that are safer.

Altered Pharmacokinetics or Pharmacodynamics in the Elderly. Most narcotics are rapidly absorbed whether given orally or by intramuscular injection, but morphine has very poor activity after oral administration. This is partly because first-pass extraction is substantial for morphine. Only about 25% of a dose of morphine administered orally reaches the systemic circulation. Codeine, oxycodone, levorphanol, and methadone have good oral effectiveness. Some narcotics are well-absorbed through rectal mucosal membranes and are employed as suppositories.

Morphine is only about one-third bound to plasma proteins in the blood. Volume of distribution for morphine is smaller in elderly persons, so that any given dose results in higher initial plasma concentrations.

Renal or hepatic dysfunction can prolong the effect of narcotics and promote accumulation if the interdose interval is not increased. Smaller doses may need to be used in either case. Since a degree of renal impairment is almost invariably present in an elderly client and some hepatic impairment may be evident, it is likely that most elderly clients need to be given lower doses when narcotics are required.

Adverse Effects and Contraindications in the Elderly.   Narcotics depress the respiratory center in the medulla oblongata of the brain and its normal responsiveness to rising levels of carbon dioxide. Narcotics cause many fatal overdoses each year due almost invariably to respiratory failure. In most instances of overdose, the individual can survive, usually none the worse for wear, if he or she reaches a clinical setting before respiratory arrest occurs. Artificial respiration and administration of a narcotic antagonist are usually all that is required to reverse effects of the overdose.

Other than the immediate risk of death from overdose, there can be no doubt that the most threatening adverse potential of narcotics is risk of dependence. Narcotics have the highest level of capability for producing both psychological and physical dependence of any class of drugs. Only the most potent stimulants can match narcotic liability for psychological dependence and only the sedative-hypnotics can match narcotics as regards risk of physical dependence. Dependence is indeed such a characteristic feature for this class of drugs that the term *narcotic,* in legal language, has come to stand for any drug with addiction liability regardless of pharmacological classification. Abuse potential is determined by dosage, dosage interval, and period of use, and need not be feared when narcotics are used short-term, even in high doses. Accordingly, when it develops, tolerance can be mild, moderate, or severe, and the associated physical dependence and subsequent withdrawal syndrome will vary likewise in severity. Severity of withdrawal can be minimized by tapering doses or switching for a period from a strong to a weak narcotic before ultimate discontinuation. Weaning programs for those with outright addictions make use of this principle.

Narcotics lower the seizure threshold, posing a risk for those with seizure disorders and those with temporarily elevated seizure liability because of withdrawal syndromes. Narcotics increase intracranial pressure—mainly a problem for those with head injury, brain tumors, or intracranial lesions.

Narcotics are essentially depressant drugs and share the potential of other central nervous system depressants for symptoms of excess depression. Depressed respiration is one manifestation mentioned already, but other possibilities include drowsiness, lethargy, disorientation, confusion, and, even, delirium. Performance of both mental and physical tasks is often impaired. Elderly individuals are especially susceptible to mental impairments caused by CNS depressants. They are more prone to falls and injury from motor impairments and they are more susceptible to automobile accidents due to impaired alertness.

Narcotics produce a characteristic dual action on the motor activity of the intestinal tract. They stimulate nonpropulsive movements, producing the sensations of cramps, sometimes painful, and they also inhibit propulsive movements, causing constipation. The constipating effect can be put to good use when these drugs are used for alleviation of persistent diarrhea.

Orthostatic hypotension is an effect of all narcotics in overdose situations and an effect of some even at therapeutic doses. Meperidine is particularly likely to cause this problem. Orthostatic hypotension is often more of a difficulty for elderly individuals because the dizziness or fainting that might occur upon abrupt standing is more likely to cause a fall for a person with impaired balance or motor control.

Many of the narcotics have weak anticholinergic activity, promoting urinary retention or hesitancy or other anticholinergic problems. These are often more troublesome for elderly persons. For example, urinary retention may add to bladder control problems caused by incontinence or prostate hypertrophy.

Many of the narcotics are weak bases and these are the kind of drugs most likely to cause histamine release from mast cells. Morphine, for example, is a potent histamine releaser and may cause anaphylactoid reactions. Histamine release is especially troublesome for elderly persons who suffer from asthma or chronic obstructive pulmonary disease or those with urticaria.

Cough suppression caused by narcotics is often used for therapeutic purposes, but at times can constitute a side effect. Suppression of productive cough is often counterproductive to sound pulmonary function. Pentazocine and butorphanol increase pulmonary artery pressure and peripheral vascular resistance. These drugs should be avoided in elderly clients who have cardiovascular problems, asthma, or other respiratory ailments.

Interactions in the Elderly.   Narcotics, as depressant drugs themselves, will add to the depressant effects of any other depressant drugs that the client requires. In practice, additive CNS depression is most likely to occur in elderly clients because they take the largest number of drugs, are most likely to be using two or more CNS depressants concurrently, and are most vulnerable to mental impairments because of declining neural function. Additive CNS depression occurs between narcotics and sedative-hypnotics, neuroleptics, antiepileptics, anxiolytics, and many other drugs.

The anxiolytic diazepam can add to cardiodepressant effects of fentanyl or hypotensive effects of alfentanil. Nitrous oxide potentiates cardiodepressant effects of both fentanyl and alfentanil. Droperidol, which is packaged with fentanyl as Innovar, can add to the hypotensive effect of fentanyl and its tendency to cause decreased pulmonary arterial pressure.

Drugs that induce liver enzymes, such as hydantoins and rifampin, speed the metabolism of certain narcotics, notably meperidine and methadone. If methadone is being used for maintenance, plasma levels may drop below the level necessary to prevent withdrawal symptoms. Monoamine oxidase inhibitors interfere with metabolism of meperidine, resulting in severe toxic reactions.

Propoxyphene increases the effects of warfarin.

Administration in the Elderly.   When injections of narcotics are required, the intramuscular route is preferred to the subcutaneous route, because the latter is associated with tissue irritation.

The traditional method of managing pain in clinical settings is based on periodical injections or oral administration as required. A drawback of this approach is that serum levels of the narcotic fluctuate widely, causing parallel variations in mental status. When the client decides that the pain is more than he or she can bear, there is often a considerable delay before a nurse can respond to the request for medication and a further delay before the drug is absorbed. An important recent trend in pain management, patient-controlled analgesia (PCA), addresses some of these difficulties. The most widely used method of PCA allows the client to operate an apparatus that provides small intravenous bolus injections of a narcotic at the client's demand. Pain relief is provided more rapidly and the client is an active participant in determining when the relief is really needed. The apparatus controls two features of administration: the **dose per administration** and a **lockout interval.** The lockout interval establishes a minimum interdose interval, preventing overly frequent administrations. Some pumps will provide a minimum baseline infusion rate to tide the client through periods of sleep so that peaks and valleys in plasma concentrations will not be overly great. Studies of PCA indicate that clients generally appreciate not having to ask for an analgesic each time pain develops and not having to wait once the need is apparent.

Strong Narcotics

ALFENTANIL   (Alfenta)

Unspecified adult analgesic dose: IV only, usually concommitant with anesthesia.

FENTANYL   (Sublimaze)

Unspecified adult analgesic dose: IV only, usually concommitant with anesthesia.

HYDROMORPHONE   (Dilaudid)

Recommended oral analgesic dose in the elderly: No specific recommendation.

Unspecified adult analgesic dose for comparison: 2 mg orally, every 4–6 hours as required.

LEVORPHANOL   (Levo-Dromoran)

Recommended analgesic dose in the elderly: No specific recommendation.

Unspecified adult analgesic dose for comparison: 2 mg PO or SC.

MEPERIDINE   (Demerol, Pethadol, and generic)

Recommended analgesic dose in the elderly: Reduce dose in clients with hepatic dysfunction.

Unspecified adult analgesic dose for comparison: 50–150 mg IM, SC, or PO, every 3–4 hours as required.

METHADONE   (Dolophine, generic)

Recommended analgesic dose in the elderly: Reduce dose in clients with hepatic dysfunction.

Unspecified adult analgesic dose for comparison: 50–150 mg IM, SC, or PO, every 3–4 hours as required.

MORPHINE

Recommended analgesic dose in the elderly: Reduce dose in clients with renal or hepatic impairment.

Unspecified adult analgesic dose for comparison: 10 mg/70 kg SC or IM.

OXYCODONE   (generic)

Recommended oral analgesic dose in the elderly: No specific recommendation.

Unspecified adult analgesic dose for comparison: 5 mg every 6 hours.

OXYMORPHONE   (Numorphan)

Unspecified adult analgesic dose: 0.5 mg IV or 1–1.5 mg SC or IM at 4–6 hour intervals.

SUFENTANIL   (Sufenta)

Unspecified adult analgesic dose: IV only, usually concommitant with anesthesia.

Intermediate-Strength Narcotics

CODEINE

Recommended oral analgesic dose in the elderly: Reduce dose in clients with hepatic impairment.

Unspecified adult analgesic dose for comparison: 15–60 mg PO every 4–6 hours.

DIHYDROCODEINE

Recommended oral analgesic dose in the elderly: No specific recommendation.

Unspecified adult analgesic dose for comparison: 32 mg PO every 4 hours.

Weak Narcotics

HYDROCODONE

Recommended oral analgesic dose in the elderly: No specific recommendation.

Unspecified adult analgesic dose for comparison: 7.5–10 mg PO every 4–6 hours.

PROPOXYPHENE   (Darvon, Dolene, Doxaphene, Profene, SK-65, generic)

Recommended oral analgesic dose in the elderly: Reduce dose in clients with hepatic dysfunction.

Unspecified adult analgesic dose for comparison: 65 mg PO every 4 hours as needed.

PROPOXYPHENE NAPSYLATE   (Darvon-N)

Recommended oral analgesic dose in the elderly: Reduce dose in clients with hepatic dysfunction.

Unspecified adult analgesic dose for comparison: 100 mg PO every 4 hours as needed.

Mixed Agonist/Antagonists

BUPRENORPHINE   (Buprenex)

Unspecified adult analgesic dose: 0.3 mg IM or slowly IV, every 6 hours as needed.

BUTORPHANOL   (Stadol)

Unspecified adult analgesic dose: 2 mg IM or 1 mg IV, every 3–4 hours as required.

NALBUPHINE   (Nubain)

Unspecified adult analgesic dose: 10 mg/70 kg (maximum 20 mg) SC, IM, or IV, every 3–6 hours as required, not to exceed 160 mg/day.

PENTAZOCINE   (Talwin)

Recommended oral analgesic dose in the elderly: Reduce dose in clients with hepatic dysfunction.

Unspecified adult analgesic dose: 50 mg PO every 3–4 hours initially, increased up to 100 mg, not to exceed 600 mg/day.

REFERENCES AND RECOMMENDED READINGS

DiGregorio GJ, Barbieri EJ: Pharmacologic management of pain. *Am. Fam. Physician* 1983; 27(5):185–188.

Foley KM: The practical use of narcotic analgesics. *Med. Clin. North Am.* 1982; 66(5):1091–1104.

Goodman CE: Pathophysiology of pain. *Arch. Intern Med.* 1983; 143:527–530.

Hayes AH Jr: Therapeutic implications of drug interactions with acetaminophen and aspirin. *Arch. Intern Med.* 1981; 141(3):301–304.

Heidrich G, Perry S: Helping the patient in pain. *Am. J. Nurs.* 1982; 82(12):1828–1833.

Langman MJS, Coggon D, Spiegelhalter D: Analgesic intake and the risk of acute upper gastrointestinal bleeding. *Am. J. Med.* 1983; 74(6A):79–82.

Levy G: Comparative pharmacokinetics of aspirin and acetaminophen. *Arch. Intern. Med.* 1981; 141:279–281.

Mar DD: The narcotic analgesics. *Am. J. Nurs.* 1981; 81(7):1364–1365.

Mar DD: The simple analgesics. *Am. J. Nurs.* 1981; 81(6):1206–1208.

McCaffery M: Patients shouldn't have to suffer: how to relieve pain with injectable narcotics. *Nursing* 1980; 10(10):34–39.

McCaffery M: How to relieve your patients' pain fast and effectively with oral analgesics. *Nursing* 1980; 10(11):58–63.

Mielke CH Jr: Influence of aspirin on platelets and the bleeding time. *Am. J. Med.* 1983; 74(6A):72–78.

Panayotoff K: Managing pain in the elderly patient. *Nursing* 1982; 12(8):53; 56–57.

Settipane GA: Adverse reactions to aspirin and related drugs. *Arch. Intern. Med.* 1981; 141:328–332.

Temple AR: Acute and chronic effects of aspirin toxicity and their treatment. *Arch. Intern. Med.* 1981; 141(3):364–369.

CHAPTER 16

Antiarthritic Drug Therapy for the Elderly

Two kinds of arthritis, rheumatoid arthritis and osteoarthritis, afflict approximately 22 million Americans and 20 million persons in the United Kingdom. By age 75, one or the other of these conditions affects about 28% of the population. Arthritic conditions account for approximately 15% of individuals seeking treatment from general practitioners. These conditions provide the main applications for antiarthritic drugs, which are either the first or second most widely used drugs by elderly people, determined in various studies.

Rheumatoid arthritis is a prototypical rheumatic disorder triggered by gradual accumulation of antigen-antibody complexes within joints. The antigen, called rheumatoid factor (RF), is produced by lymphocytes in the affected joints. Both RF and the matched antibody are most likely immunoglobulins. The presence of the antigen-antibody complexes activates phagocytes, causing them to release lysosomal enzymes that attack the joint tissues, causing, in sequence, pannus formation, cartilage destruction, osteoporosis, and finally ankylosis. The inflammation is usually symmetrical and occurs most often in the small joints of the hands and feet, wrists, elbows, and ankles. Common complaints include pain and stiffness in the joints upon arising in the morning, early afternoon fatigue, and mental depression. Rheumatoid arthritis affects approximately 7 million Americans, women two or three times more frequently than men. Although it occurs in all age groups, only 0.2% of the population under age 25 is afflicted, compared to 1% for the total population.

Osteoarthritis, or degenerative joint disease, is a family of disorders of joints characterized by development of fissures, cracks, and general thinning of joint cartilage, bone damage, hypertrophy of the cartilage, and synovial inflammation. Ultimately the cartilage is calcified and ossified, impairing mobility. Osteoarthritis occurs in about 16 million Americans and its frequency increases with age. It is rare before age 40, but afflicts 60% of Americans by age 60. Obesity and joint trauma also increase liability. Women are more often afflicted than men. Onset shortly after menopause is common among women.

Treatment of rheumatoid arthritis depends on severity. In current practice, the least toxic nonsteroidal anti-inflammatory drugs (NSAIDs) are used first, along with nondrug measures including rest, heat, and therapeutic exercise. If a second level of intervention is required, more potent NSAIDs may be substituted, steroids may be given by intra-articular injection, or antimalarials or analgesics might be added. Additional nondrug measures at this stage might include orthopedic devices (splints, bars, or a cane) or intensive physical or occupational therapy. More difficult cases requiring a third level of intervention might entail use of gold salts, oral steroids, surgery, or hospitalization. Last resort treatments include immunosuppressives, reconstructive surgery, or placement in a rehabilitation center. Treatments for osteoarthritis include rest, weight loss, heat, exercise, and drug therapy. The drugs used are largely limited to the NSAIDs for osteoarthritis. Steroids are not felt to have any place in treatment of this form of arthritis.

NONSTEROIDAL ANTI-INFLAMMATORY DRUG USE IN THE ELDERLY

Because aspirin was for many years the principal drug in this class and because it remains the prototype, the NSAIDs are often referred to simply as the aspirin-like drugs. Drugs in this family have a rather remarkable range of pharmacological actions and a corresponding diversity of clinical uses. All of the drugs also possess antipyretic (fever-reducing) capability and analgesic activity (as discussed in Chapter 15). The common link in these three seemingly disparate actions of NSAIDs is that fever, pain, and inflammation are all promoted by a family of substances called prostaglandins, found in the body. Aspirin itself has additional values as an antithrombotic drug (see Chapter 13) and was once used as a uricosuric for gout, but these effects are not shared by other drugs in the NSAID class. Acetaminophen, a nonnarcotic analgesic discussed in Chapter 15, has too little anti-inflammatory value to warrant discussion here as an NSAID.

Prostaglandins are produced in the body by a set of enzymes collectively referred to as **prostaglandin synthetase.** This enzyme group also produces various other mediators of inflammation, including thromboxane A2 and leukotrienes. The aspirin-like drugs inhibit production of prostaglandins and thromboxane A2, but do not suppress production of leukotrienes. Leukotrienes also contribute to inflammation and can play a role in hypersensitivity reactions to aspirin-like drugs, so it is hoped that someday inhibitors of leukotriene production will be added to the arsenal of drugs available clinically for suppression of inflammation.

In contrast to steroidal anti-inflammatory drugs, the NSAIDs do not alter activity of the phagocytic cells (macrophages and leukocytes) that recognize, engulf, and kill microorganisms. Thus, the advantage of NSAIDs is that they suppress inflammation without significantly diminishing the body's capacity to fend off infection.

Aspirin has been in widespread use since the beginning of the twentieth century. It is a derivative of salicylate, which occurs naturally in willow bark. New NSAIDs have been developed at a relentless pace over the last two decades. Aspirin, the pyrazolone derivatives (e.g., phenylbutazone), and indomethacin are the ones that have been available longest for clinical practice and comprise the first-generation drugs. The first-generation drugs are as efficacious or more so than newer drugs, but they also have a higher propensity for adverse effects. The newer drugs have improved on the incidence of side effects, but they have not added therapeutic potential. Some of the newer drugs also provide the added convenience of less frequent administration made possible by a longer half-life. The currently available NSAIDs (see Table 16.1) are grouped into several families:

1. salicylates
2. propionic acid derivatives
3. acetic acid derivatives
4. fenamates
5. pyrazolone derivatives
6. oxicams

Table 16.1 Comparisons of Nonsteroidal Anti-Inflammatory Drugs

Drug	Daily Maximum Dosage (mg)	Anti-Inflammatory Effectiveness	Overall Toxicity
Salicylates			
Aspirin	3,900	++	++
Diflunisal	1,500	++	+
Propionic Acid Derivatives			
Ibuprofen	3,200	++	+
Fenoprofen	3,200	++	+
Ketoprofen	300	++	+
Naproxen	1,100	++	+
Suprofen	800	+	+
Fenamates			
Meclofenamate	400	++	+++
Parachlorobenzoic Acid Derivatives			
Indomethacin	50	++++	++++
Sulindac	400	+++	+++
Tolmetin	1,800	+++	+
Pyrazolone Derivatives			
Phenylbutazone	600	++++	++++
Oxyphenbutazone	600	++++	++++
Oxicams			
Piroxicam	20	++	+

+, lowest degree of effectiveness or toxicity; ++++, highest degree of effectiveness or toxicity.

Clinical Indications in the Elderly.   NSAIDs are indicated for inflammation and pain associated with rheumatic arthritis, osteoarthritis, systemic lupus erythematosus, and rheumatic variants, including ankylosing spondylitis, Reiter's syndrome, and psoriatic arthritis. For rheumatoid arthritis or systemic lupus erythematosus, NSAIDs are often part of a multidrug regimen. NSAIDs have little value for nonrheumatic types of inflammatory disorders such as psoriasis, contact dermatitis, polyarteritis, or ulcerative colitis.

Altered Pharmacokinetics or Pharmacodynamics in the Elderly.
NSAIDs are rapidly absorbed after oral administration and most are completely absorbed. Malabsorption, which is common among the elderly, might be expected to alter absorption of NSAIDs, but studies thus far on half a dozen NSAIDs have indicated no decrement in absorption in relation to malabsorption. NSAIDs are absorbed more rapidly from the intestines than the stomach, in spite of their acid structures, because of the much larger surface area for absorption in the intestines. Taking one of these drugs, formulated as an ordinary tablet or capsule, with a meal will predictably retard drug absorption due to the prolonged gastric emptying time, but will not diminish ultimate extent of absorption. Enteric-coated preparations taken with meals are less well-absorbed than on an empty stomach. Concurrent administration of antacids has variable effects on different NSAIDs. Most, including piroxicam, tolmetin, and phenylbutazone, are unaffected, but absorption of indomethacin is impaired, while that of aspirin or naproxen is increased. The increased absorption of aspirin caused by antacids may be offset by more rapid excretion in the urine if systemic absorption of the antacid is sufficient to cause alkalinization of the urine.

Some of the NSAIDs, notably aspirin and diclofenac, undergo substantial first-pass elimination after oral administration. As a result, only about 65% of an aspirin dose taken orally reaches the systemic circulation. Nevertheless, the aspirin metabolite initially formed in the liver is also pharmacologically active, so the action of aspirin is less affected by first-pass extraction than that of other drugs subject to this influence. The normal decline in hepatic function with aging does not significantly impact on most NSAIDs, for whatever reason. Aspirin and phenylbutazone, however, both have a significantly prolonged half-life in elderly clients. These drugs are used at concentrations that are close to those required to saturate hepatic metabolizing capacity in young adults and they more readily saturate the diminished hepatic capacity of an elderly client.

The most unequivocal age-dependent change in pharmacokinetics of NSAIDs, as with so many other drugs, relates to renal excretion. Renal function declines in elderly individuals, even without renal disease. Elimination is significantly impaired for aspirin and diflunisal, for example. On the other hand, pharmacokinetic studies have indicated that diclofenac, piroxicam, and fenbufen can be given to clients who have decreased renal function without dosage reduction.

Adverse Effects and Contraindications in the Elderly.   Some of the adverse effects of NSAIDs are shared more or less for all drugs in the class.

The reason that such side effects occur with all the drugs is that these adverse effects, like the therapeutic ones, all relate to actions of one or another prostaglandin. The most universal problem with NSAIDs, an irritant effect on the gastrointestinal mucosa with potential bleeding, is more common for people over 60 and equally common for men and women. Many of the NSAIDs inhibit platelet agglutination, adding to bleeding tendencies. Fifteen percent of individuals taking aspirin for inflammation lose over 10 ml of blood per day from occult bleeding in the alimentary tract. Another 70% lose between 5 and 10 ml daily. The incidence is highest with plain aspirin, slightly lower with effervescent formulations, and considerably lower with enteric-coated products. Clients may develop anemia from such daily losses of blood. Perforation or hemorrhage can occur and both pose a threat to life. The elderly have higher susceptibility to gastric irritation from NSAIDs because of declining mucosal integrity with advancing years. Some of the newer drugs in this class produce less bleeding at therapeutic doses than does aspirin, yet none are completely devoid of this problem. Indomethacin, aspirin, and phenylbutazone are high-risk drugs for gastrointestinal problems and should be avoided for use in the elderly. As many as 3% of individuals taking indomethacin regularly develop peptic ulcers. All NSAIDs should be avoided or used with great caution in clients with clotting abnormalities or those receiving anticoagulants. NSAIDs need to be discontinued one week prior to elective surgery, even minor oral surgery, to prevent excess bleeding. Elderly clients taking potassium supplements in conjunction with diuretic therapy are especially prone to combined irritant effects on the gastric mucosa from the potassium salt and NSAIDs.

Histamine H_2-receptor antagonists (e.g., ranitidine) and gastric acid pump inhibitors (e.g., omeprazole) fail to protect against the ulcergenic influence of NSAIDs, but misoprostol provides significant protection against both gastric and duodenal ulcers induced by NSAIDs. Misoprostol is a nonabsorbable, synthetic prostaglandin developed expressly for this application. It counters gastrointestinal effects of NSAIDs without impairing their systemic values.

Prostaglandins play a role in the uterine contractions of labor and menstruation. Therefore, aspirin-like drugs often demonstrate good ability to relieve pain associated with menstrual cramps, but use of an aspirin-like drug for whatever purpose during the last trimester of pregnancy may delay onset of labor and prolong labor dangerously. Moreover, aspirin-like drugs tend to promote bleeding in a fetus or neonate, as in others.

Nephrotoxicity is another common potential with NSAIDs and the elderly, with already diminished renal function, are more susceptible to this problem. Apparently inhibition of prostaglandin synthetase in the kidneys promotes renal ischemia and a reduction in glomerular filtration rate. Aspirin, phenylbutazone, sulindac, and indomethacin thereby promote fluid retention and edema. Most, if not all, NSAIDs mildly elevate blood pressure and can potentially antagonize antihypertensive drug therapy. The frequency of significant interactions with antihypertensive drug regimens is about 1%, but is higher for elderly and blacks. This can be especially problematic for elderly clients, complicating any tendency they may have toward congestive heart failure.

Dermatological side effects are not uncommon with NSAIDs. Problems can include rash, urticaria, pruritis, and increased sweating. Though rare, life-threatening erythema multiforme has occurred after treatment with various NSAIDs, including aspirin, phenylbutazone, and diflunisal.

Overdose toxicity is seldom a problem in elderly clients except when aspirin is used for a suicide attempt. In overdoses, aspirin and other salicylates cause hyperpnea (rapid respiration), which leads to alkalosis. Neurological toxicities may develop, including tinnitus or deafness. Older people are more susceptible to the risk of deafness or ringing of the ears and may develop this problem in response to plasma concentrations at the upper limit of the therapeutic range. Indomethacin causes more frequent neurological problems, such as headache, dizziness, or giddiness, than other NSAIDs and these are more frequent and more troublesome for older clients.

Pyrazolones have a special risk of bone marrow suppression, enough so that one drug in this family, oxyphenbutazone, was withdrawn in the United Kingdom (though it remains available for use in the United States) and the remaining drug, phenylbutazone, is largely limited to closely supervised use in young people with ankylosing spondylitis. Pyrazolones should not be used in elderly clients because they have elevated risk of aplastic anemia.

Interactions in the Elderly.   Many of the NSAIDs interact with warfarin, the major oral anticoagulant drug. What makes this particularly important is that warfarin concentrations must be carefully regulated to ensure an adequate anticoagulant effect without undue risk of hemorrhage. Aspirin, diclofenac, pyrazolones, and propionic acid derivatives are substantially bound to plasma proteins in the blood and displace warfarin from these sites, potentiating its effect. Aspirin compounds the displacement problem by also adding its own antithrombotic action and an inhibition of synthesis of vitamin K-dependent clotting factors. Pyrazolones also pose a problem with warfarin by inhibiting its metabolism. Although indomethacin has no direct interaction with warfarin, caution must still be exercised when using it or any NSAID with warfarin because of the risk of occult bleeding associated with NSAIDs.

Since hypertension and arthritis are the two most common drug-treated conditions among the elderly, there is a great deal of concern about the possibility that NSAIDs antagonize antihypertensive drug regimens. The extent to which this occurs varies with the specific drugs selected. For example, sulindac antagonizes the antihypertensive effect of the beta-blocker, propranolol, but piroxicam does not. Neither sulindac, piroxicam, nor diclofenac prevents the blood pressure lowering effect of calcium channel blockers. Aspirin, phenylbutazone, and indomethacin are poor choices for use in elderly persons with hypertension.

Many of the NSAIDs are weak organic acids that compete with other acids for a renal secretory mechanism. Aspirin, phenylbutazone, and diclofenac have all been reported, for example, to inhibit renal clearance of methotrexate. Probenecid slows renal clearance of some of the NSAIDs, such as naproxen and indomethacin, by the same interaction. Several of the

NSAIDs, including diclofenac and indomethacin, inhibit renal excretion of lithium, increasing its toxic potential.

Pyrazolones are potent inducers of hepatic microsomal enzymes and can speed metabolism of a variety of other drugs as a result. Pyrazolones can, on the other hand, competitively inhibit metabolism of other drugs that require hydroxylation.

Administration in the Elderly. The profound import of recognizing the need for dosage reduction in the elderly is well-illustrated by a highly publicized incident that occurred with a new NSAID introduced in the United Kingdom in 1980. Benoxaprofen was introduced with a recommended dosage of 600 mg daily based on pharmacokinetic studies conducted, according to the accepted practice of the day, in young adults. The clinical trials, likewise conducted using young adults, had indicated low toxicity, especially a low incidence of gastrointestinal bleeding. As an NSAID, benoxaprofen was clearly going to be used after approval mainly in elderly clients and the manufacturer sensibly directed its marketing campaign to that audience. A study sponsored by the manufacturer and completed prior to marketing had reported that the half-life of benoxaprofen averaged 111 hours in a small group of elderly clients, as opposed to the 19–26 hours in young adults, but this finding was overlooked or ignored. Within the first 12 months after its introduction, benoxaprofen was involved in over 3000 adverse drug reactions. In one study, 69% of subjects over age 70 had side effects serious enough to require discontinuation of the drug. Phototoxicity, jaundice, and renal failure were some of the problems. When benoxaprofen was ultimately withdrawn in August of 1982, it had already been prescribed to a half-million recipients, causing 61 deaths, mainly in elderly persons. More than any other single episode in drug testing, this incident has contributed to establishing an important new principle of drug testing: **a drug must be tested in the subject population that will be its primary market if approved.**

Although therapeutic benefits are theoretically little affected by the selection of a particular brand of aspirin, product formulation can impact on the risk of gastric irritation. Poorly formulated aspirin tablets disintegrate slowly and result in clumps lying against portions of the gastric mucosa, which can contribute to local irritation and erosive action.

In selecting a particular NSAID for an elderly client, it is best to avoid the more toxic drugs (pyrazolones, indomethacin, and aspirin) because of the elderly person's greater liability for gastric bleeding, fluid retention, and neurological side effects, or, in the case of the pyrazolones, bone marrow suppression. Ibuprofen and fenoprofen may be slightly less efficacious than aspirin, but they cause much fewer side effects. Naproxen matches the efficacy of aspirin with far fewer side effects. Overall, propionic acid derivatives, diclofenac, and piroxicam appear to provide the best balance between benefit and adverse effects (see Table 16.1). Adherence to prescribed regimens can sometimes be improved by selection of a drug that is appropriate for once-a-day administration, such as diclofenac or ketoprofen.

Combinations of two or more NSAIDs provide no additional benefit, but they increase risk of adverse reactions in comparison with an optimized dosage of a single drug. Products that combine aspirin with caffeine or acetaminophen provide no additional benefit for arthritis over aspirin alone and are more expensive.

Salicylates

ASPIRIN

Recommended initial oral dose in the elderly: Reduce dose for hepatic or renal dysfunction.

Young adult initial dose in arthritis for comparison: 3.2–6 g/day in divided doses.

CHOLINE SALICYLATE   (Arthropan)

Recommended initial oral dose in the elderly: No specific recommendation.

Young adult initial dose in arthritis for comparison: 5–10 ml (870 mg/5 ml) up to 4 times daily.

DIFLUNISAL   (Dolobid)

Recommended initial oral dose in the elderly: Reduce for renal dysfunction.

Young adult initial dose in arthritis for comparison: 500 mg to 1 g daily in 2 divided doses.

MAGNESIUM SALICYLATE   (Doan's, Magan, Mobidin)

Recommended initial oral dose in the elderly: No specific recommendation.

Young adult initial dose in arthritis for comparison: 3.27–4.1 g/d in 3 to 6 divided doses.

SALSALATE   (Amigesic, Disalcid, Salflex, generic)

Recommended initial oral dose in the elderly: No specific recommendation.

Young adult initial dose in arthritis for comparison: 3000 mg/d in divided doses.

SODIUM SALICYALTE

Recommended initial oral dose in the elderly: No specific recommendation.

Young adult initial dose in arthritis for comparison: 325–650 mg every 4 hours.

Propionic Acid Derivatives

CARPROFEN   (Rimadyl)

Recommended initial oral dose in the elderly: Begin with reduced doses.

Young adult initial dose in arthritis for comparison: Approved but not yet marketed.

FENOPROFEN   (Nalfon)

Recommended initial oral dose in the elderly: Begin with reduced doses.

Young adult initial dose in arthritis for comparison: 300–600 mg 3 or 4 times daily.

FLUBIPROFEN   (Ansaid)

Recommended initial oral dose in the elderly: Begin with reduced doses.

Young adult initial dose in arthritis for comparison: 200–300 mg 2, 3, or 4 times daily.

IBUPROFEN   (Motrin, Rufen, generic)

Recommended initial oral dose in the elderly: Begin with reduced doses.

Young adult initial dose in arthritis for comparison: 1.2–3.2 g/day in 3 or 4 divided doses.

KETOPROFEN   (Orudis)

Recommended initial oral dose in the elderly: Begin with reduced doses.

Young adult initial dose in arthritis for comparison: 75 mg 3 times daily or 50 mg 4 times daily.

NAPROXEN   (Naprosyn, Anaprox)

Recommended initial oral dose in the elderly: Begin with reduced doses.

Young adult initial dose in arthritis for comparison: 250–500 mg twice daily (Naprosyn); 275–550 mg twice daily (Anaprox, which is the sodium salt of naproxen).

OXAPROZIN   (Daypro)

Recommended initial oral dose in the elderly: Begin with reduced doses.

Young adult initial dose in arthritis for comparison: 1200 mg once daily.

Acetic Acid Derivatives

DICLOFENAC   (Voltaren)

Recommended initial oral dose in the elderly: Begin with reduced doses.

Young adult initial dose in arthritis for comparison: 100–150 mg/day in divided doses for osteoarthritis, or 150–200 mg/day in divided doses for rheumatoid arthritis. Liver function tests are mandatory.

ETODOLAC   (Lodine)

Recommended initial oral dose in the elderly: Begin with reduced doses.

Young adult initial dose in arthritis for comparison: 800–1200 mg/day in divided doses.

INDOMETHACIN (Indocin, generic)

Recommended initial oral dose in the elderly: Begin with reduced doses.

Young adult initial dose in arthritis for comparison: 25 mg 2 or 3 times daily.

NABUMETONE (Relafen)

Recommended initial oral dose in the elderly: No difference in efficacy or safety reported in older or younger clients.

Young adult initial dose in arthritis for comparison: 1000 mg as a single dose with or without food.

SULINDAC (Clinoril)

Recommended initial oral dose in the elderly: Begin with reduced doses.

Young adult initial dose in arthritis for comparison: 150 mg twice daily.

TOLMETIN (Tolectin)

Recommended initial oral dose in the elderly: Begin with reduced doses.

Young adult initial dose in arthritis for comparison: 400 mg 3 times daily.

Fenamates

MECLOFENAMATE (Meclomen)

Recommended initial oral dose in the elderly: No specific recommendation.

Young adult initial dose in arthritis for comparison: 200–400 mg/day in 3 or 4 divided doses.

Pyrazolone Derivatives

PHENYLBUTAZONE   (Azolid, Butazolidin)

Recommended initial oral dose in the elderly: Not recommended for use in the elderly.

Young adult initial dose in arthritis for comparison: 300–600 mg divided into 3 or 4 doses.

OXYPHENBUTAZONE

Recommended initial oral dose in the elderly: Not recommended for use in the elderly.

Young adult initial dose in arthritis for comparison: 300–600 mg divided into 3 or 4 doses.

Oxicams

ISOXICAM   (Maxicam)

Investigational.

PIROXICAM   (Feldene)

Recommended initial oral dose in the elderly: Begin with reduced doses.

Young adult initial dose in arthritis for comparison: 20 mg once daily.

STEROIDAL ANTI-INFLAMMATORY DRUG USE IN THE ELDERLY

Inflammatory responses are many times health-maintaining reactions on the part of the body that protect against incursions of pathogens or damaging effects of toxins. Sometimes, however, inflammation runs amok, causing more damage to host tissue than protection. Under these circumstances, anti-inflammatory drugs can help by holding down an overly vigorous inflammatory process. Steroids inhibit inflammatory responses in a different manner than the NSAIDs. Steroids suppress the activity of phagocytic cells at several steps. Steroids inhibit migration of phagocytic cells to the site of inflammation, they inhibit the recognition of potential objects of phagocytosis by these cells, and they inhibit the ability of phagocytic cells to use their potent chemical mediators (lysosomal enzymes and superoxides) that destroy engulfed substances but sometimes also damage tissue. The anti-inflammatory benefit of steroids therefore comes at the cost of impaired resistance to infection.

Some steroidal anti-inflammatory drugs are natural hormones of the adrenal gland—one of the five classes of steroids released by the adrenal cortex. Hence, these drugs are often referred to as corticosteroids or glucocorticoids. Some steroidal anti-inflammatory drugs are synthetic derivatives, which typically provide a longer duration of action.

Clinical Indications in the Elderly.   Steroidal anti-inflammatory drugs used systemically are mainstays for the many kinds of the nonrheumatic inflammatory disorders, because these are largely nonresponsive to NSAIDs. Steroids are used, for example, as the main mode of therapy for carditis, polyarteritis, dermatomyositis, multiple sclerosis, ulcerative colitis, and contact dermatitis. They are used for brief periods in bursitis or tendonitis. They are used together with other drugs for severe systemic or discoid lupus erythematosus. Systemic glucocorticoids are used for certain kinds of cancer, including acute lymphocytic leukemia and lymphomas, usually in combination with other anticancer drugs (see Chapter 17). Steroidal anti-inflammatory drugs are not useful for osteoarthritis, but provide a secondary drug intervention for rheumatoid arthritis, especially when active rheumatoid arthritis threatens the mobility needed for self-reliance of an elderly person. Systemic steroid therapy is a potentially high-benefit, high-risk example of drug use and requires careful weighing of the advantages and disadvantages likely to accrue.

Topical dosage forms of steroidal anti-inflammatory drugs are widely used for various kinds of inflammations of the skin: atopic dermatitis, seborrheic dermatitis, and localized neurodermatitis.

Altered Pharmacokinetics or Pharmacodynamics in the Elderly.
Most steroids are readily absorbed after oral administration. Synthetic steroids are used in preference to the natural ones for oral administration, because metabolism of natural steroids is overly rapid after this route. Intramuscular injection also provides a rapid route of systemic administration. When this route is selected, esters or suspensions can provide extended action, whereas water soluble drugs in this family provide rapid, short-lasting effects.

Steroids distribute widely throughout the body, but their volume of distribution is smaller in elderly clients because of reduced muscle mass and plasma volume. Lower doses should be considered when these factors are present and elderly clients should be monitored every six months during steroid therapy for changes in blood pressure, blood glucose, or electrolytes. Hydrocortisone is highly bound to plasma proteins, but synthetic steroids are not.

Steroids are metabolized in both the liver and peripheral tissues with liver metabolism providing approximately 70% of inactivation. Steroid metabolites are then excreted in the urine. Dexamethasone and betamethasone have long half-lives providing biological activity for 36–54 hours. Prednisone is a prodrug that must be metabolized to prednisolone before it becomes active. Both of these compounds as well as methylprednisolone and triamcinolone have intermediate durations of activity, from 18–36 hours. Cortisone and hydrocortisone, two natural steroids, have short action, from 8–12 hours.

Adverse Effects and Contraindications in the Elderly.

Adverse effects of glucocorticoids depend ever so much on how they are used, route of application (topical or systemic), and duration of therapy. Topical administration is generally associated with a much lower risk of adverse reactions, though some systemic absorption ultimately occurs from most sites of application. Short-term use (up to 2 or 3 weeks) of glucocorticoids, even in rather high doses, is likewise associated with a relatively low level of risk. After all, glucocorticoids are produced each day by the adrenal gland, so a certain level of glucocorticoid action is part and parcel of every day life. Escalating that activity for a short period for medical benefits entails minimal risk. Toxicity is therefore most evident when steroidal anti-inflammatory drugs are used systemically for prolonged periods, particularly when doses are moderate or high. Under these circumstances, glucocorticoids can cause a wide range of serious problems that have to be given significant weight in benefit/risk analysis. The adverse effects generally fall into three categories: (1) excess glucocorticoid actions, (2) mineralocorticoid actions, and (3) withdrawal symptoms (see Table 16.2). The first set is sometimes referred to as Cushing's syndrome because the symptoms resemble those of Cushing's disease caused by hyperplasias or tumors of the adrenal gland.

All steroidal anti-inflammatory drugs possess glucocorticoid activity, but the various drugs differ markedly in the extent to which they possess mineralocorticoid (aldosterone-like) activity as well. The natural glucocorticoids, cortisone and hydrocorticone, have a lot of mineralocorticoid action. Prednisone and prednisolone have a lesser mineralocorticoid action, while dexamathasone and betamethasone have none. Mineralocorticoid activity, if the drug possesses it, causes sodium and fluid retention but potassium depletion—all clearly problematic for elderly clients already suffering from hypertension, fluid retention, edema, or congestive heart failure. Clients receiving glucocorticoids with mineralocorticoid activity should be taught to weigh themselves daily as a means of monitoring for fluid retention. Diet might need to be adjusted to provide reduced sodium and increased potassium intake. Synthetic steroidal anti-inflammatory drugs that lack mineralocorticoid activity should be used preferentially for clients already suffering from hypertension or fluid retention.

Glucocorticoids get their name from their action on glucose homeostasis. Glucocorticoids are released, along with adrenaline, as part of the body's response to stressful circumstances. The job of the glucocorticoid in stress is to ensure adequate energy supply for a burst of physical activity by elevated blood glucose levels. This action, when caused day after day by exogenously

Table 16.2 Adverse Effects of Prolonged Glucocorticoid Therapy

Excess Glucocorticoid Activity	Excess Mineralocorticoid Activity	Withdrawal
Carbohydrate Metabolism	***Electrolyte Imbalance***	Fever
Hyperglycemia	Hypernatremia	Myalgia
Glycosuria	Hypokalemia	Arthralgia
Diabetes Mellitus	Alkalosis	Malaise
Blood Cells	Hypervolemia	Depression
Lymphocytopenia	Hypercalcemia	Fatigue
Monocytopenia		Hypotension
Eosinopenia	***Cardiovascular Effects***	Anorexia
Neutrophilia	Hypertension	Nausea
Involution of lymph tissue	Congestive Heart Failure	Vomiting
Ocular		
Increased intraocular pressure		
Cataracts		
Ulcers (possibly)		
Psychological dependence		
Growth suppression in children		
Suppression of Pituitary/ Adrenal Axis		
Cushing's Syndrome		
Psychosis		
Irritability		
Susceptibility to infection		
Easy bruisability		
Acne		
Redistribution of Fat		
Moon face		
Buffalo hump		
Pendulous abdomen		
Striae		
Negative Nitrogen Balance		
Muscle wasting		
Osteoporosis		

administered glucocorticoids, will be most obviously problematic for clients with diabetes mellitus, who will probably require an increase in their daily insulin dosage to counter the added serum glucose. The hyperglycemic influence of glucocorticoids, given enough time, can even be the cause of diabetes in previously healthy persons by driving the pancreas to exhaustion.

Steroids increase secretion of hydrochloric acid in the stomach and, with prolonged use, can bring on peptic ulcers. Antacid therapy may need to be instituted. Use of other ulcergenic substances, such as tobacco, caffeine, and alcohol, should be discontinued. More frequent, smaller meals and bedtime snacks sometimes stave off development of peptic ulcers for a while. Clients should be taught to observe for evidences of occult bleeding, such as tarry stools, cold, clammy skin, or easy fatigueability. Glucocorticoids may be taken with milk or food to reduce gastric irritation.

Another big liability for elderly clients receiving glucocorticoids is muscle wasting. Elderly people tend to lose muscle mass as they age and become less active, all the more so if their mobility is impaired by arthritis. Glucocorticoids can worsen this problem because they cause a negative nitrogen balance or catabolic effect. Clients receiving chronic glucocorticoid therapy need to maintain a high protein diet to help prevent muscle wasting.

Glucocorticoids often promote a gradual redistribution of fat stores, reducing stores in the extremities while simultaneously building stores on the torso and face. The result is a thinning of the limbs but often conspicuous expansion of the fat pad over the back of the shoulders (creating a "buffalo hump"), face ("moon face"), and abdomen.

Glucocorticoids used chronically promote several types of ocular problems. Intraocular pressure increases, promoting or aggravating glaucoma. Cataracts are more likely.

Osteoporosis, already a problem for many elderly people and especially small-framed postmenopausal women, is worsened by glucocorticoids. Glucocorticoids inhibit calcium absorption from the gut, gradually break down the protein matrix of bone, and inhibit osteoblast activity. When serum calcium levels drop, the body has to respond by releasing parathyroid hormone. This helps to keep up the critically important serum level of calcium, but at the cost of calcium stores in bone and teeth. Daily exercise will help slow development of osteoporosis, but not indefinitely.

Although neutrophil counts are increased by chronic exposure to exogenous glucocorticoids, all other classes of white blood cells decline in number. The result is an impaired ability to combat infections. Clients who must receive prolonged glucocorticoid treatment need to intensify personal hygiene and guard against contact with those carrying active infectious diseases. It will be harder to identify infection early on for the client receiving glucocorticoids, because the normal inflammatory response is absent. Clients who have latent infectious problems, such as herpes simplex virus or latent tuberculosis, should not be given glucocorticoids as these will reactivate the infectious disorder. Glucocorticoids also increase the risk of thromboembolic disorders.

Psychiatric side effects are frequent when steroidal anti-inflammatory drugs must be used systemically for more than a few weeks. Clients may experience mood swings from mania to depression. Symptoms resembling those of schizophrenia may develop. Before Cushing's disease was recognized by Cushing as an endocrine problem, it was viewed as a psychiatric disorder, which illustrates the potential prominence of psychiatric side effects with these drugs. The elderly have higher risk of mental disturbances from steroidal anti-inflammatory drugs. Use should be avoided whenever possible in clients with a history of psychiatric problems.

A major risk of long-term glucocorticoid administration is suppression of endogenous production by the adrenal gland. Given daily, exogenous glucocorticoids will suppress pituitary secretion of corticotropin by stimulating the feedback control mechanism. If the medication is discontinued later, endogenous production may recover only after several weeks, if ever. Glucocorticoids must not be withdrawn abruptly after long-term use except for medical emergency. Instead, doses need to be tapered over several weeks. An appropriate rate of withdrawal for prednisone, for example, is a reduction of 2.5 mg every 4–10 days. Rates for other drugs can be calculated by dosage equivalence. If withdrawal is abrupt, symptoms will include fever, muscle and joint aches, malaise, depression, fatigue, hypotension, and gastrointestinal upset. Giving glucocorticoids on an alternate day schedule greatly reduces the risk of suppressing the hypothalamic-pituitary-adrenal system and the likelihood of withdrawal symptoms.

Interactions in the Elderly.   The ulcergenic effect of glucocorticoids is additive with that of other ulcergenic drugs, including caffeine, alcohol, nicotine, aspirin, indomethacin, and virtually all NSAIDs. The catabolic effect of glucocorticoids counters and is countered by the anabolic effect of anabolic steroids. Steroid metabolism is increased by and their action is decreased by inducers of liver enzymes, including most antiepileptics, barbiturates, most antihistamines, and rifampin.

Glucocorticoids reduce the therapeutic effects of several kinds of drugs often required by elderly clients. For example, they counter beneficial effects of antihypertensive drugs and diuretics to the extent that they have mineralocorticoid properties. Glucocorticoids not only block beneficial effects of diuretics, but they also aggravate the hypokalemia to the extent that the drug possesses mineralocorticoid activity. Glucocorticoids necessitate dosage increases for insulin or oral hypoglycemic medications required for diabetes mellitus because of their hyperglycemic action. The aggravation of osteoporosis caused by steroidal anti-inflammatory drugs counters beneficial effects of vitamin D and calcium salts in forestalling progression of osteoporosis.

Administration in the Elderly.   A special kind of topical administration of steroids, intra-articular injection, can be valuable in rheumatoid arthritis. This technique entails insertion of a needle directly into the arthritic joint, aspiration of fluid, and injection of the steroid. This method of application increases the benefit/risk ratio by ensuring that most of the drug acts at the desired locus and systemic adverse effects are reduced.

Glucocorticoids for oral administration are available as tablets. These are best taken with meals to minimize gastrointestinal irritation. Single daily doses for long-acting drugs are best taken in the morning to simulate the natural steroid rhythm.

BETAMETHASONE   (Celestone)

Recommended initial oral dose in the elderly: See Cortisone.

Unspecified adult initial dose for comparison: 0.6–7.2 mg/day.

CORTISONE (generic)

Recommended initial oral dose in the elderly: Consider risk/benefit factors. Consider lower dose if muscle mass or plasma volume has declined. Monitor blood pressure, electrolytes, and blood glucose every 6 months.

Unspecified adult initial dose for comparison: 25–300 mg/day.

DEXAMETHASONE (Decadron, Dexone, Hexadrol, generic)

Recommended initial oral dose in the elderly: See Cortisone.

Unspecified adult initial dose for comparison: 0.75–9 mg/day.

DEXAMETHASONE SODIUM PHOSPHATE (Dalalone, Decaject, Dexone, Solurex, generic)

Recommended initial oral dose in the elderly: See Cortisone.

Unspecified adult initial dose for comparison: 0.5–9 mg daily orally; intra-articular, large joints 2–4 mg; small joints 0.8–1 mg.

HYDROCORTISONE, CORTISOL (Cortef, and generic)
Hydrocortisone Cypionate (Cortef)

Recommended initial oral dose in the elderly: See Cortisone.

Unspecified adult initial dose for comparison: 20–240 mg/day.

HYDROCORTISONE SODIUM PHOSPHATE (generic)

Recommended initial oral dose in the elderly: See Cortisone.

Unspecified adult initial dose for comparison: 15–240 mg/day.

HYDROCORTISONE SODIUM SUCCINATE (A-Hydrocort, Solu-Cortef)

Recommended initial oral dose in the elderly: See Cortisone.

Unspecified adult initial dose for comparison: 100–500 mg repeated at 2, 4, or 6 hour intervals.

METHYLPREDNISOLONE (Medrol, generic)

Recommended initial oral dose in the elderly: See Cortisone.

Unspecified adult initial dose for comparison: 4–48 mg/day or twice the usual daily dose on alternate days.

PREDNISONE (Deltasone, Meticorten, Orasone, generic)

Recommended initial oral dose in the elderly: See Cortisone.

Unspecified adult initial dose for comparison: 5–60 mg/day.

PREDNISOLONE (Delta-Cortef, Prelone, generic)

Recommended initial oral dose in the elderly: See Cortisone.

Unspecified adult initial dose for comparison: 5–60 mg/day.

PREDNISOLONE TERBUTATE (Hydeltra, generic)

Recommended initial dose in the elderly: See Cortisone.

Unspecified adult initial intra-articular dose for comparison: 20 mg for large joints (e.g., knee); 8–10 mg for small joints.

TRIAMCINOLONE (Aristocort, Atolone, Kenacort, generic)

Recommended initial oral dose in the elderly: See Cortisone.

Unspecified adult initial oral dose for rheumatic disorders for comparison: 8–16 mg.

TRIAMCINOLONE HEXACETONIDE (Aristospan)

Recommended initial dose in the elderly: See Cortisone.

Unspecified adult initial intra-articular dose for comparison: 10–20 mg for large joints; 2–6 mg for small joints.

SECONDARY ANTIARTHRITIC DRUGS FOR THE ELDERLY

Gold salts can be a useful alternative to steroidal and nonsteroidal anti-inflammatory drugs. Gold salts accumulate in joints, but the mechanism of their beneficial effect in arthritis is unknown. These salts appear to work best in the early stages of rheumatoid arthritis, so they are less likely to be of benefit for older clients. Gold salts are indicated for cases of moderate severity because they do not work in severe cases and are not required for mild cases. Clinical response is slow, requiring at least 6–8 weeks, and sometimes months. Adverse responses are more frequent among elderly clients, partly because elderly excrete gold salts more slowly and partly because they require higher doses for benefit. Doses must be individualized in elderly clients because blood levels in response to a given dose will vary more widely than for younger clients. Thus, gold salts have less of a role for treating rheumatoid arthritis among the elderly than in younger clients.

The antimalarials hydroxychloroquine and chloroquine are secondary antirheumatic drugs that are effective in about one-third of treated clients. Hydroxychloroquine provides the best benefit/risk combination because of less frequent toxicity, particularly retinal damage associated with chloroquine. Antimalarials should not be continued for more than 3 months for rheumatoid arthritis.

The immunosuppressives methotrexate (Rheumatrex), cyclophosphamide (Cytoxan), and azathioprine (Imuran) find occasional use for rheumatoid arthritis, but only for clients refractory to alternative treatments. Only methotrexate has FDA approval for this application.

REFERENCES AND RECOMMENDED READINGS

Baxter JD, Rousseau GG (eds): *Glucocorticoid Hormone Action*. New York, Springer-Verlag, 1979.

Clive DM, Stoff JS: Renal syndromes associated with nonsteroidal anti-inflammatory drugs. *N. Engl. J. Med.* 1984; 310:563–572.

Conner CS: Oral gold in arthritis. *Drug Intell. Clin. Pharm.* 1984; 18(10):804–805.

Cupps TR, Fauci AS: Corticosteroid-mediated immunoregulation in man. *Immunol. Rev.* 1982; 65:133–154.

Dixon R, Christy N: On the various forms of corticosteroid withdrawal syndrome. *Amer. J. Med.* 1980; 68:224–230.

Gall EP: The use of drugs in rheumatic diseases. *Primary Care* 1984; 11(2):369–380.

Hart FD, Huskisson EC: Non-steroidal anti-inflammatory drugs. Current status and rational therapeutic use. *Drugs* 1984; 27:232–255.

Kantor TG, Kaplan H, Ward JR: NSAID therapy made a little simpler. *Patient Care* 1984; 30(1):123.

Lamb C: Corticosteroid misuse and ill effects. *Patient Care* 1981; 15:69–72.

LoDolce D, et al.: Alternate programs of steroid administration for patients on long-term therapy. *J. Neurosurg. Nurs.* 1980; 12:187–194.

Melby JC: Clinical pharmacology of systemic steroids. *Annu. Rev. Pharmacol. Toxicol.* 1977; 17:511–527.

Miller SB: NSAIDs: examining therapeutic alternatives. *Geriatrics* 1982; 37(3):70–78.

Nuki G: Drug therapy for rheumatic diseases in the elderly, in K. O'Malley and JL Waddington (eds): *Therapeutics in the elderly*. New York, Elsevier Sci. Publ., 1985, pp. 127–142.

O'Duffy JD, Luthra HS: Current status of disease-modifying drugs in progressive rheumatoid arthritis. *Drugs* 1984; 27:373–377.

Settipane GA: Adverse reactions to aspirin and related drugs. *Arch. Intern. Med.* 1981; 141:328–332.

Strand CV, Clark SR: Adult arthritis: drugs and remedies. *Am. J. Nurs.* 1983; 83(2):266–269.

Streeten DHP: Corticosteroid therapy. 1. Pharmacologic properties and principles of corticosteroid use. *JAMA* 1975; 232:944–947.

Vernoski B, Chernow B: Steroids: use and abuse. *Crit. Care Q.* 1983; 6(3):28.

CHAPTER 17

Cancer Chemotherapy
for the Elderly

Cancer is a malignant hyperproliferation of cells that results in one or more cellular masses, called tumors or neoplasms, or a hyperproliferation of free-floating blood cells. Cancer is the second leading cause of death in the United States, causing more than 400,000 deaths per year. Elderly people are more likely to have concurrent chronic diseases that are affected by cancer or that modify response to cancer treatments. Elderly people have different rates of response to treatment for some kinds of cancer but not for others. Adverse effects of antineoplastic drugs affect the elderly more than younger people, but not, perhaps, as great a difference as exists for many other classes of drugs or is commonly presumed by medical practitioners.

INCIDENCE OF CANCER IN THE ELDERLY

Cancer disorders include more than a hundred different types, but the three major sites in each gender account for the majority of both occurrences and deaths. For males those three sites are the lungs, colon and rectum, and prostate, whereas for women the three leading sites are the lungs, breast, and colon and rectum. The ranking of these three leading sites for each gender change with age. Lung cancer drops to third after age 85 and prostate cancer moves into second rank for men after age 75 and first rank after age 85.

Approximately half of cancers are first diagnosed in people over age 65 and more than 60% of deaths from cancer occur after age 65. The abnormal proliferation characteristic of cancer cells appears to be the result of damaged chromosomes, called oncogenes. Among the factors that contribute to such damage are environmental agents (radiation, ultraviolet light, mutagenic drugs, industrial pollutants, cigarette smoke), diet (nitrates, low fiber, high fat, aflatoxin B, alcohol), oncogenic viruses (e.g., Epstein-Barr virus), parasitic infections, genetic predisposition, mechanical or thermal trauma, and aging. Chromosomal stability declines with aging. DNA from the lymphocytes of elderly people exhibits more breaks and errors. Chromosomes of elderly people are reportedly more susceptible to rearrangements in response to radiation or carcinogenic chemicals. The elderly may also be more susceptible because of senescence of the immune system, resulting in less vigorous defense against foreign antigens combined with more frequent autoimmune reactions.

CLINICAL MANIFESTATIONS

Symptoms are often not evident during the early stage of tumor development. As long as the tumor remains small, it may not interfere significantly with function of body systems. This is especially likely to be the case if the tumor is located in a distensible region, such as the abdomen, but less likely to be true in the cranium. As the tumor expands, symptoms ultimately develop when the tumor either constricts blood flow to a tissue, compresses soft tissue, or activates immune or inflammatory response. Bowel compression by a tumor might result in obstruction and constipation or, conversely, compensatory hypermotility. Pressure against the bronchioles might result in atelectasis. Pain might develop due to pressure exerted on pain receptors. Pain that is continuous and gradually increasing in intensity is a hallmark of neoplasms. Tissue irritation will develop once immune or inflammatory response comes into play. In clients with leukemias or lymphomas, the metabolic demands related to hyperproliferation of blood cells may cause symptoms of fatigue or lethargy.

For many kinds of cancer, early detection is a major determinant of survival rates. Unfortunately, the elderly often suffer in this regard because complaints such as fatigue, aches and pains, or constipation are less likely to arouse suspicion when voiced by an elderly person. All too often medical personnel and family members attribute such complaints simply to aging.

As cancer progresses, symptoms become more severe and less likely to be ignored. Nausea, anorexia, weight loss, and malaise are often early systemic manifestations. Neurological symptoms may follow next, including ataxia, weakness, spasticity, sensory loss, or even dementia. Anemia or coagulation defects may develop. Metabolic problems of acidosis or hyperlipidemia are possibilities. Most kinds of cancer appear to progress at about the same pace in elderly individuals as in younger people. Three exceptions are malignant melanoma, thyroid cancer, and breast cancer in women, which are all more aggressive in elderly clients. Thyroid carcinoma, for example, is more likely to culminate in death in males over 40 and females over 50 than in younger individuals by a factor of 6 (27% fatality rate versus 4%).

COMPARATIVE RESPONSIVENESS TO TREATMENT IN ELDERLY AND YOUNGER INDIVIDUALS

The three modes of treatment for cancer are surgery, radiation, and chemotherapy. Surgery is the most effective means of curing cancers that have not metastasized at the time of diagnosis. Older patients, however, are more vulnerable to mortality from surgical procedures for cancer. Careful attention to preoperative and postoperative care can help reduce mortality in elderly individuals who require surgery. Surgery is of little value for the third or so of instances of cancer that have already metastasized at the time of initial diagnosis. Surgical resection is the only form of treatment for lung cancer that affords any hope of cure, and elderly clients have mortality rates from this procedure that are twice those of younger patients.

Radiation, administered by x-rays or, less often, radioactive drugs, is another valuable tool for cancers that are localized and poses less risk for elderly clients than chemotherapy. However, elderly clients are more susceptible to injury of skin or mucosal membranes from radiation exposure than are younger individuals. There appears to be no difference in response rates to radiation therapy for prostate cancer in elderly men and younger men.

Chemotherapy is the main method of treatment for cancers that have metastasized. Prognosis is always poorer when cancer has metastasized than when it has not, so, not surprisingly, success rates are much lower for chemotherapy than for surgical or radiation therapies. The relative rates of response for elderly clients versus younger individuals to cancer chemotherapy varies with the type of cancer. Response rates for older people in colorectal cancers would be only slightly lower than in younger individuals were it not for the fact that the condition is often diagnosed when in a more advanced state in elderly persons.

Cure rates for prostate cancer appear to be independent of age but substantially dependent upon the stage at which the condition is diagnosed, regardless of age. If the condition is advanced at the time of treatment, estrogen therapy with diethylstilbestrol is the usual treatment. Elderly men are more likely to experience cardiovascular problems from estrogen therapy than are younger men. In elderly men with preexisting cardiovascular disease, mortality rates are double. In high risk clients such as these, orchiectomy provides equal response rates and far less risk.

Five kinds of cancer in which age correlates adversely with survival rates are lymphoma, Hodgkin's disease, thyroid cancer, malignant melanoma, and acute nonlymphocytic leukemia. Elderly have higher mortality rates from acute nonlymphcytic leukemia because the aged immune system is less resistant to the adversities caused by both the disease and the drugs required to treat the disease. The bone marrow of the elderly client is less able to withstand the drug suppression that is required to achieve cure. The 5-year cure rate for this condition in elderly individuals of 50% is well below the level for younger people.

Breast cancer in women exhibits some distinctive age-related trends. The incidence increases with age and more than half of cases develop after age 65. It is well-established that responsiveness of women with breast cancer is dependent on hormonal status and presence or absence of estrogen receptors (ERs) in the tumor cells. Sixty-six percent of tumors that are ER-positive based on biopsy are likely to respond to estrogen therapy—the favored method of cancer chemotherapy. Responsiveness is better if the woman is also postmenopausal and still better if she is 10 years or more postmenopausal. Moreover, only 40% of breast tumors in women who are premenopausal are ER-positive, while more than 75% of those in women over age 75 are. In the event of relapse, older women with ER-positive tumors are also more likely to respond to secondary treatments such as antiestrogens, androgens, or adrenalectomy. ER-negative tumors seldom respond to estrogen therapy. Oophorectomy (removal of the ovaries), if the woman is premenopausal, or mastectomy may be required. When breast cancer has already metastasized at the time of diagnosis, chemotherapy will be required. Responsiveness in this event to chemotherapy appears to be similar for older and younger women except that older women are much more likely to receive reduced and subeffective doses. Many elderly post-menopausal women were found, in one study, to receive doses of the standard protocol (cyclophosphamide, methotrexate, and fluorouracil) that were less than 75% of optimal doses for responsiveness. This may be one instance of medical practice that runs directly counter to the most recurrent theme of this book—the need to reduce doses of many drugs for elderly clients.

ALTERED PHARMACOKINETICS FOR ANTICANCER DRUGS IN THE ELDERLY

Very little has been specifically determined regarding altered pharmacokinetics for anticancer drugs in the elderly. What is relevant mainly pertains to alterations required in relation to hepatic or renal dysfunction, and even there information is sketchy. As discussed in Chapter 4, elderly people invariably exhibit a decline in renal function even in the absence of specific renal disease and much more so if renal disease is present. Elderly people exhibit a lesser decline in liver function unless hepatitis or cirrhosis has developed. Thus, restrictions on drug use relating to renal or hepatic impairment often pertain to elderly people. Some warnings regarding doses for anticancer drugs are listed in Table 17.1 for renal impairment and in Table 17.2 for hepatic dysfunction.

SENSITIVITY OF ELDERLY PERSONS TO COMMON ADVERSE EFFECTS OF ANTICANCER DRUGS

Antineoplastic drugs are drugs that are toxic to cells as they proliferate. Tumor cells proliferate faster than most healthy tissue cells and the hope is that the toxicity exerted by the antineoplastic drug will therefore fall more heavily on the cancerous cells than normal cells. This strategy is least successful with respect to those tissue cells that have a naturally rapid rate of cell proliferation: the bone marrow, epithelial cells of the alimentary tract, hair follicles, and gonadal cells. These tissues are therefore the main ones subject to injurious effects from almost any antineoplastic drug.

Most antineoplastic drugs suppress the bone marrow, though they vary in the severity of this effect and on the relative propensity for affecting the various classes of blood cells: granulocytes, thrombocytes, red blood cells, or lymphocytes. Most readers will recognize that these various cells are involved in quite different functions, so that the impact on health will vary

Table 17.1 Some Anticancer Drugs with Warnings Relating to Renal Dysfunction

Drug	Nature of Warning
Aldesleukin	Reduced renal function may delay elimination and increase risk of adverse events.
Cladribine	Use caution when administering to patients with known or suspected renal dysfunction. Data insufficient.
Cyclophosphamide	Serum metabolite levels are elevated in patients with renal dysfunction, but there is no evidence of increased toxicity or need for dosage reduction.
Carboplatin	Reduce doses if creatinine clearance is less than 60 ml/min.
Daunorubicin	Evaluate renal function prior to treatment using standard tests.
Fludarabine	Administer cautiously. Renal impairment predisposes to increased toxicity. Monitor closely for excessive toxicity and adjust dosage accordingly.
Goserelin	Serum half-life increased to 12.1 hours when creatinine clearance was less than 20 ml/min compared to 4.2 hours with clearance greater than 70 ml/min. There was no evidence of increased toxicity in clients with renal impairment.
Hydroxyurea	Use caution in patients with marked renal dysfunction.
Idarubicin	Evaluate renal function before treatment. Consider dose reduction if creatinine clearance is not normal.
Mercaptopurine	Start with smaller doses due to possibly slower drug elimination and accumulation.
Methotrexate	Impaired renal impairment may result in accumulation to toxic levels. Exercise caution. Reduce dosage or discontinue drug if renal impairment occurs in response to methotrexate. Consider relatively low doses. Adequate renal function (creatinine clearance greater than 60 ml/min) must be documented before initiating therapy.
Mitomycin	Do not give to patients with serum creatinine > 1.7 mg/dl.
Pentostatin	Treat only if potential benefit justifies potential risk. Two clients with impaired renal function achieved complete response without unusual adverse events.
Plicamycin	Use extreme caution. Monitor renal function before, during, and after treatment.
Procarbazine	Undue toxicity may occur in patients with known renal impairment. Consider hospitalization for the initial course of treatment.

accordingly. The timing of bone marrow suppression by various anticancer drugs all varies as regards onset, peak suppression, and recovery time. Those working directly with clients during cancer chemotherapy will need to be aware of the likely period of bone marrow suppression, so that appropriate precautions can be taken. During the period of bone marrow suppres-

Table 17.2 Some Anticancer Drugs with Warnings Relating to Hepatic Dysfunction

Drug	Nature of Warning
Aldesleukin	Reduced hepatic function may delay elimination and increase risk of adverse events.
Cladribine	Use caution when administering to patients with known or suspected hepatic dysfunction. Data insufficient.
Cyclophosphamide	Use cautiously.
Cytarabine	Use with caution and at reduced doses in patients with poor hepatic function.
Daunorubicin	Evaluate hepatic function prior to treatment using standard tests.
Doxorubicin	Evaluate hepatic function before treatment using AST, ALT, alkaline phosphate, and bilirubin.
Idarubicin	Evaluate hepatic function before treatment. Consider dose reduction if bilirubin is not normal.
Mitotane	Administer with care to patients with liver disease. Drug accumulation might occur.
Paclitaxel	Use caution when administering to patients with severe hepatic impairment.
Plicamycin	Use extreme caution.
Procarbazine	Undue toxicity may occur in patients with known hepatic impairment. Consider hospitalization for the initial course of treatment.
Teniposide	Plasma clearance is decreased if serum alkalin phosphate or gamma glutamyl-transpeptidase is elevated. Exercise caution if teniposide is administered to clients with hepatic dysfunction.
Vinblastine, Vincristine	Fifty percent reduction in the dose is recommended for clients having a direct serum bilirubin value greater than 3 mg/dl.

sion, the client needs to be protected from stress or trauma, to avoid contact with infected persons, to examine the skin and mucous membranes for signs of infectious overgrowths, and to observe for and report episodes of sore throat, fever, chills, or respiratory infections. If the drug is one that suppresses thrombocytes, clients will also need to watch for signs of occult bleeding, such as tarry stools, petechiae, ecchymoses, blood in vomitus, bleeding nose or gums, or ease of bruising. If the drug is one that suppresses red blood cells, clients need to be alert for increased fatigue or pallor. The elderly are more susceptible to the hematological toxicities of anticancer drugs than younger persons. Indeed, this elevated liability is probably the most important difference in potential for adverse reactions between elderly and younger individuals. Increased risk of hematological toxicities has been most clearly demonstrated to date with respect to methotrexate, lomustine, and carmustine (see Table 17.3), but probably applies generally to antineoplastic drugs, given the changes that occur in the vitality of the bone marrow with aging.

The epithelium of the mucosal cells that line the alimentary tract are especially vulnerable to cytotoxic actions of anticancer drugs because of their high rate of turnover. Nausea and vomiting are routine features of cancer chemotherapy and often require pharmacological intervention. Chlorpromazine and prochlorperazine are often used for suppression of nausea and vomiting in connection with cancer chemotherapy. Dronabinol, which is tetrahydrocannabinol (the active constituent of marihuana), is also approved exclusively for this application. Nausea may be so discomforting for some clients, with a drug like cisplatin, for example, that they may flatly refuse further treatment. Whenever feasible, drug administration should be scheduled so that peak nausea and mealtimes do not coincide. Other helpful tactics for coping with the nausea of cancer chemotherapy include smaller, more frequent meals, emphasis on cold foods, and added emphasis on attractive presentation of food so that it has an appealing influence on appetite. If normal food intake can still not be maintained, dietary supplementation may be necessary. Sometimes adverse gastrointestinal responses to anticancer drugs are severe to the point of stomatitis, gastrointestinal bleeding, ulcers, or desquamation. Prolonged vomiting may cause electrolyte depletion and nutritional deficits. Oral hygiene needs to be intensified to protect oral membranes from irritation and superinfection.

Another adverse effect common to most antineoplastic drugs is alopecia (hair loss). It is almost always reversible but, for elderly persons, may grow back more slowly or with a change of color. Hair is an important part of self-image for many people, so alopecia can be an important drawback of cancer chemotherapy emotionally.

Anticancer drugs suppress proliferation of reproductive cells, causing inhibition of spermatogenesis in men or anovulation in women. These effects as well as the potential for teratogenicity may be less an issue for older clients.

Table 17.3 Adverse Responses to Antineoplastic Drugs That Are More Common for the Elderly

Nature of Toxicity	Drugs
Greater incidence of leukopenia	Carmustine Hydroxyurea Lomustine Methotrexate
Greater incidence of thrombocytopenia	Lomustine
Greater incidence of pneumonitis	Bleomycin
Greater incidence of nephrotoxicity	Cisplatin Hydroxyurea Methotrexate Vincristine
Greater risk of cardiac myopathy	Doxorubicin

If the anticancer drug is successful in promoting cytolysis of tumor cells, there may be a sharp increase in production of uric acid with resultant hyperuricemia. Some clients may experience joint or flank pain as a consequence. Many antineoplastic drugs exert toxic effects on the liver, kidney, lungs, or brain, though these problems are not as universal to all antineoplastic drugs as the foregoing effects. Hepatic toxicity is most likely with methotrexate, mercaptopurine, and azathioprine. If the elderly client has preexisting hepatic dysfunction, the risks of drug-induced exacerbation will be great. Renal toxicity is most often an occurrence with cyclophosphamide, cisplatin, streptozocin, and methotrexate. Nephrotoxicity is more common for elderly clients than their younger counterparts with cisplatin, hydroxyurea, methotrexate, and vincristine. Elderly clients under the best of circumstances have diminished renal function and some suffer from specific renal disorders, thus any nephrotoxicity occurring as a result of cancer chemotherapy will be superimposed on preexisting deficits. Pulmonary toxicity occurs most often with cyclophophamide, busulfan, methotrexate, and bleomycin. Elderly clients with chronic obstructive pulmonary disease would be at extra risk. Finally, neurotoxic effects are most prevalent when the regimen includes vincristine, vinblastine, procarbazine, L-asparaginase, fluorouracil, methotrexate, or cytarabine. Elderly persons with preexisting mental impairments, such as organic brain syndrome, are at risk of added cognitive deficits from such drugs.

REFERENCES AND RECOMMENDED READINGS

American Cancer Society: *Cancer Facts & Figures*. New York, American Cancer Society, 1986.

Carter SK: Cancer chemotherapy: new developments and changing concepts. *Drugs*, 1980; 20:375–397.

Chabner B: *Pharmacologic Principles of Cancer Treatment*. Philadelphia, W. B. Saunders, 1982.

Daeffler R: Oral hygiene measures for patients with cancer (parts 1 and 2). *Cancer Nurs.* 1980; 3(5):347–356, 3(6):427–432.

Elbaum N: With cancer patients, be alert for hypercalcemia. *Nursing* 1984; 14(8):58–59.

Hopefl AW: Cancer in the elderly, in Delafuente, Stewart: *Therapeutics in the Elderly*. Baltimore, Williams & Wilkins, 1988, pp. 285–293.

Horton J, Hill E (eds.): *Clinical Oncology*. Philadelphia, W. B. Saunders, 1977.

Hughes CB: Giving cancer drugs: some guidelines. *Am. J. Nurs.* 1986; 86(1):34–38.

Koch PM: Thrombocytopenia. *Nursing* 1984; 14(10):54–57.

Lurn JLJ et al.: Nursing care of oncology patients receiving chemotherapy. *Nurs. Res.* 1978; 27:340–346.

Miller SA: Nursing actions in cancer chemotherapy administration. *Oncology Nursing Forum* 1980; 7:8–16.

Smith FP, McCabe MS: Preventing chemotherapy-induced alopecia. *Am. Fam. Physician* 1983; 28(1):182–184.

Thomas NP et al.: Preparing cancer patients to administer medication. *Patient Counsel. Health Educ.* 1982; 3(4):137–143.

Valentine AS, Stewart JA: Oncologic emergencies. *Am. J. Nurs.* 1983; 83(9):1282–1285.

Wroblewski SS, Wroblewski SH: Caring for the patient with chemotherapy-induced thrombocytopenia. *Am. J. Nurs.* 1981; 81:746–749.

Index